Design and Shielding of Radiotherapy Treatment Facilities

IPEM Report 75, 2nd Edition

Series in Physics and Engineering in Medicine and Biology

About the Series

Series in Physics and Engineering in Medicine and Biology will allow IPEM to enhance its mission to "advance physics and engineering applied to medicine and biology for the public good."

Focusing on key areas including, but not limited to:

- clinical engineering
- diagnostic radiology
- informatics and computing
- magnetic resonance imaging
- nuclear medicine
- physiological measurement
- radiation protection
- radiotherapy
- rehabilitation engineering
- ultrasound and non-ionising radiation.

Design and Shielding of Radiotherapy Treatment Facilities

IPEM Report 75, 2nd Edition

Patrick Horton
Royal Surrey County Hospital, Guildford, UK

David Eaton
Mount Vernon Cancer Centre, London, UK

IOP Publishing, Bristol, UK

IPEM Report 75 2nd Edition is an update of IPEM Report Number 75, a report produced by the Institute of Physics and Engineering in Medicine

ISBN 978-0-7503-1440-4 (ebook)
ISBN 978-0-7503-1441-1 (print)
ISBN 978-0-7503-1442-8 (mobi)

DOI 10.1088/978-0-7503-1440-4

Version: 20170701

IOP Expanding Physics
ISSN 2053-2563 (online)
ISSN 2054-7315 (print)

British Library Cataloguing-in-Publication Data: A catalogue record for this book is available from the British Library.

Published by IOP Publishing, wholly owned by The Institute of Physics, London

IOP Publishing, Temple Circus, Temple Way, Bristol, BS1 6HG, UK

US Office: IOP Publishing, Inc., 190 North Independence Mall West, Suite 601, Philadelphia, PA 19106, USA

Contents

Preface

Soon after the discovery of x-rays, it became clear that these 'healing rays' could also cause harm. Early pioneers of radiology and radiotherapy gave little thought to radiation protection, and their own health paid the price. Current units are governed by strict legislation, which in the UK requires the involvement of a radiation protection advisor (RPA) in the design and verification of radiation facility shielding.

National and international guidance on best practice supports the RPA in these endeavours, and the publication of IPEM Report 75 in 1997 provided a solid foundation for many years of safe and effective shielding. However, there have been significant developments in treatment techniques and room design recently, which have provided one impetus for this updated report. Other international reports are available (NCRP 2005, IAEA 2006), but these are not always comprehensive in their scope and also lack the latest developments. In particular, the introduction of intensity modulated radiotherapy (IMRT), with longer radiation beam-on times, has directly affected greater secondary bunker shielding, and flattening-filter-free (FFF) beams with higher dose rates have questioned the need for increased primary barrier protection. Variable use of instantaneous and time-averaged dose rates gives the potential for shielding to be excessive. Specialist applications have altered the usual proportion of primary and secondary shielding. At the same time, new and reliable higher density shielding materials have come onto the market, and new bunker designs using doors instead of mazes have been built based on the desire to save space and cost, as popularised in North America. Finally, the increase in the accuracy and speed of Monte Carlo simulation makes it an attractive complement, or even replacement, for empirical calculation for shielding design and visualisation.

Specific updates in this report include:

- radiation protection requirements, related to current and successor legislation based on the European Community Basic Safety Standards,
- the effect of modern treatment techniques such as IMRT, volumetric intensity modulated arc therapy, stereotactic body radiotherapy and FFF linear accelerators on the radiation protection of facilities,
- Monte Carlo simulation and visualisation of x-ray and neutron scatter in linear accelerator bunkers for comparison with established shielding calculation methods,
- current brachytherapy techniques,
- new shielding materials and bunker designs,
- specialised techniques such as TomoTherapy®, Gamma Knife® and CyberKnife®,
- current kilovoltage practice, including novel electronic brachytherapy devices and
- shielding for particle therapy (proton and carbon ion) facilities, since such facilities are becoming increasingly widespread, including in the UK.

The concept of updating IPEM Report 75 first originated from an IPEM Scientific Meeting in 2009 entitled *Current Developments in the Design of Radiotherapy Treatment Room Facilities*, and showed even then how much treatment techniques and bunker design had developed since Report 75. The second impetus for a new report was to capture the extensive experience gained by medical physicists in the UK through the expansion of NHS radiotherapy facilities through the National Opportunities Fund and subsequent initiatives. The original IPEM working party for this report comprised P W Horton (chair), E G Aird, W P M Mayles, D J Peet and R M Harrison. With the help of IPEM's Radiotherapy Special Interest Group, the number of contributors has been expanded considerably in order to achieve a comprehensive scope. In addition to writing their original contribution, everyone has played a part in developing the overall report. Almost all the contributors are from the UK, but the breadth of the scope, and depth of the detailed worked examples, will hopefully be of benefit to those in all countries. The report is primarily intended for Qualified Experts in radiotherapy physics and radiation protection, such as RPAs, but will also be of use to administrators, planners, architects, constructors and others involved in the design of radiotherapy facilities.

P W Horton
Perth
February 2017

D J Eaton
London

Acknowledgments

A full list of contributors is given. The editors are most grateful to them for their contributions and the time and effort they have put into reviewing all parts of the report. The editors are also extremely grateful to the two external general referees, Dr D Temperton and Mr J Thurston, and the specialist external referee for chapter 11, Dr R Lüscher, for their thorough reviews and constructive comments which enhanced the final report. The editors and contributors are also grateful to Accuray Incorporated, Elekta Instruments AB and Varian Medical Systems for permission to use their illustrations and diagrams.

(PWH) Many thanks to my wife, Roberta, who has been living with this project almost as long as I have. (DJE) Many thanks to Pat, my co-editor, for persevering with this project since its inception seven years ago. Thank you to Rosie, my wife, for correcting my errant ideas on radiation protection, and to my beautiful children, Deborah and Jonathan, for making me smile every day. *Soli de gloria.*

Author biography

Patrick Horton

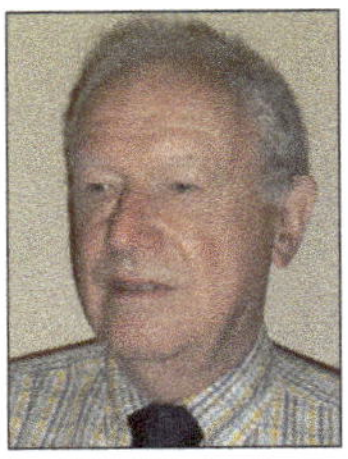

Professor Horton has a BSc in Physics from Imperial College, London and a PhD from the University of Manchester. He began his medical physics career in the Department of Clinical Physics and Bio-engineering of the West of Scotland Health Boards, initially as a Senior Physicist in Radiotherapy and latterly as a Principal Physicist in Nuclear Medicine, both at the Western Infirmary in Glasgow. He was next appointed as the first Head of Department of the Department of Medical Physics and Bio-engineering at the Riyadh Armed Forces Hospital in Saudi Arabia, where he established a new department which played a key role in the introduction of radiotherapy, nuclear medicine and complex radiology. He returned to the UK to become Head of the Department of Medical Physics at the Royal Surrey County Hospital, Guildford and Honorary Professor of Medical Physics at the University of Surrey. He was also Quality Assurance Director of the NHS Breast Screening Service in the South East (East) Region, for 14 years, responsible for the breast screening centres in Kent, Surrey and Sussex. Since retiring from the NHS he has worked as a consultant to construction companies building new cancer centres in the UK and abroad, on projects for the European Community and the International Atomic Energy Agency and lectured at the European School of Medical Physics on installation shielding in radiotherapy. Publications include one book, several book chapters and 115 scientific papers and reports on medical physics topics. He is a Fellow of the Institute of Physics and Engineering in Medicine, the Institute of Physics and the Institution of Engineering and Technology. He is also a member of the British Institute of Radiology and the American Association of Physicists in Medicine.

David Eaton

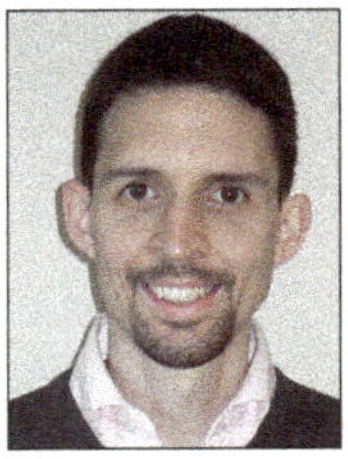

David Eaton received his undergraduate degrees (MA MSci) in natural sciences (physical) from Gonville and Caius college, Cambridge in 2003, returning to collect his PhD in intraoperative radiotherapy physics several years later. He trained as a clinical scientist at Addenbrooke's hospital, Cambridge, then worked as a radiotherapy physicist at the Royal Free Hospital in London. Currently, he is the lead clinical scientist for the UK radiotherapy trials quality assurance group (RTTQA), based at Mount Vernon hospital in London. He has published widely on intraoperative radiotherapy, kilovoltage dosimetry and clinical trials QA, with about 30 papers and book chapters, and 50 conference abstracts. As well as writing and reviewing for a range of journals, he is an associate editor for the *British Journal of Radiology* and the Indian *Journal of Medical Physics*. He is a fellow of the Institute of Physics and Engineering in Medicine (IPEM), a recipient of their president's prize and founders' award, and chair of the IPEM radiotherapy special interest group, who commissioned this report.

Contributors

Edwin G Aird
Mount Vernon Cancer Centre, Northwood, UK

Richard Amos
University College Hospital, London. UK

Mary Costelloe
Oxford University Hospitals, UK

David J Eaton
Mount Vernon Cancer Centre,
Northwood, UK

Francesca Fiorini
CRUK and MRC Oxford Institute for Radiation Oncology,
Department of Oncology,
University of Oxford,
Oxford, UK

Zamir Ghani
Neutron and Gamma Diagnostics,
UK Atomic Energy Authority,
Culham Centre for Fusion Energy,
Abingdon UK

Stuart Green
Medical Physics,
University Hospitals Birmingham NHS Foundation Trust,
Queen Elizabeth Hospital,
Birmingham, UK

Tony Greener
Guys and St Thomas' NHS Hospital Foundation Trust,
Cancer Centre,
Guys Hospital,
London, UK

Mark J Hardy
Radiotherapy Physics Group,
Christie Medical Physics and Engineering
The Christie NHS Foundation Trust,
Manchester, UK

Roger M Harrison
University of Newcastle, UK

Patrick W Horton
Medical Physics, Royal Surrey County Hospital, Guildford, UK

Colin J Martin
University of Glasgow, UK

Richard Maughan
University of Pennsylvania, Philadelphia, USA

W Philip M Mayles
Clatterbridge Cancer Centre NHS Foundation Trust, UK

Debbie J Peet
Medical Physics Department,
Leicester Royal Infirmary,
Leicester, UK

David Prior
Brighton and Sussex University Hospitals NHS Trust, Brighton, UK

Jill Reay
Aurora Health Physics Services Ltd, Didcot, UK

Tracey Soanes
Medical Physics and Clinical Engineering, Sheffield Teaching Hospitals, UK

Michael J Taylor
Division of Molecular and Clinical Cancer Sciences,
The University of Manchester,
Manchester, UK

Chris Walker
Northern Centre for Cancer Care,
Newcastle upon Tyne,
Hospitals NHS Foundation Trust, UK

Lee Walton
Medical Physics and Clinical Engineering, Sheffield Teaching Hospitals, UK

IOP Publishing

Chapter 1

The design and procurement process

P W Horton

1.1 Introduction

The need for new equipment, the upgrading of an existing facility or the development of a new radiotherapy facility can arise from a number of circumstances. These include:

- the need to replace unreliable equipment,
- the need to have new equipment with features enabling current accepted clinical practice,
- the need for additional equipment to increase treatment capacity to meet increasing demand or treatment complexity and keep waiting times for treatment to specified standards,
- the need for a new cancer centre to replace an outdated facility for a variety of reasons,
- provision of a satellite treatment unit to an existing centre to increase treatment capacity and provide more local patient treatments or
- the need to meet the NHS England Radiotherapy Service Specifications (NHS Commissioning Board 2013).

In many instances, the first and second needs will both apply. Expenditure on new facilities or new equipment is termed a capital project within the NHS. Similar arrangements will apply in private hospitals and charitable institutions.

The stages in progressing a capital project are set out in table 1.1. The stages outlined in the table may not be followed exactly, but some elements of each stage will be required. The NHS Trust or organisation should appoint a senior member of staff as the project officer and he/she will be responsible for the overall management of the project. This will include preparation of the business case for the funding and the project brief and, in the case of major schemes, the appointment of an external project manager (often the architect or the organisation employing him/her) or a

doi:10.1088/978-0-7503-1440-4ch1

Table 1.1. Stages in the introduction of new equipment.

Strategic proposal
Business case
Strategic Outline Programme (SOP)
Strategic Outline Case (SOC)
Outline Business Case (OBC)
Full Business Case (FBC)
Design and design team
Tenders and contracts
Buildings and services
Equipment
Construction
Acceptance and handover
Buildings and services
Equipment
Commissioning
Clinical services
Equipment
Evaluation

private consortium for a public private partnership (PPP). A realistic timetable must be agreed for design, equipment selection, letting contracts, construction, equipment installation, and acceptance and equipment commissioning for clinical use, with a contingency built in to allow for unavoidable slippage in the project, e.g. poor crane utilisation due to high winds. Gantt charts are invaluable to show the timetabling and interaction of the individual activities within the project and to help ensure that each takes place on a logical and timely basis. A more detailed discussion of the stages follows below.

The roles and responsibilities of the medical physicists available to the development will vary according to local circumstances and the expertise of the individuals available. At minimum there must be a medical physics expert (MPE) in radiotherapy and a radiation protection adviser (RPA). Medical physics involvement in all of the following activities (in the order in table 1.1) is essential for a successful project:

- Participation in the design of the radiation facility.
- Specification of the necessary radiation protection.
- Writing the specification for the equipment required.
- Scientific and technical advice during the selection of the equipment.
- Monitoring of the construction of the facility to ensure that the radiation protection requirements and the service requirements for the selected equipment are met.
- Liaison with the equipment supplier and co-ordination of the equipment installation.

- Acceptance testing of the equipment with the supplier's installation engineers.
- Responsibility for the radiation survey of the new facility and electrical safety of the installed equipment.
- Commissioning of the equipment prior to clinical use.
- Establishment of quality assurance regimes, documentation and training.

Medical physicists may also undertake additional roles, e.g. some of the project management.

1.2 Strategic proposal and business case for a new development

Due to the capital cost and possibly revenue costs, the project will require a business case for its approval in the public sector; similar needs will apply in the private and charitable sectors. In many organisations a strategic proposal can be submitted at the start of the annual capital planning cycle, sometimes using a standard pro-forma to help ensure that all the relevant information to enable a decision is available. The proposal may include the following topics for a successful development, depending on its magnitude:

- The purpose of the application.
- The strategic context.
- The case for change, including the difficulties or deficiencies that currently exist, their cause(s) and the proposed solution. It is important to include substantiated evidence to show the existence and the extent of the problem.
- Benefits, both service and financial.
- Risks.
- Available options (including 'do nothing') and their consequences.
- Preferred option.
- Procurement route.
- Anticipated costs—capital and revenue.
- Management arrangements, both organisational and financial.

Business cases are a mandatory part of the planning, approval, procurement and delivery of investments in the public sector. A good business case provides an organisation with the evidence to support its decision making and provides assurance to other stakeholders, e.g. service commissioners, that it has acted responsibly. The 'Five Case Model' of the Office of Government Commerce (2013) is the recommended standard for the preparation of business cases and is used extensively in the public sector. The Five Case Model comprises the following five key components:

- *The strategic case.* This sets out the strategic context and the case for change, together with the investment objectives for the scheme.
- *The economic case.* This demonstrates that the organisation has selected the choice for development which best meets the existing and future needs of the service and optimises value for money.

- *The commercial case*. This outlines the content of the proposed deal.
- *The financial case*. This confirms the funding arrangements and explains any effects on the balance sheet of the organisation, i.e. affordability.
- *The management case*. This demonstrates that the scheme is achievable and details the plans for the successful delivery of the scheme to cost, time and quality standards.

The business planning process using the Five Case Model is an iterative process using the five headings above with increasing detail as the proposal progresses through four phases, each requiring approval before proceeding to the next. These phases are:

- Strategic Outline Programme (SOP).
- Strategic Outline Case (SOC).
- Outline Business Case (OBC).
- Full Business Case (FBC).

Guidance on the process and detailed templates for the four phases above are available from the Office of Government Commerce (2013). More information on the approval process in England is available from NHS England (2013; *NHS Business Case Approval Process—Capital Investment, Property, Equipment and ICT*) which also has pro-formas and checklists. For radiation users this guidance is also available in the RCR (2012) publication *Writing a Good Business Case*, intended for non-financial persons and having a good explanation of the terminology. In 2014, the NHS Trust Development Authority modified the Five Case Model (*Capital Regime and Investment Business Case Approvals—Guidance for NHS Trusts*) and inserted *the clinical quality case* between the *strategic* and *economic cases* above. This sets out the clinical and patient benefits of the proposal more clearly than might previously have been the situation as part of the *strategic case*.

Depending on the financial rules of the organisation, a proposal may be classified as a *minor capital* scheme if the costs are not high and there are no wide implications, e.g. replacement of a kilovoltage treatment unit, or a *major capital* scheme if the costs are high and there are wider implications such as building or additional staffing costs. The funding of a new project can come from a number of sources. Within the NHS these include:

- An internally generated cash surplus by the NHS Trust at year end from unspent capital, depreciation, disposal of assets, revenue surplus, etc.
- Capital Investment Loans from the Department of Health on which the NHS Trust pays a fixed rate of interest for the period of the loan and repays the capital at regular intervals.
- Central programme capital for central initiatives.

The capital plans of NHS Trusts must be agreed with the NHS Trust Development Authority who review them to ensure they are affordable, achievable and fit with local and strategic priorities. All plans are then agreed with the Department of Health to ensure they are affordable within the overall NHS capital programme.

A major development such as a new cancer centre may necessitate a PPP because of the large capital cost. The most common form of PPP has been the *private finance initiative* (PFI), where the capital investment is provided by the private sector on the strength of a contract with the NHS Trust over a long period to provide agreed services and the cost of providing the service is borne wholly or in part by the NHS. The private sector recovers its costs over the contract period (often 25 years or more) and assumes a financial, technical and operational risk in the project. Commonly the private sector is a consortium of a construction company, a maintenance company and a bank lender to develop, build, maintain and operate the asset for the period of the contract. At the end of the contract period, the asset either remains with the private sector contractor or is returned to the NHS, depending on the terms of the contract. The purpose of the PFI is to increase private sector involvement in the provision of public services with the perceived benefits of bringing in private sector expertise and lower costs to the taxpayer.

Some organisations may choose to lease the equipment or use a managed equipment service company to reduce the capital outlay.

1.3 Design team

1.3.1 General

The wide range of professionals who may be involved in the planning, construction and commissioning of a radiotherapy treatment facility is shown in table 1.2. The actual number involved will depend on the magnitude of the project and the contractual arrangements.

1.3.2 Minor capital schemes

For a minor capital scheme, the main activities are most likely to be the selection of the equipment and the adaptation of an existing room to take the new equipment. A small design team is sufficient and can be usually drawn from hospital staff. The team should include:

- a representative of the Planning Department (who may also be the project leader),
- a radiotherapy physicist,
- a radiographer,
- a medical physics technical officer and
- a member of the Works Department.

The selection of the equipment may be undertaken by a wider group of radiotherapy physicists, radiographers and technical officers, including the radiotherapy physicist and radiographer on the project team.

When the new equipment has been chosen and the installation and adaptation requirements are clear, the project team should also include:

- selected representatives of the hospital's approved contractors, e.g. for building and electrical work,
- the supplier's representative and
- the RPA.

Table 1.2. Persons involved in the design and construction of radiotherapy treatment facilities.

Hospital/Trust representatives
Finance officer
Oncology business manager
Planning officer
Estates/works officer
RPA
IT specialist(s)
Patient and public voice partner
Users
Radiation oncologists
Radiotherapy physicists
Therapy radiographers, including Radiation Protection Supervisor
Medical physics technical officers
External design team
Architect
Structural engineer
Electrical engineer
Mechanical engineer
Quantity surveyor
Design consultant
Contractors
Construction company
Electrical work sub-contractor
Mechanical work sub-contractor
Specialised shielding and component (e.g. doors) sub-contractors
Treatment equipment manufacturer
Installation co-ordinator
Delivery and rigging sub-contractor
Installation engineers

1.3.3 Major capital schemes

For a major capital scheme, e.g. involving the installation of linear accelerator(s) in a new or modified building, there will be more complex issues around the design, construction or alteration of the building and its integration into existing facilities and services. This will require additional expertise from outside the hospital and will usually include an architect, a structural engineer, an electrical engineer and a quantity surveyor. These may all come from the same organisation, depending on the contract arrangements. The project may well be managed at two levels: a smaller project team and a larger design and execution team. The effects of the works and the introduction of new equipment on the maintenance of clinical services will also have to be assessed and any adverse effects minimised. The project team might comprise the following:

- a senior member of the Finance Department (who may be the project officer),
- a radiation oncologist,
- a senior radiotherapy physicist (MPE),
- the radiotherapy patient services manager,
- a representative of the Planning Department,
- a member of the Estates Department and
- the selected architect.

The larger design team will report to the project team at regular intervals through one of its members who serves on both teams. The design team will include:

- the selected architect (who may be the project manager) and his/her supporting staff,
- the representative of the Planning Department,
- the senior medical physicist,
- relevant radiotherapy physicists,
- radiotherapy patient services manager,
- relevant senior radiographers,
- a medical physics technical officer,
- a member of the Estates Department,
- the RPA,
- IT specialist(s) and
- patient and public voice (PPV) partners.

When the building design and the selection of the equipment has been finalised and construction is underway, progress meetings of the design team should also include:

- representatives of the construction company,
- the structural engineer,
- the electrical engineer,
- the mechanical engineer and
- the equipment supplier's representative.

All project and planning team meetings should be minuted and any changes in the design (variation orders) carefully costed and agreed, as these are often the source of additional expenditure and budget overruns.

The role of the IT specialist(s) is important with modern complex radiotherapy management systems and the sharing of images and large amounts of data between treatment planning and treatment systems. He/she may come from medical physics or the hospital's IT Department, or preferably one from both. The requirements of the equipment vendor's management software should be clearly understood so that it is not compromised by the hospital's general IT requirements. Common practice is to confine the heavy radiotherapy data flows to a separate network (linking the treatment units, planning systems and CT simulators) with a firewall to the hospital network for the import/export of patient administrative information and the import of images from hospital imaging facilities.

1.3.4 Public private partnership

As stated earlier, a major development may entail a PPP to design, construct and operate the facility through a PFI. This requires comprehensive and substantial teams such as those outlined above for a major capital scheme in both the hospital and the construction components of the partnership. The role of the hospital team is to specify the objectives of the new facility, particularly with regard to the range of services to be provided, their volume and expected growth, and check that the completed scheme meets these objectives. The role of the construction company together with its appointed architect will be to design and construct the facility to meet the hospital's objectives for the cost agreed. Whilst construction companies are familiar with mechanical, electrical and structural matters, they are much less familiar with the requirements of radiotherapy and radiation protection legislation and should have a radiotherapy expert and an RPA available to their design and construction teams. It is beneficial to the project if the contractual arrangements allow a dialogue between the hospital's radiotherapy team and RPA and the contactor's expert and RPA so that details of the design, e.g. the planned radiation workload for individual linear accelerators, and radiation protection policy are available to the design team from the earliest possible stage. It is essential that the final design of any radiation facilities, together with the radiation protection calculations to meet the hospital's radiation protection policy, are approved by the hospital's RPA before construction starts. At the conclusion of the project, there must be agreement with the hospital's RPA on the performance of the radiation survey of the new facility and the wide availability of survey results to ensure that the design criteria have been met and the facility is safe for clinical use. The hospital's RPA may also need to notify the Health and Safety Executive if it is a new radiation facility. The maintenance company in the PPP will be familiar with building maintenance but usually less familiar with the technical support usually provided in radiotherapy by medical physics technical officers to ensure high levels of equipment availability for treatment. This issue needs to be discussed long before clinical services commence and a sub-contract with the hospital team may be necessary due to the very specialised nature of the work.

1.4 Process, tenders and contracts

1.4.1 Minor capital schemes

For a minor capital scheme, the starting point will be a specification for the new equipment. This will be drawn up by radiotherapy physicists and radiographers, in conjunction with the radiation oncologists, to meet the clinical need. Prior to finalising the specification it is advisable to have preliminary discussions with manufacturers to ensure that the proposed specification reflects current possibilities. The specification may be in the form of an output based specification which describes what the equipment has to achieve or a detailed specification of the equipment and its performance, or a combination of the two. Specifications must not be written so that only one manufacturer can comply. After approval by the hospital, the specification can be sent to potential suppliers and must be advertised with a clear closing date for offers in the Official Journal of the European Union (OJEU) if it is expected to cost more than a prescribed limit. Current thresholds valid from 1 January 2016 to 3 December 2017 are £106 047 for NHS Trusts and £164 170 for NHS Foundation Trusts. Although these thresholds are based on thresholds in euros, they remain unchanged during this period independent of currency fluctuations. Alternatively, the hospital can use the radiotherapy equipment framework agreement negotiated by the NHS Supply Chain. Using the framework it is possible to set up a mini-competition between suppliers without advertising in the OJEU. Additions to the baseline specification can be agreed between the suppliers and the purchaser. In some circumstances it is possible that a new model of equipment may not be available in the framework.

To evaluate the offers in a uniform and objective manner, the users should develop an option appraisal pro-forma in which each of the identified performance parameters is given a weight according to its relative importance. Each performance parameter can then be scored over a set range for each supplier's equipment on the basis of how closely it matches the desired performance and a weighted total score calculated to indicate which supplier's equipment most closely approaches the ideal solution. It will also be necessary to look at other issues, such as operator and physicist training, maintenance arrangements and costs, reliability (as determined from other users), compatibility with existing equipment, installation requirements and cost, and to include these in the decision on the first choice. Visits to other users of the proposed equipment can be valuable for assessing ease of use, reliability and the standard of service support. A purchase order can then be issued for the equipment. At this stage, the installation issues should be clear and a specification for the building and electrical works can be drawn up by the Estates Department. This can be issued to contractors approved by the hospital and quotations invited by a given date. Site visits by potential equipment suppliers and contractors are important to ensure the quality of quotations. These can be evaluated by the project team, contracts issued to the successful contractors and the first meeting of the larger team convened to draw up a timetable for the development, taking account of delivery dates and the possible need to modify the clinical service. The progress of the project should be monitored at regular intervals through project team meetings with reports to the responsible hospital officer. Contact persons must be available to the supplier and contractors to respond to technical issues and to minimise any interference with ongoing clinical services.

1.4.2 Major capital schemes

For a major capital scheme, a more complex procedure employing external expertise is necessary. The project team will need to draw up a design brief with an outline of the scheme including the building, equipment and siting requirements, together with an overall indication of cost. Expressions of interest to design and manage the project will be invited from suitably experienced organisations through an advertisement in OJEU. These expressions of interest are evaluated by the project team and a shortlist (usually three organisations) is invited to make presentations to the project team with more details of their design, proposed management of the project, professional expertise available and fee structure. The hospital will then enter into a contract with the successful organisation and in all probability their architect will become the project manager and lead the design team. The design will begin with general layouts which will be evaluated for their workability, relationship to existing facilities and appearance. Having selected an optimal layout, the design details will be developed into plans and room data sheets by the design team. These will be supported by structural, mechanical and electrical plans developed by the architect's team and consulting engineers. Once the plans and data sheets are finalised, expressions of interest can be invited from construction companies to construct the facility though an OJEU announcement. Again these expressions of interest are evaluated by the project team together with the architect, and a tender to build the facility can be issued to a shortlist (usually three) of companies with a closing date. Presentations by the shortlisted companies are very helpful in assessing previous experience in this specialised area, quality and commitment. The tenders returned will be evaluated by the larger project team for quality and price, and the construction contract issued to the successful bidder.

A specification for the equipment can be developed in parallel with the building design. This must clearly state the key features of the desired equipment and any accessories required. Expressions of interest and tenders can again be invited from equipment suppliers through an OJEU announcement or by using the framework agreement negotiated by the NHS Supply Chain. Presentations by the suppliers are helpful to learn more about the equipment and options available and for the supplier to inspect the proposed site. The tenders returned by the closing date will be evaluated by the radiotherapy and medical physics members of the larger project team for compliance with the specification. Again, the users should develop an option appraisal pro-forma in which each of the identified performance parameters is given a weight according to their relative importance. Each performance parameter can then be scored over a given range for each equipment supplier on the basis of how closely it matches the desired performance and a weighted total score calculated to indicate which supplier's equipment most closely approaches the ideal solution. It will also be necessary to look at other issues such as operator training, maintenance training, reliability (as determined from other users), compatibility with existing equipment, installation requirements and cost, and to include these in the decision on the first choice. Again, visits to other users of the proposed equipment can be valuable for assessing ease of use, reliability and the standard of service support. A purchase order can then be issued for the equipment. In some instances, the equipment will be supplied as part of a wider national initiative. There is usually some flexibility within these arrangements to ensure that the recipient receives equipment which meets the local requirements and is compatible with existing equipment. In these circumstances, a pro-forma should be used for an option appraisal of the alternatives from different suppliers in order to reach an objective conclusion. This can be a helpful summary of the reasons for the first choice if unsuccessful suppliers ask for the reasons why they were unsuccessful. In general, it is desirable to complete the selection of the equipment before the design and room data sheets are finalised, so that any detailed requirements relating to specific equipment, e.g. the position of primary shielding in relation to the treatment isocentre, may be incorporated into the latter before tenders are issued.

1.4.3 Public private partnership

For a PFI, the Trust project team will need to draw up a comprehensive brief for the services to be provided by the new facility. This will require estimates of future growth to ensure that the facility remains clinically sufficient over the long period of the contract, but should be as accurate as possible to minimise costs and future charges. Similarly equipment requirements should be realistic and not excessive. Expressions of interest to design, construct and manage the project will be invited from suitably experienced consortia through an advertisement in the OJEU. These expressions of interest are evaluated by the project team and a shortlist (usually three consortia) is invited to make presentations to the project team with more details of their design, proposed management of the project, professional expertise available and costs. The hospital will then enter into negotiation with the preferred consortium to finalise all aspects of the project. If this is successful, a contract will be awarded to the successful bidder and in all probability their architectural practice will become project manager and lead the design work. The design will need to be evaluated for its ability to meet the specification now and in the future, its relationship to existing facilities and compliance with a wide range of regulations. Having selected an optimal layout, the design details will be developed into plans and room data sheets by the design team. These will be supported by structural, mechanical and electrical plans developed by the architect's team and consulting engineers. The equipment supplier will in all probability be a sub-contractor to the construction element of the consortium and it is important to ensure that the equipment requirements are clearly understood by the supplier and not altered in the supply chain.

1.5 Construction

The steps in the construction of a facility, the selection of equipment, and its installation and commissioning for safe clinical use are shown in figure 1.1.

In a *major capital scheme*, regular design team meetings with the building contractor are essential during construction, in particular as the construction nears completion and more questions on detail arise. Attention to radiation protection issues is important during the construction of shielding. During the pouring of concrete bunkers for linear accelerators, samples will be taken at regular intervals for analysis, usually to check mechanical properties. It is also important to have the density of these samples measured to ensure that the density of the concrete is not less than that assumed in the shielding calculations. It is also important to check that the shielding is not compromised by joints in the concrete or block work, ducts for services or the position of shuttering bolts. These matters are dealt with in greater detail in chapter 7. As construction nears completion it is important to check that

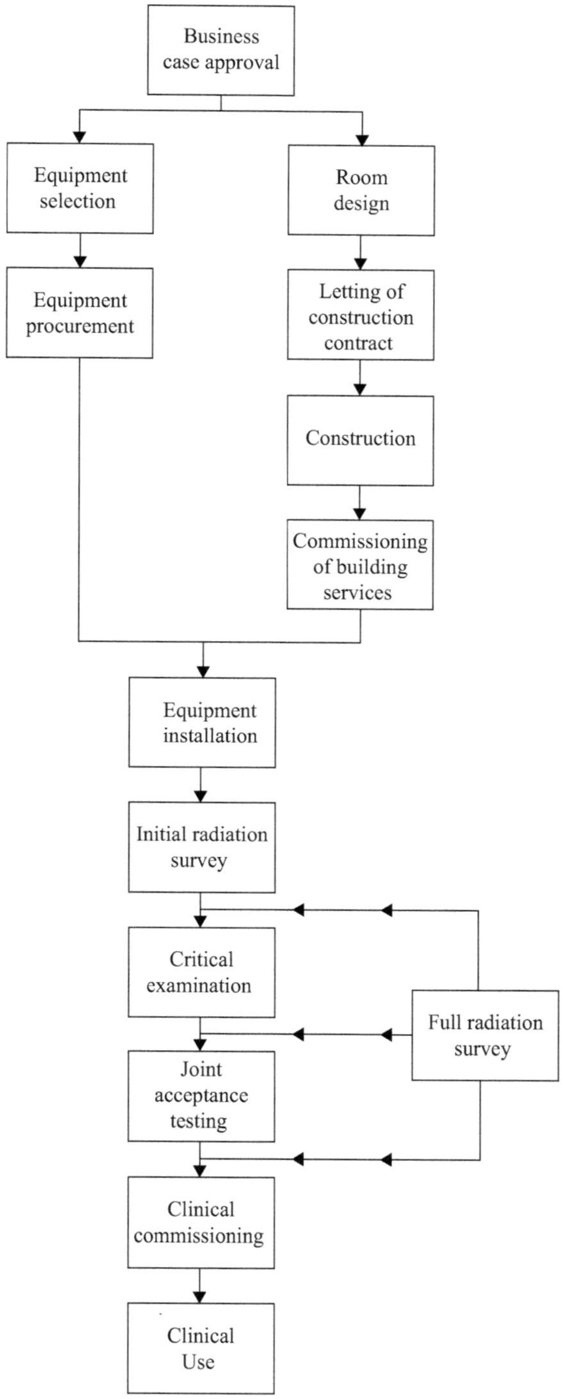

Figure 1.1. Flow chart showing the stages in building and equipment procurement and commissioning for clinical use.

engineering controls and warning signs are sited according to the plans. At this stage, the details for the delivery of the equipment can be finalised with the supplier's representative. For a new linear accelerator, the base frame will be installed as construction nears completion, but all suppliers will only deliver the accelerator and other components to a virtually complete and clean bunker to avoid problems caused by dust, etc. Once the site is clean, the equipment can be installed and connected by the supplier's engineers and the programme to make the equipment operational started. During construction, it is also important to have a day-to-day link with the patient services manager to ensure that the construction work is phased to minimise any impact on ongoing clinical services.

For a *PFI project*, the responsibility for construction will lie with the construction company and compliance with the plans will be the responsibility of the design team and consultants, but will have the same emphasis as that outlined above.

1.6 Acceptance and handover

1.6.1 Buildings and services

For a *major capital scheme*, acceptance of the building and services will be undertaken by a hospital team including senior staff who will be working in the new facility. 'As built' plans of the facility must be handed to the hospital. A detailed inspection of the facility should take place and be compared with the plans and room data sheets. A snagging list of all defects should be drawn up and a timetable to remedy them agreed with the construction company.

Similar arrangements apply for a *PFI scheme*. However, whereas in a major capital scheme the maintenance of the new facility will be by the hospital's Estates Department, in a PFI scheme the responsibilities will be borne by an external maintenance contractor. Details such as the warranties on service equipment, e.g. air conditioning plant, need to be passed to the appropriate organisation.

1.6.2 Radiotherapy treatment facilities

The acceptance of radiotherapy treatment facilities will be undertaken by the RPA, checking the adequacy of the radiation protection for staff and members of the public, and an MPE radiotherapy physicist, with the assistance from other members of the radiotherapy physics team, checking the performance of the equipment against its specification.

Acceptance should begin with a basic radiation protection survey by the RPA of the shielding provided by the facility when the installation engineer states that the installation can produce radiation. At this stage, although installation is complete and the equipment operational, its radiation performance will not be optimised to match the specification. This survey should ensure that external dose rates are acceptable over a range of equipment orientations and that the facility is safe to operate for an extended series of tests. Engineering controls and warning signs should also be checked for correct operation. Electrical safety tests should also be performed at this stage to ensure that the equipment does not present an electrical hazard to the acceptance team. The latter testing may be done by the clinical engineering section of the medical physics department or by the hospital's electro-medical equipment maintenance department.

A more detailed radiation protection survey should be performed following the acceptance procedure, when it is confirmed that the equipment performance, in particular beam energies and dose rates, matches the specification. External dose rates should be measured over a range of equipment orientations with and without scatter material in the radiation beam at the isocentre. Measured dose rates can then be compared to those in the radiation protection calculations to assess compliance with the calculations and any assumptions. More details on performing a radiation survey are given in chapter 12.

During the acceptance, a *critical examination* as required by the *Ionising Radiation Regulations* (IRR 1999) should be carried out by the supplier to confirm that the intended radiation protection and safety features incorporated into the equipment and its operation are satisfactory in the current installation. The examination may be performed by a representative of the equipment supplier or by the RPA at the request of the supplier.

In PFI projects, the radiation protection surveys may be undertaken by the construction company's RPA as part of their contract with the company. Alternatively, they can be done by the hospital's RPA to a protocol agreed with the constructor's RPA and with the constructor's approval. The latter is often more convenient if surveys are done at short notice. In either situation, the results of surveys should be approved by both RPAs and be generally available to show that the facility complies with national regulations and the hospital's policy on radiation protection.

Following acceptable outcomes for the basic radiation protection survey and electrical safety testing, acceptance testing of the mechanical and radiation performance of the equipment can then commence safely. Joint acceptance testing with the equipment supplier's installation engineer using the supplier's test pro-forma is commonplace. This will cover a wide range of parameters and the acceptable tolerances will be given in the pro-forma. As each test is passed within tolerance, it should be signed off by the supplier's engineer and the radiotherapy physicist. This is better than gathering a large amount of data for subsequent analysis and approval. If the equipment fails a test, further adjustment will be necessary, which may impact on tests already performed and render them invalid. Ideally all tests should be done as a complete set with no intervening adjustments to settings. At the conclusion of testing, the equipment may be accepted as meeting the specification, accepted subject to a small list of remedial actions, or not accepted because of non-compliance with a performance parameter of major importance or a long list of faults requiring remedial action. In the second case, time scales should be agreed for correcting the defects. In the third case, a new joint acceptance procedure is necessary after the installation engineer has corrected the problem(s). The final section of the joint acceptance pro-forma should reflect this situation and must be signed by both the installation engineer and responsible physicist. Following successful acceptance, this section will be the basis for further payment to the supplier for the equipment.

1.7 Commissioning

1.7.1 Clinical services

Following handover of the facility, reconfiguration of clinical services may be necessary. This should be done by the senior oncology staff involved taking into account all the relevant factors and a clear timetable developed to make all staff aware of the changes and their role in them.

1.7.2 Equipment commissioning

Following acceptance of the equipment, further commissioning will be necessary before it enters clinical use. This includes the gathering of detailed information on equipment characteristics and radiation beams for treatment planning systems, absolute calibrations of radiation output, establishment of quality assurance protocols, establishment of clinical treatment protocols and operator training. It should be understood that in the interests of patient safety, commissioning cannot be shortened to make up for any earlier delays in construction, etc.

1.8 Project evaluation

NHS Trusts are required to evaluate and learn from their projects. This is mandatory for projects over £1M and a report must be made to the Department of Health for projects over £20M. An initial evaluation should be performed 6–12 months after commissioning and a long term evaluation two years after commissioning. The evaluation should cover the following areas:

- Brief description of project.
- Accuracy of the original strategic context.
- Correctness of option appraisal.
- Review of procurement process including comparison with estimated costs.
- Review of project management including compliance with the planned timetable.
- Realisation of benefits.
- Outcome and impact.
- Lessons for future projects.

More details on project evaluation are given in (NHS Trust Development Authority 2014).

References

IRR 1999 *The Ionising Radiations Regulations* SI 1999/3232 (London: The Stationery Office)

NHS Commissioning Board 2013 www.england.nhs.uk/commissioning/spec-services/npc-crg/group-b/b01/ (Accessed: 23 January 2017)

NHS England 2013 *NHS Business Case Approvals Process–Capital Investment, Property, Equipment and ICT* (London: NHS England)

NHS Trust Development Authority 2014 *Capital Regime and Investment Business Case Approvals—Guidance for NHS Trusts* (London: NHS Trust Development Authority)
Office of Government Commerce 2013 *Public Sector Business Cases Using the Five Case Model* (London: HM Treasury)
RCR (Royal College of Radiologists) 2012 *Writing a Good Business Case* (London: RCR)

Chapter 2

The design of radiotherapy facilities

P W Horton

2.1 General

A typical radiotherapy facility will comprise a number of shielded treatment rooms, each with an adjacent control room/area. The number of treatment rooms will depend on the population served and the availability of specialised treatment techniques. This service will be supported by pre-treatment facilities for patient imaging and treatment planning and by general facilities for patient changing and waiting. Medical physicists will require laboratories for equipment calibration and technical staff will require workshops for equipment repair and preparation of individual patient shielding devices. It may also be necessary to have a secure store for radioactive sources and a mould room for the preparation of patient immobilisation devices. If part of a cancer centre, there will also be facilities for chemotherapy, outpatient clinics and ward accommodation for inpatients. Accommodation will be required for oncologists, radiographers, medical physicists, dosimetrists, technical officers, administrative and clerical staff. The general requirements for cancer services have been comprehensively described in the Department of Health's *Cancer Treatment Facilities: Planning and Design Manual (Version 1.1: England)* (DH 2011) and *Health Building Note 02-01: Cancer Treatment Facilities* (DH 2013). Features on radiotherapy from these two sources of guidance are included in the sections which follow.

2.2 Linear accelerators

Linear accelerators are now the most common treatment units in radiotherapy departments in cancer centres and units. They produce high energy x-ray and electron beams. Most models of linear accelerators produce two or three beams of x-rays and typically five electron beams, each with a different energy to facilitate a range of patient treatments. As a consequence of the penetrating nature of the x-ray beam they need to be sited in a shielded bunker to reduce the external dose rates and annual doses

doi:10.1088/978-0-7503-1440-4ch2

to meet the constraints imposed by national legislation (see chapter 3). The two common arrangements for safely housing a linear accelerator are shown in plan in figure 2.1(a) and (b). Both layouts show the increased thickness of shielding (*primary shielding*) needed to attenuate the x-ray beam when it falls directly on a wall after passing through the patient. An increased thickness in shielding will also be required in the roof of the bunker in the area directly irradiated by the x-ray beam and in the floor if the treatment units are sited above occupied areas. The layouts also show the thinner shielding (*secondary shielding*) required in the other walls to attenuate the lower energy leakage radiation from the treatment head of the linear accelerator and the radiation scattered by the patient and from the directly irradiated walls. Calculation of the necessary wall thicknesses to attenuate primary and secondary radiation to the dose constraints imposed by national legislation is described in chapters 5 and 6. Further practical considerations to help achieve the dose constraints and to help ensure the integrity of the shielding during construction are described in chapter 7.

In figure 2.1(a), an acceptable dose rate at the entrance to the bunker is achieved by using a *maze* down which the intensity of the scattered x-radiation is attenuated by distance from the source and multiple scatter interactions with its walls. To prevent inadvertent entry during patient treatment when the beam is on, engineering controls are used at the entrance to the maze. This can be a simple interlocked gate or a light beam. If the gate is opened or the light beam broken, production of the beam stops. In general terms the dose rate at the maze entrance will be reduced by greater length and more bends in the maze. Clearly such an arrangement requires additional space for the maze. If space is limited, the arrangement shown in figure 2.1(b) can be adopted with a shielded door at the entrance to the bunker to attenuate the external dose rate to an acceptable level. Such doors are heavy and need to be power operated. They require additional safety features compared with the simple gate or light beam interlock described above. A direct door can also lead to a claustrophobic atmosphere in the bunker for the patient being treated. A short maze (figure 2.1(c)) can be very helpful in this situation to both reduce the claustrophobic feeling and to reduce the weight of the door. For endpoint energies of 8.5 MV and above[1], consideration should also be given to neutron scatter down the maze, although this scatter may not be significant with 10 MV operation. 15 MV x-ray beams produce a much higher neutron fluence. An acceptable dose rate at the maze entrance can be achieved with a suitably long maze or a shorter maze lined with neutron absorbent material and/or an absorbent door operating at the higher x-ray energies. Empirical methods for calculating the x-ray and neutron scatter down the maze, together with the calculation of appropriate door thickness, are described in chapter 5. However, these methods have uncertainties and Monte Carlo simulations have been used to increase the accuracy of these calculations, in particular neutron scatter down the maze. In the past the accuracy of these calculations was limited due to the long calculation times needed to include a sufficient number of events for statistical certainty. However, with modern powerful computers, there is no reason (apart from the expertise required)

[1] This report adopts the commonplace practice of defining the end point energy in MV when it should strictly be in MeV. Alternatively it can be considered as the effective accelerating potential in MV.

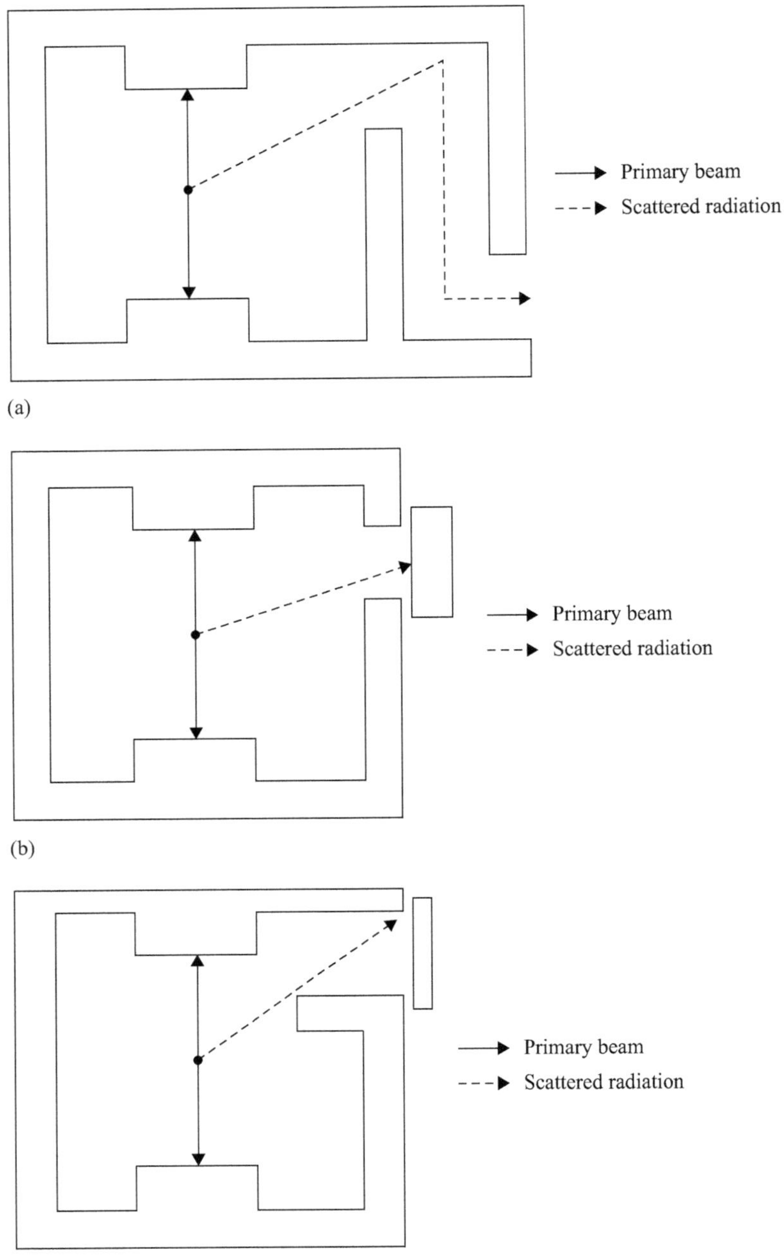

Figure 2.1. (a) Linear accelerator bunker with a maze. (b) Linear accelerator bunker with a direct door. (c) Linear accelerator bunker with a direct door and a short maze.

Table 2.1. Typical linear accelerator bunker wall thicknesses. *Primary shielding* (top). The thicknesses for concrete, steel and lead are calculated using the TVL_1 and TVL_e values in table 5.1 and the thicknesses in magnetite are calculated from the measured TVL values in table 7.3. *Secondary shielding* (bottom). The thicknesses for concrete are calculated using the TVL_1 and TVL_e values in table 5.2, the thicknesses in magnetite are calculated from the measured TVL values in table 7.3 and the thicknesses of steel and lead are calculated using the primary TVL_1 and TVL_e values in table 5.1.

Material	Density (kg m^{-3})	Thickness (m) x-ray beam energy 6 MV	10 MV	15 MV
Concrete	2350	2.11	2.36	2.61
Magnetite	3800	1.16	1.38	1.59
Steel	7900	0.63	0.69	0.69
Lead	11 340	0.36	0.36	0.36

Note: these thicknesses are based on a dose rate of 6 Gy min^{-1} at the isocentre, a distance of 5 m from the x-ray focus to the exterior surface of the wall and an instantaneous dose rate limit of 7.5 μSv h^{-1} at the exterior surface.

Material	Density (kg m^{-3})	Thickness (m) x-ray beam energy 6 MV	10 MV	15 MV
Concrete	2350	0.97	1.03	1.12
Magnetite	3800	0.53	0.59	0.81
Steel	7900	0.33	0.36	0.36
Lead	11 340	0.19	0.19	0.19

Note: these thicknesses are based on a dose rate of 6 Gy min^{-1} at the isocentre, head leakage of 0.1%, a distance of 5 m from the isocentre to the exterior surface of the wall and an instantaneous dose rate limit of 7.5 μSv h^{-1} at the exterior surface.

that the design of entire bunkers cannot be optimised using Monte Carlo simulations of the photon and neutron pathways. These techniques, together with the available Monte Carlo calculation codes and computer packages to visualise the scatter paths and flux densities within the bunker, are described in chapter 6.

Table 2.1 shows some typical thicknesses for primary and secondary shielding for different materials for linear accelerators operating at 6, 10 or 15 MV calculated using the attenuation data in chapters 5 and 7. However, these figures are for indicative purposes only and may be used in the initial planning of the overall layout of a radiotherapy facility. To ensure that statutory dose constraints are met, individual bunker shielding must always be calculated using a methodology such as that described in chapters 5 or 6, taking into account the proposed layout and patient workload. These calculations will determine the final design which should be approved by the Radiation Protection Adviser.

The *Cancer Treatment Facilities: Planning and Design Manual* (DH 2011) recommends that new treatment bunkers with linear accelerators should provide adequate shielding for x-rays up to a maximum of 15 MV. This is felt to be the highest energy required for modern clinical practice. Such an arrangement means that any replacement linear accelerator with an x-ray energy up to 15 MV can be accommodated without the need for additional shielding, although the manual notes that additional neutron protection may be required with accelerators operating with x-rays above 8.5 MV. Such a future-proofing arrangement also needs to consider possible variations in the position of the isocentre, as this varies with different models of accelerator and will affect the position (and possibly the width) of the primary shielding. A broader width of primary shielding (than that required for a particular accelerator) may be necessary to cope with a variety of models over the life of the bunker. In a large cancer centre, the need to make all bunkers adequate for 15 MV x-rays is excessive and will add to space and cost. In this situation, the number of 15 MV bunkers should be sufficient to meet the clinical need and allow replacement of 15 MV accelerators without loss of 15 MV treatment capacity. Other bunkers need to be designed for 10 MV x-ray operation for future flexibility. The provision of 15 MV bunkers at a satellite facility will depend on the local clinical need and the existing provision of 15 MV bunkers at the centre. A minimum of two accelerators with the same configuration of x-ray and electron energies should be available in a centre or satellite to ensure continuity of treatment during planned maintenance or breakdowns (*Guidance on the Management and Governance of Additional Radiotherapy Capacity* (RCR 2013)).

The treatment room should be large enough to allow full extension of the treatment couch in all directions, with room for the radiographers to walk round it, but not excessive to minimise the distance between the control room and the patient. Storage space will need to be provided for electron applicators, electron beam cut-outs and patient immobilisation devices, and these should be conveniently sited for treatment use to minimise manual handling. Identical layouts in all treatment rooms will help staff to work efficiently. The introduction of dynamic wedges and multi-leaf collimation has removed the need for mechanical wedges and shielding blocks. Room illumination should be adjustable with subtle lighting during patient treatment, dim lighting to see treatment marks on the patient during treatment set-up and bright lighting for maintenance and other tasks. The lighting level and the operation of the alignment lasers should be convenient to operate from a hand set on the patient couch. Modern radiotherapy management systems have in-room monitors showing the patient details and the condition of the linear accelerator in relation to the next treatment. These should be sited for easy viewing from the area of the treatment couch during treatment set-up. Consideration needs to be given to the siting of the radiation warning sign, last person out button (to allow an uninterrupted view of the whole treatment room) and the emergency off buttons (see chapter 3). The room will require one or two washbasins in compliance with local infection control practice. It will also require electrical sockets for ancillary and medical physics equipment and data points connected to the IT network. The treatment room should be ventilated with at least three air changes per hour to remove ionisation products (NCRP Report 151 (NCRP 2005)). Linear accelerator manufacturers often require more changes, e.g. six, to remove heat generated by the accelerator and architects often specify more changes, e.g. 15, for environmental reasons. The passage of air conditioning ducts in the bunker walls and maze must not compromise the radiation protection of the bunker (see chapter 7). Sprinkler fire systems should not be used in treatment rooms to avoid damage to electrical systems. More information on treatment room design is given in chapter 4.

The entry into the treatment room (including bends in the maze) must be sufficiently wide and high enough for the passage of the components of the linear accelerator during installation, for patient beds, trolleys or wheelchairs and items of equipment required for maintenance or quality assurance. Corner and wall protection should be provided against damage by equipment, beds, etc. The maze will not be large enough for the passage of the magnet for magnetic resonance image guided linear accelerators and the magnet will need to be introduced though a hole in a bunker wall or roof, which is subsequently filled. The entrance to the treatment room will also require radiation warning signs and lights (see chapter 3).

The linear accelerator requires a base frame in the floor to ensure that it is mounted accurately in relation to the patient couch, which is also mounted on the base frame. Lifting eyes may be located over the accelerator for the possible removal of the treatment head. The route from the off-loading point to the site of the linear accelerator should have floor loadings sufficient to take the heaviest component of the accelerator. Cable ducts will be required in the floor to connect the components of the accelerator and link it to the control area. A cable route (or permanently wired connection) that does not compromise the radiation protection of the barrier through which it passes will be required between the bunker and the control room for dosimetry purposes (see chapter 7). The accelerator will require stabilised mains electrical power, compressed air for some models and chilled water for cooling; these services will need to be brought to the rear of the accelerator stand. The plant may be sited in the roof space and consideration given to controlling access during accelerator operation if dose and dose rate constraints are not met during operation. Computer systems will require uninterruptible power supply (UPS) systems to enable an orderly shutdown in the event of mains electrical failure. Consideration may have to be given to connecting some accelerators to the emergency power supply to maintain key patient treatments during an extended loss of mains power. Rigid ceiling and wall mountings will be required for the alignment lasers, in-room monitors and respiratory gating cameras. Mountings may also be required for specialised patient localisation and imaging systems. The linear accelerator manufacturer's requirements regarding access, environment and services are often conveniently combined in an Installation Data Package (IDP).

Linear accelerators that are to be used for total body irradiation (TBI) of patients will require a larger bunker in the plane of the radiation beam and will need to be offset with respect to the midline of the room (see figure 2.2). To irradiate a 2 m long patient, the minimum distance from the isocentre to the primary shielding will be such that the diagonal (set horizontally) of the largest radiation field encompasses the length of the patient placed close to the primary barrier; this distance is 2.5 m for

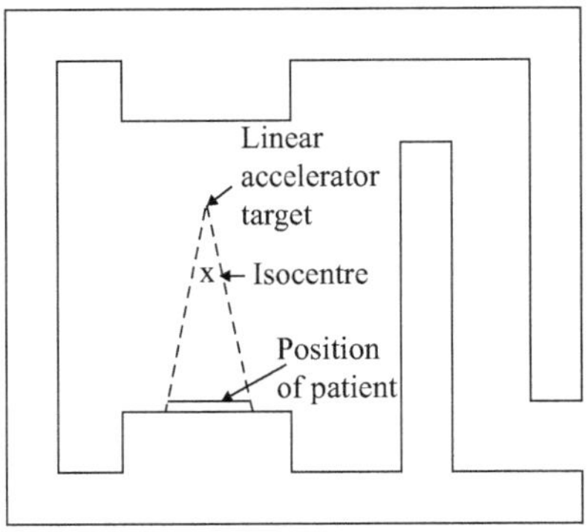

Figure 2.2. Linear accelerator bunker with a maze, with an offset isocentre for TBI.

a 40×40 cm field at the isocentre. Without collimator rotation, the distance needs to be increased to 4 m for a horizontal 40 cm wide field at the isocentre; in this configuration the vertical field width can be reduced to that necessary for the beam to cover the patient. The widths and thicknesses of the primary barriers may be different in such a bunker.

In designing a facility with adequate shielding, it is important that the designer has clear information from the users about the proposed clinical practice. This requires clear information on the number of patients per day, x-ray energies, proportion of intensity modulated radiotherapy (IMRT) or volumetric modulated arc therapy (VMAT) patients at each energy and the dose per patient per day. A pro-forma is useful to help ensure a comprehensive picture is obtained (see chapter 4).

The control area should be sited as close as possible to the treatment room entrance to provide the shortest route into the treatment room and enable monitoring of the entrance for unauthorised entry of persons by the staff in charge of the unit. To maintain the privacy of patient information, the interior should not be easily visible to patients and their carers. Modern linear accelerators require a number of visual display units (VDUs) to operate them and for patient imaging, and adequate bench space must be provided for ergonomic operation and monitoring. Bench space can be saved if keyboard video monitor (KVM) switches are used so that a VDU can be used to display more than one function. Closed circuit television (CCTV) will be required for patient monitoring during treatment with pan and zoom cameras in the treatment room. The latter should be sited well away from areas where the treatment beam can point and preferably have a resistance to ionising radiation damage. An intercom for the radiographers to speak to the patient is also required and should have a privacy facility so that conversation in the control area cannot be overheard. Adequate power and data points need to be provided. More information on control room design is given in chapter 4.

Consultation with experienced radiography staff is essential during the design of treatment rooms and control areas to ensure that they are as practical and as pleasant as possible to work in. A check list of key requirements for a treatment facility with a linear accelerator is set out in table 2.2. This can also be used as the basis for a check list for any external beam facility but not all the requirements may be necessary.

Table 2.2. Checklist of requirements for a treatment facility with a linear accelerator.

Access
For equipment installation and maintenance
For calibration and quality assurance equipment
For patients on trolleys
Dosimeter cable route
Equipment services
Stabilised electrical supply
Chilled cooling water
Compressed air (for some linear accelerators)
UPS for computers
IT network connections
Health and safety
Shielding
Maze and/or shielding door
Radiation warning signs
Radiation warning lights
Emergency stop buttons
Door/barrier interlock
Last person out button
Treatment room
Laser alignment devices
In-room monitors
Lighting level control
Mount for gating camera
Connections to IT network
Wash basin(s) and water supply
Treatment room storage
Immobilisation devices
Applicators
Electron beam cut outs
Control area
Connections to IT network
Dosimeter cable route to treatment room
Control area storage
Patient notes and radiographs
Clinical procedures
Safety procedures
Quality assurance procedures and records
Equipment fault log
Dosimetry charts
Patient communication
CCTV
Voice intercommunication
General
Patient changing facilities
Patient waiting area
Other storage requirements
Equipment performance and maintenance records
Quality assurance equipment
Spare parts and test equipment

Both TomoTherapy® and CyberKnife® employ linear accelerators producing 6 MV x-rays but have specific requirements for beam orientation and utilisation that are different from those for linear accelerators[2]. The shielding requirements for these special cases are discussed in chapter 8. Engineering controls and general arrangements are similar to those above for linear accelerators.

2.3 Cobalt-60 units

Cobalt-60 teletherapy units have largely been replaced by linear accelerators due to the latter's higher dose rate and smaller penumbra for radiation fields. However cobalt-60 is still used for external beam radiotherapy in the Gamma Knife®.[3] This equipment employs a large number of Co-60 sources mounted in a 'helmet' for the radiosurgery or radiotherapy of brain lesions. The special shielding requirements, engineering controls and general arrangements for this equipment are described in chapter 8.

2.4 Kilovoltage units

The *Cancer Treatment Facilities: Planning and Design Manual* (DH 2011) describes superficial/orthovoltage treatment units as optional, but most centres have one such unit. This might be an orthovoltage unit operating at x-ray energies up to 300 kV or a superficial unit operating at two or three x-ray energies up to a maximum of 150 kV for the treatment of superficial and near surface conditions.

The manual shows a typical example of a treatment room with the control room immediately outside; the main features are shown in figure 2.3. For a new facility, the walls may be of concrete and of sufficient thickness to meet the dose constraints at the highest operating x-ray energy. The x-ray unit is mounted away from the door, usually on a ceiling suspension, and the generator is sited within the treatment room. The room must be of sufficient size to allow any area of the patient to be treated in a seated or lying position. There should also be room for a wash-hand basin and for storage of applicators and lead cut-outs for irregular treatment areas. A supply of chilled water for cooling the x-ray tube will be required. Radiation warning signs and lights must be provided in the treatment room and at its entrance.

There should be an interlocked door between the control and treatment rooms; a sliding door reduces the space required. The door should be lead lined with good overlaps and will need to be power-operated because of its weight. The door should preferably be out of the main beam to reduce its radiation protection requirements. CCTV for patient monitoring during treatment and an intercom for the radiographers to speak to the patient are required. The control room should have benching sufficient for the treatment control unit and computer equipment, etc, together with power and data points. A cableway needs to be provided between the control and treatment room for dosimetry purposes that does not compromise the radiation

[2] TomoTherapy and CyberKnife are registered trademarks of Accuray Incorporated.

[3] Gamma Knife is a registered trademark of Elekta.

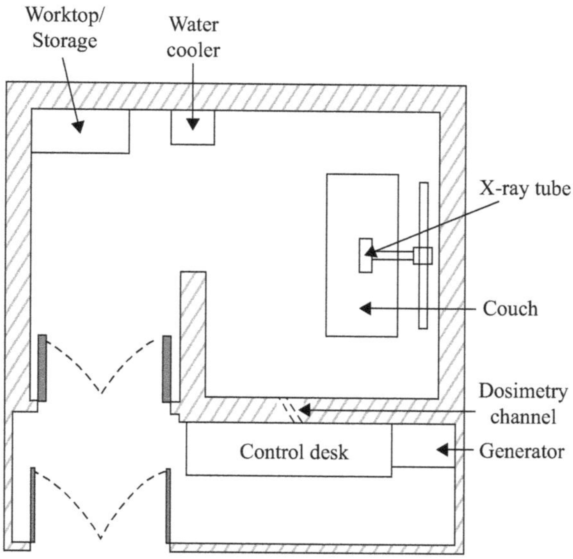

Figure 2.3. Sample room layout for kilovoltage treatment unit (after DH 2011).

protection provided by the barrier. The requirements and shielding information for kilovoltage treatment units are discussed in greater detail in chapter 9.

2.5 Brachytherapy

The *Cancer Treatment Facilities: Planning and Design Manual* (DH 2011) describes a brachytherapy suite as optional, but most centres provide one or more brachytherapy services.

Brachytherapy using radioactive sealed sources is now largely confined to automatic high dose rate (HDR) afterloading of high activity sources, pulsed dose rate (PDR) afterloading of medium activity sources, the temporary external placement of plaques containing a radioactive source or the permanent interstitial implantation of small sealed sources ('seeds'). A recent innovation has been the introduction of intraoperative radiotherapy (IORT) using miniature x-ray sources or mobile linear accelerators producing electron-only beams (IOERT) to deliver the radiation dose to tissue surrounding the tumour following surgical removal of the tumour. This has been termed electronic brachytherapy. The facilities for each are considered in outline below.

HDR afterloading employs a computer controlled afterloader containing a small high activity source, e.g. 370 MBq of iridium-192. This is introduced into the patient, who may be anesthetised, through transport tubes into one or more applicators positioned earlier without the radioactive source present. The position and dwell time of the source are accurately controlled by the computer according to the treatment plan to build up the required dose distribution in the patient. Patient treatment times are short, lasting minutes. The procedure takes place in a shielded room in which the walls, floor and ceiling all provide primary shielding when the

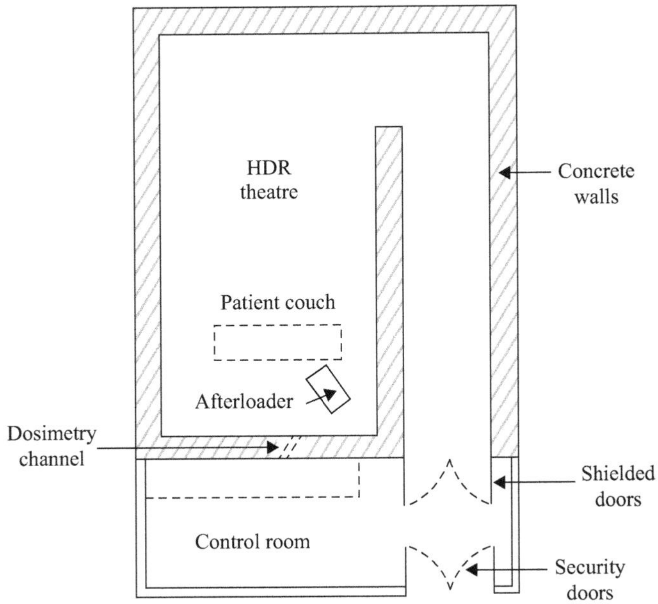

Figure 2.4. Layout of a typical HDR brachytherapy suite.

source is within the patient. The room will require a door providing adequate shielding to meet dose constraints and a short maze is effective in reducing the shielding in the door. A typical layout is shown in figure 2.4. The door should be interlocked with the afterloader so that inadvertent entry to the room causes the source to return to the safe in the afterloader. The afterloader will be fitted with a battery electrical supply to return the source to the afterloader in the event of mains failure and a manual means of retracting the source if it sticks in the expose position. The position of the afterloader in the room will need to be restricted so that the source in the expose position in the patient cannot be near the inner entrance to the maze. Such restraint may also serve to meet the requirements for source security. The room will need to be large enough to hold the afterloader, patient couch, anaesthetic trolley if necessary and a crash trolley in an emergency. It should be supplied with piped medical gases. The room may also need to be large enough to accommodate a C-arm x-ray unit for orthogonal images of the applicators. Colour CCTV should be provided to enable monitoring of the anaesthetised patient during treatment. Radiation warning signs and lights need to be provided at the entrance to the shielded room and the warning light should remain on from the start of treatment, i.e. from the source leaving the afterloader safe to enter the first applicator, to the end of treatment, i.e. when the source returns to the safe from the last applicator. It should not go out when the source returns to the safe between intermediate applicators. A radiation monitor with an audible alarm should be installed in the treatment room as an independent means of knowing that the source has returned safely to the safe after treatment is complete. A cableway needs to be provided between the control and treatment room for dosimetry purposes that does not compromise the radiation protection provided by the barrier. Consideration needs to be given to the siting of the last person out button (to allow an uninterrupted view of the whole treatment room) and the emergency off buttons. The room will also require a washbasin, electrical sockets for ancillary and medical physics equipment, and data points connected to the IT network. The control room should be adjacent to the entry door to control access and for prompt access to the patient. It should have sufficient bench space for the console controlling the afterloader and be fitted with power and data points. Spaces for the induction and recovery of anaesthetised patients will be required near the treatment room, together with clean and dirty utility areas.

In designing the shielded room, it is important that the designer has clear information from the users about the proposed clinical practice. This requires clear information on the number of patients per day undergoing each afterloading procedure, the typical dose per patient and the source exposure time to reach that dose for a specified source activity. Treatment times will increase as the source decays.

PDR afterloading has largely replaced low dose rate (LDR) afterloading. The latter was commonly used to treat gynaecological cancers using three trains of caesium-137 or cobalt-60 sources with inert spacers to give the required dose distribution. The three applicators were accurately positioned without radioactivity present and the trains were transferred by the afterloader into the applicators at the start of treatment. Treatment lasted for about two days and the sources were withdrawn at the end of treatment or temporarily during nursing care. The radiobiological effect of HDR afterloading is different from LDR afterloading and adjustment has to be made to the total dose delivered. PDR afterloading was introduced to combine the benefit of a reliable single source delivery system with a lower overall dose rate. Using a higher activity source (typically 37 MBq of iridium-192), the same total dose is given to the patient over the same period of time (e.g. two days) but the patient is only irradiated for a predetermined period in each hour, e.g. for 10 min h^{-1}. The technique also employs a computer controlled afterloader to control the dwell times of the source in the applicators. It requires a suitably shielded room in which the patient is confined to bed whilst connected to the afterloader. The walls, floor and ceiling all provide primary shielding when the source is within the patient. The room will require a door providing adequate shielding to meet dose constraints and a short maze is effective in reducing the shielding in the door. The door should be interlocked with the afterloader so that inadvertent entry to the room causes the sources to return to the safe in the afterloader. The afterloader will be fitted with a battery electrical supply to return the source to the afterloader in the event of mains failure and a manual means of retracting the source if it sticks in the expose position. The position of the afterloader in the room will be restricted by the position of the patient bed. An external means of interrupting treatment and returning the sources to the safe in the afterloader is sited at the entrance to the treatment room to enable nursing care during the long period of treatment or safe access to the patient in an emergency; routine care can usually take place in the interval between the hourly irradiations. Radiation warning signs and lights need to be provided at the entrance to the shielded room. A radiation monitor with an audible alarm should be installed in the treatment room as an independent means of knowing that the source has returned safely to the safe when treatment is interrupted or is complete. CCTV should be provided to enable observation of the patient during treatment from the nursing station. The console controlling the afterloader needs to be sited in a secure area adjacent to the treatment room. The treatment room is best sited near the oncology wards to facilitate nursing care.

The commonest use of external brachytherapy sources is now the temporary attachment of radioactive plaques to the surface of the eye. The plaques contain either ruthenium-106 (maximum β-particle energy 3.54 MeV and half-life 374 days) or iodine-125 (28 keV x-rays and half-life 60 days) sources. These do not require substantial radiation protection measures except when being handled. Treatment may last a few days and the patient should be nursed in a single room with appropriate systems of work. A small clean laboratory is also required for the preparation of the plaques and their sterilisation.

Interstitial radiotherapy commonly uses iodine-125 or palladium-104 sterile seeds, which are permanently implanted in the patient for the treatment of prostate cancer. Both are low energy x-ray emitters (28 and 21 keV respectively) and do not require substantial radiation protection measures. The seeds may be inserted in the patient at specific positions either using a 'gun' loaded with a magazine of seeds or hollow needles pre-loaded with seeds positioned in the needles according to a prepared treatment plan. Both are done with the aid of ultrasound imaging. The former technique requires real time treatment planning taking the positional information of inserted seeds from the ultrasound images to guide the positioning of subsequent seeds to achieve the required dose distribution. Space needs to be provided in the treatment room for the staff and treatment planning computer. The latter technique requires a separate clean room for the loading of the seeds into the needles before patient insertion. Insertion of the seeds takes place under general anaesthetic and the treatment room must have space for an anaesthetic trolley and the appropriate theatre staff. Spaces for the induction and recovery of the anaesthetised patient will be required near the treatment room, together with clean and dirty utility areas. The treatment room must also be large enough to accommodate a C-arm x-ray unit for orthogonal images of the completed insertion to check its quality and audit the number of seeds inserted. Because of the anaesthetic requirement, seed insertions can be done in the shielded room used for HDR brachytherapy if one is available or in an operating theatre with suitable radiation protection measures; the former is preferred because it is a dedicated radiation facility.

The shielding and radiation protection arrangements for sealed source brachytherapy are considered in greater detail in chapter 10.

Electronic brachytherapy usually takes place in an operating theatre following excision of the tumour. Treatment units typically produce 30 keV x-rays (IORT) or electrons in the energy range 4–12 MeV (IOERT). Satisfactory standards of radiation protection can usually be achieved with standard room construction and temporary shields, good operating procedures and training. However, it should be noted that dose rates can be high and access may need to be restricted beyond the operating theatre. Electronic brachytherapy may also be employed to treat skin lesions in departments, e.g. dermatology, where staff are less familiar with radiation hazards and substantial training is required. The radiation protection requirements for IORT and IOERT are considered further in chapter 9.

2.6 Particle therapy

Particle radiotherapy employs protons or carbon ions. The clinical benefit in principle is that the beam energy is deposited in tissue at a limited range of depths around the Bragg peak. Whilst treatment facilities are not common, they are becoming increasingly widespread. The Particle Therapy Co-Operative Group website (http://www.ptcog.ch) says that 66 facilities are operational, 42 under construction and 18 more are planned worldwide (as of November 2016); six centres are planned for the United Kingdom. Particle therapy usually takes place in a separate building at a large oncology centre. PTCOG Report 1 (PTCOG 2010) outlines ten such facilities. A facility typically comprises a particle injector, a cyclotron or synchrocyclotron accelerator, a high energy beam line and up to three treatment rooms; the treatment rooms can have a fixed gantry with one beam position or a rotational gantry with 360° rotation of the beam. Protons with energies of 230–250 MeV and carbon ions with energies of 320–430 MeV amu^{-1} are used clinically. Dose rates range from 1 to 2 Gy min^{-1} for large 30 cm × 30 cm treatment fields to 15–20 Gy min^{-1} for the small fields used in treating ocular cancers. Recently single treatment room systems using a synchrocyclotron have been developed, suitable for smaller oncology centres.

The dominant product of any beam interactions is high energy neutrons (and their reaction products) and substantial shielding (2–4 m thick) is required to reduce the dose rates to acceptable levels. These interactions take place in the beam line (to a limited extent) and in the beam shaping devices, energy or range shifters, and the patient in the treatment room. Neutron production is reduced if pencil beam scanning is employed to shape the treatment area instead of passive scattering devices. Since, at the energies concerned, much of the neutron production is in the forward direction, the shielding of a fixed beam room will require the wall in the direction of the beam to be much thicker than the other walls, whilst a room with a 360° rotational beam will require substantial shielding in all beam directions. Less local shielding is required with synchrocyclotrons as these can accelerate the particles to the exact energy required and avoid the need for energy shifters, which are a source of neutrons. Empirical methods can be employed to calculate the shielding required for particle therapy facilities. However Titt and Newhauser (2005) and Newhauser *et al* (2002) have shown that these can overestimate actual dose rates by a factor 15. Monte Carlo simulations are more accurate and may overestimate by a factor of 2. Monte Carlo simulation is essential for the calculation of the shielding of particle therapy facilities and the MCPNX and FLUKA codes (see chapter 6) have been used for this purpose. An introduction to the shielding of particle therapy facilities, together with a list of the information required for the design of adequate shielding for such a facility, is given in chapter 11.

References

DH (Department of Health) 2011 *Cancer Treatment Facilities: Planning and Design Manual 9075*: Version 1.1: England (London: Department of Health)

DH (Department of Health) 2013 *Cancer Treatment Facilities* Health Building Note 02-01 (London: Department of Health)

NCRP (National Council on Radiation Protection and Measurements) 2005 *Structural Shielding Design and Evaluation for Megavoltage X- and Gamma-Ray Radiotherapy Facilities* Report 151 (Bethesda, MD: NCRP)

Newhauser W D, Titt U, Dexheimer D, Yan X and Nill S 2002 Neutron shielding verification measurements and simulations for a 235 MeV proton therapy centre *Nucl. Instrum. Methods Phys. Res.* A **476** 80–4

PTCOG (Particle Therapy Co-Operative Group) 2010 *Shielding Design and Radiation Safety of Charged Particle Therapy Facilities* Report 1 http://ptcog.web.psi.ch (Accessed: 11 November 2016)

RCR (Royal College of Radiologists) 2013 SCoR (Society and College of Radiographers), IPEM (Institute of Physics and Engineering in Medicine), *Guidance on the Management and Governance of Additional Radiotherapy Capacity* (London: RCR)

Titt U and Newhauser W D 2005 Neutron shielding calculations in a proton therapy facility based on Monte Carlo simulations and analytical models: criterion for selecting the method of choice *Radiat. Prot. Dosim.* **115** 144–8

Chapter 3

Radiation protection requirements

D J Peet

3.1 Introduction

Radiation protection considerations in a radiotherapy department include the following:

- Design of radiation facilities including:
  - a safe design,
  - specification of shielding required,
  - consideration of engineering controls and
  - safety features for routine operation.
- Involvement in the licensing or permitting of the premises.
- Risk assessments of the radiation hazard including those for pregnant staff.
- Development of contingency plans in the event of a radiation emergency.
- Commissioning facilities to confirm the radiation protection requirements are in place and operate correctly. This will include:
  - a critical examination on behalf of the installer and
  - a shielding survey.
- Operational radiation protection during routine operation including involvement in the drafting of local rules and procedures.
- Analysis and advice on any incidents.
- Guidance and assistance with inspections by regulatory authorities.
- Personal monitoring.
- Environmental monitoring.
- Audit of radiation protection arrangements including compliance with conditions of licenses or permits.
- Teaching and training related to radiation protection.
- Consideration of the end of life of the facility, radiation equipment or radioactive source.

doi:10.1088/978-0-7503-1440-4ch3

Radiation protection requirements and the complexity of those requirements depend on the type of radiation source, the nature of the hazard and the level of risk as a result of that hazard. If radioactive material is involved, sealed or unsealed, the complexity of radiation protection requirements can increase significantly.

A Radiation Protection Adviser (RPA) as described in the *Ionising Radiation Regulations* 1999 (IRR 1999) should be involved with all the elements above, but the design will have the best outcome if a multidisciplinary team is involved and works cooperatively (see chapter 2). In addition RPAs are involved in a critical examination of the safety features and warning devices in any new installation on behalf of the installer of any equipment; the RPA may be from the installer or the user (IRR 1999, IPEM 2012).

The decisions made as part of the design process are likely to be an integral part of the risk assessments for the facility and should be recorded. A prior risk assessment is also required before work starts with ionising radiation. The design criteria and decisions can be used as part of that assessment.

It should be noted that the greatest risks in radiotherapy in a correctly designed facility are to the patient. Patient safety and treatment accuracy are not part of this report. There are many documents detailing the radiation protection requirements for patient safety and risk assessment (HSE 2000, IRMER 2000, RCR 2008a, RCR 2008b, ICRP 2009).

3.2 Quantities and units

An understanding of the quantities and units used in radiation protection is required to apply the regulations and requirements for facility design and operation. These are outlined below.

3.2.1 Radiation exposure and dose

3.2.1.1 Exposure

The basic quantity that can be measured using an ionisation chamber is exposure with the derived SI unit C kg^{-1}. This is not a particularly helpful unit for radiation protection where the dose to an individual or organ is usually required. The following quantities are all measures of absorption of energy.

3.2.1.2 Air kerma

Environmental dose measurements can be made using suitable conversion factors or calibrations of air kerma (or absorbed dose in air) with the unit of the gray (Gy). This quantity can be calculated and compared with chamber measurements, e.g. during a shielding survey.

3.2.1.3 Absorbed dose in organs

In radiotherapy organ dose is well understood and has the same units as air kerma, i.e. the gray (Gy).

3.2.1.4 Equivalent dose

The quantity air kerma or organ dose multiplied by the radiation weighting factor (table 3.1) is known as the equivalent dose with the units of J kg^{-1}, termed the sievert (Sv). This is the determinant used in this report for the specification of shielding. The radiation weighting factor used to be known as the quality factor. The choice of the correct weighting factor to use for neutron fluences in radiotherapy facilities can be difficult when the energy spectrum of neutrons in a linear accelerator maze and at the maze entrance is uncertain. A factor of 10 is usually used if the energy spectrum is not known. Dose limits for individual organs are set in terms of terms of equivalent dose.

3.2.1.5 Effective dose

The sum of the weighted equivalent doses for individual organs multiplied by the tissue weighting factors (table 3.2) for those organs is the effective dose, again with the unit of the sievert (Sv).

Table 3.1. Radiation weighting factors (ICRP 2007).

Radiation	Weighting factor
X-rays, gamma rays, electrons	1
Protons	2
Neutrons	Continuous function dependent on energy

Table 3.2. Tissue weighting factors (ICRP 2007).

Tissues	Tissue weighting factor
Bone-marrow (red), colon, lung, stomach, breast, remainder tissues	0.12 for each
Gonads	0.08
Bladder, oesophagus, liver, thyroid	0.04 for each
Bone surface, brain, salivary glands, skin	0.01 for each

Effective dose is not a quantity that can be directly measured but is derived from measurements of exposure or air kerma with corrections for the weighting factor of the radiation type and tissue weighting factors when the exposure of an individual is not uniform. Whole-body dose limits and dose constraints for staff and members of the public are set in terms of effective dose.

3.2.2 Operational quantities

Other radiation protection quantities and units are also used, known as operational quantities. These are as follows.

3.2.2.1 Ambient dose equivalent H(d)*

Many dose rate meters, for example, are calibrated to display the ambient dose rate equivalent, which relates to the dose equivalent at a defined depth in the 300 mm tissue equivalent International Commission on Radiation Units and Measurements sphere (ICRP 1996). For most practical purposes in the measurement of gamma rays and x-ray photons this quantity and the air kerma rate are likely to be numerically equivalent.

3.2.2.2 Personal dose equivalent Hp(d)

Personal monitors are calibrated to give the personal dose equivalent from exposure to gamma rays and photons at a prescribed depth of 0.07 mm (Hp(0.07)) or 10 mm (Hp(10)). It should be noted that Hp(10) is indicative of effective dose. For most energies and geometries, Hp(10) is a conservative estimate of effective dose (Zankl 1999).

3.2.3 Dose rate

Measurements and calculations in and around radiotherapy installations are often of dose rate. Dose can be air kerma or ambient dose equivalent as described above. The dose rate can be that at a particular moment in time, i.e. instantaneous dose rate (IDR), or averaged over a period of time. In this case the quantity is known as the time averaged dose rate (TADR), typically over 8 or 2000 h, e.g. $TADR_{2000}$. These quantities and their application in the design of radiotherapy facilities are discussed more fully in section 3.7.

3.3 System of radiation protection

The international system of radiation protection is based on the basic principles of radiation protection laid down by the International Commission of Radiological Protection (ICRP 2007). Justification, optimisation and dose limitation form the basis of all standards and regulatory systems worldwide.

The European Commission (2013) and the International Atomic Energy Agency (IAEA 2014) have both developed a Basic Safety Standard from ICRP statements. The former is a Directive for the basis of radiation legislation in European Union countries and the latter is international guidance for countries without their own legislation in this area. The latest revisions of these documents incorporate annual dose limits for radiation workers and members of the public and a new lower figure for the lens of the eye from the ICRP (2012). New regulations are to be made in the UK in 2018 which are anticipated to include the new limits.

The international system and the Basic Safety Standards have three descriptions for radiation exposure: planned, existing or emergency exposure situations. Radiotherapy is generally a planned exposure situation, although emergency situations also need to be considered. Existing exposure situations may occur in areas of high natural background or if the building material used could cause such a background.

Within each of these situations, there are three categories of exposure: occupational, public and medical. The design of a radiotherapy facility requires consideration of occupational and public exposures. The prescription of medical exposures is outside the scope of this publication but a knowledge of the number of patients, the patient doses and types of exposure is essential for accurate estimation of the radiation workload in the facility (see chapter 4) and to enable a realistic design.

3.4 Regulatory framework in the UK

Regulations in the UK are based on the EC Basic Safety Standard (see above) and each set of regulations has a regulatory authority and a local expert adviser who may have to hold a certificate of competence. These are set out in table 3.3.

The IRR (1999) are designed to protect staff and the public from exposure to ionising radiation arising from work with radiation. They do not apply exclusively to work in the medical sector, although there are some regulations applying to equipment used for medical exposures.

The *Ionising Radiation (Medical Exposure) Regulations* (IRMER 2000) are designed to ensure that the patient receives the prescribed dose from ionising radiation.

The *Environmental Permitting Regulations* (EPR 2016) supersede and combine a number of amendments made since these regulations were implemented in 2010 (EPR 2010). These are designed to protect the environment from the impact of the use of radioactive material. There is some overlap with the IRR in terms of source control and regulatory requirements for the management of sources. These incorporate the requirements originally laid down in the *High Activity Sealed Source Regulations* (HASS 2005), which relate to high activity sealed sources and apply in many radiotherapy centres with high dose rate (HDR) brachytherapy.

The *Carriage of Dangerous Goods and Transportable Pressure Equipment Regulations* (HSE 2009) and subsequent amendments cover the transport of radioactive material by road, rail, sea and air. They reflect the requirements of the ADR

Table 3.3. Statutory regulations impacting on radiotherapy.

Regulation	Regulatory authority	Expert adviser
IRR99	HSE	RPA
IR(ME)R2000	DH/CQC	MPE
RSA/EPR	Environment Agencies	RWA/CTSA
Transport	ONR	RPA/DGSA
REPPIR	HSE	RPA
MARS	DH/ARSAC/CQC	MPE

Key: RPA—Radiation Protection Adviser; MPE—Medical Physics Expert; RWA—Radioactive Waste Adviser; DGSA—Dangerous Goods Safety Adviser; CTSA—Counter Terrorism Security Adviser; HSE-Health and Safety Executive; DH-Department of Health; CQC-Care Quality Commission; ONR-Office of Nuclear Regulation; ARSAC-Administration of Radioactive Substances Advisory Committee

(*Accord Europeen relative au transport international des marchandises dangereuses par route*) (UNECE 2017) which are updated every two years.

The *Radiation (Emergency) Preparedness and Public Information Regulations* (REPPIR 2001) relate to the emergency arrangements in the event of incidents involving large amounts of radioactive material. Emergency plans required under these regulations are not generally required by hospitals.

The *Medicines (Administration of Radioactive Substances) Regulations* (MARS 1978) relate to the administration of radioactive material to humans. They apply to oncologists practising brachytherapy but will not be discussed further here.

It is necessary to consult an RPA on a range of matters under the regulations listed above and the appointment of an RPA is required in centres carrying out radiotherapy. They are required to have suitable and sufficient knowledge of radiotherapy facilities and practice to be able to advise appropriately. A certificate of competence from RPA2000 is a recognition of competence but not necessarily suitability. Medical RPAs are expert in the regulations but perhaps not always in the practice of radiotherapy.

Medical Physics Experts (MPEs) are required to be appointed in radiotherapy. They are likely to be an integral part of the radiotherapy department and have expert knowledge of radiation dosimetry and clinical radiotherapy practice. Certification of these experts is expected to be required following new regulations in 2018.

A Radioactive Waste Adviser (RWA) to advise on radioactive waste and other radiation protection matters is required to be appointed by an employer holding permits under the Environmental Permitting Regulations (EPR 2016). A certificate of competence under RPA2000 is a recognition of competence but employers are required to ensure the RWA has suitable experience to give advice on the employer's specific practice.

A Dangerous Goods Safety Adviser is required under the Carriage of Dangerous Goods Regulations (HSE 2009) when transporting radioactive material. Many centres employ transport companies to transport radioactive material if needed, although a derogation currently exists to allow professionals to transport material without the external warning signs in private cars provided suitable insurance is in place and a range of other conditions are met. Some UK insurance companies will not cover this activity.

The employer is ultimately responsible for ensuring that all regulations are complied with. A Chief Executive Officer (CEO) of an organisation is unlikely to be able to directly implement the requirements and it is normal for them to delegate tasks to others in the organisation through the management chain. These persons in turn need to feedback through that chain to assure the CEO that the regulations are being implemented satisfactorily. When the experts are also employees, there may need to be careful division between roles when expert advice is being given and when the employer has delegated tasks to the expert to complete on their behalf to meet the requirements of the regulations.

Other roles on a more operational level include the Radiation Protection Supervisor (responsible for ensuring radiation protection policy and procedures are being followed in their area of responsibility), those supervising the use of sealed radioactive sources (sometimes called 'source custodians'), those supervising the use and disposal of unsealed radioactive material, and managers in individual areas.

Following the publication of the new EC Basic Safety Standard Directive (European Commission 2013) in 2013, the UK regulators have reviewed IRR99, IRMER2000, and the REPPIR and MARS regulations. These reviews will result in new regulations to be enacted in 2017 and 2018. It is expected that there will be some additional requirements for radiotherapy centres to address. These are expected to include some form of registration under the new IRR and changes relating to the use of radioactive material in radiotherapy treatment.

3.5 Basic radiation protection principles in radiotherapy

3.5.1 Justification

All radiation exposures are required to be justified. Justification of staff and public exposure resulting from radiotherapy is covered by the EC Basic Safety Standard (European Commission 1996) and includes a requirement for some form of registration of the facility. IRR (1999) contains a generic authorisation covering the use of electrical equipment to produce x-rays for the purpose of the exposure of persons for medical treatment, i.e. linear accelerators or kilovoltage units in radiotherapy. This situation is expected to change when the new regulations are made in 2017/18 and registration under the new regulations is likely to be required. Currently there is a requirement to notify the regulatory authority (the Health and Safety Executive in the UK) when working with ionising radiation for the first time or when changing the use of the facility, e.g. adding the use of radioactive material. Any notifications made under IRR (1999) will not be valid under the new regulations and a new notification or registration as described above will need to be made.

When radioactive material is used, the UK has had a system of licensing premises since 1993 under the Radioactive Substances Act (RSA 1993). This has been superseded in England and Wales by the Environmental Permitting Regulations (EPR 2016).

If permits are required, early engagement with the regulators/licensing authorities is recommended. There are often conditions associated with licenses which may affect the design of the facility, e.g. the standards of doors for security purposes. Some requirements may also affect the basic layout of the facility.

3.5.2 Optimisation

Optimisation in terms of radiation protection is realised by keeping doses as low as reasonably achievable (ALARA). For radiotherapy installations, this is achieved by setting dose constraints at the planning stage to calculate the level of shielding required and the specification of appropriate engineering controls for an installation both in terms of operational capability and location. As there are few occasions when workers remain with a patient during treatment, optimisation of staff protection is largely performed at the design stage of the facility.

3.5.3 Dose limitation

The system of dose limitation has remained unchanged since the levels set by ICRP Report 60 in 1991 (ICRP 1991) apart from the dose limit for the lens of the eye which has been reduced in ICRP Report 118 (ICRP 2012). There are dose limits for workers, the public and young people, but not for patients undergoing medical exposures. These are listed in table 3.4. Classification is required when 3/10 of a dose limit may be reached. Classification of workers in radiotherapy is now relatively rare as whole-body doses are unlikely to reach even the dose limits for members of the public. The reduced limit for the lens of the eye means that classification will be required if 15 mSv is likely to be exceeded. It is not anticipated that this dose could be exceeded in radiotherapy in current routine circumstances.

3.6 Controlled areas

Areas in radiotherapy where radiation treatment is carried out are always designated as controlled areas. A controlled area is defined as one where special measures are needed to restrict exposure in either a planned or emergency exposure situation.

It is common to define the controlled area as the room, i.e. the boundaries are specified by the walls, floor, ceiling and doors. There may be some points within this area where special measures are not required, but for simplicity of physical definition, description and access control the physical boundaries are used. Areas outside treatment rooms are not normally controlled areas, although the roofs of linear accelerators can be an exception during operation, when access needs to be controlled. Treatment rooms may not be treated as controlled areas when the equipment is not powered to provide radiation beams. Installation of new equipment into existing facilities will require new risk assessments in the areas outside treatment rooms. Some centres designate controlled areas outside treatment rooms on the basis of dose rates and or anticipated doses per annum from the use of the equipment.

Table 3.4. Dose limits in 2016, anticipated new eye dose limit for employees in brackets (IRR 1999, European Commission 2013).

	Annual dose limits (mSv)		
Site	Employees	Trainees (under 18)	Others
Whole body	20	5	1
Lens of eye	150 (20)	50	15
Skin (1 cm^2)	500	150	50

Other limits

Abdomen of women of reproductive capacity 13 mSv in 3 months.
Other persons exposed as a result of someone else's medical exposure (but not a comforter and carer) 5 mSv in 5 years.

When an assessment is made that an area need not be designated as a controlled area but that the situation needs to be kept under review, then the area concerned should be designated a supervised area. Signs and demarcation are not required for these areas but they should be identified as such in the Local Rules. Supervised areas are the exception in radiotherapy.

3.7 Optimisation in the design process

Some basic assumptions are made to enable the shielding to be calculated. Radiation workload is covered in individual chapters but the principles below are applied in all modalities.

3.7.1 The radiation protection working year

As radiotherapy equipment is increasingly operated over extended working days, up to seven days a week, it is important that shielding is not over specified as a result. It is recommended that no matter what the working pattern of the equipment is, it is the work pattern of staff (and the associated equipment use during that time) that should be considered. Usually this is based on eight hour shifts, a five day working week and a working year of 50 weeks. On this basis 2000 hours per year is the accepted conservative figure for the work pattern. Under exceptional circumstance, e.g. in the case of residential property adjacent to the facility, consideration of the total dose during the entire operation of the facility should be considered.

3.7.2 Occupancy factors

The occupancy factor is the time spent by critical groups of people at the location in question. Factors in the report *Radiation Shielding for Diagnostic Radiology* (Sutton *et al* 2012a) are shown in table 3.5 and the factors in NCRP Report 151 (NCRP 2005) in table 3.6.

The appropriate value of the occupancy factor can be contentious. For control areas and offices a factor of 100% should be used. For a neighbouring linear accelerator bunker 50% is reasonably conservative for positions 300 mm from the wall of that bunker. A higher figure might be used in the centre of the room where staff might spend more time.

Ranges are suggested in table 3.5 so that the local situation can be reflected against the knowledge of factors generally used elsewhere. This can be particularly applicable to corridors, some of which are heavily used and others rarely. Values outside the suggested ranges can of course be used. UK values tend to be higher than US values (table 3.6). A reasonable compromise is 10% for corridors, 50% for staff rooms, 20% for the entrance to the maze, 10% for patient waiting areas and 5% for car parks. When assigning a low occupancy factor it is important to consider where the persons concerned might be for the rest of the time.

Where low occupancy values have been assumed it is important that this is clearly documented so that if the use of the area changes an appropriate reassessment can be made. The report *Radiation Shielding for Diagnostic Radiology* (Sutton *et al* 2012a) recommends that occupancy should never be less than 5%. Use of a lower occupancy

Table 3.5. Occupancy factors from the report *Radiation Shielding for Diagnostic Radiology* (Sutton *et al* 2012a).

Occupancy factors provided for general guidance	
Occupancy and location	Suggested range (%)
Full occupancy	100
Control rooms	
Reception areas, nurses' stations	
Offices, shops, living quarters, children's indoor play areas, occupied space in nearby buildings	
Partial occupancy	2–50
Staff rooms	
Adjacent wards, clinic rooms	
Reporting areas	
Occasional occupancy	5–12.5
Corridors	
Store rooms, stairways	
Changing rooms, unattended car parks	
Unattended waiting rooms	
Toilets, bathrooms	

Table 3.6. Suggested occupancy factors from NCRP Report 151 (NCRP 2005).

Location	Occupancy factor
Full occupancy areas (areas occupied full-time by an individual), e.g. administrative or clerical offices, treatment planning areas, treatment control rooms, nurse stations, receptionist areas, attended waiting rooms, occupied space in nearby building	1
Adjacent treatment room, patient examination room, adjacent to shielded bunker	0.5
Corridors, employee lounges, staff rest rooms	0.2
Treatment room doors	0.125
Public toilets, unattended vending rooms, storage areas, outdoor areas with seating, unattended waiting rooms, patient holding areas, attics, janitor's closets	0.05
Outdoor areas with only transient or vehicular traffic, unattended parking lots, vehicular drop off areas (unattended), stairways, unattended elevators	0.025

with an annual dose constraint of 0.3 mSv implies that the area concerned could have an exposure greater than 6 mSv per year and should be a controlled area.

Care is needed if shielding is sited close to a party boundary. The use of the adjacent land may change, which may affect the design assumptions used, particularly if an occupancy factor has been applied.

3.7.3 Annual dose constraints

IRR99 Regulation 8 (IRR 1999) describes many ways in which exposures should be restricted and doses kept to levels as low as reasonably achievable, i.e. optimisation of exposure. The use of dose constraints when planning facilities can be used to meet this requirement. The Approved Code of Practice to IRR99 (HSE 2000) describes the use of a constraint for members of the public from a single source to be a maximum of 0.3 mSv per annum. This figure is the accepted value for the design of linear accelerator bunkers in the UK[1]. The same constraint of 0.3 mSv per annum can be recommended for members of staff, but it is acceptable to design to a higher constraint. 1 mSv per annum is often chosen if 0.3 mSv per annum is not deemed appropriate.

3.7.4 Time averaged dose rate

The TADR over 2000 h for an annual dose constraint of 0.3 or 1 mSv per annum is 0.15 or 0.5 μSv h^{-1}, respectively. This would be the dose rate if the exposure was continuous throughout that period. The occupancy and orientation factors (see chapter 4) should both be applied to calculate the TADR.

3.7.5 Instantaneous dose rate

Equivalent dose rate (taking account of the radiation weighting factor) has been used to decide on the designation of areas, as described in section 3.6 above. Whilst there are circumstances where the IDR must be noted, a value of 7.5 μSv h^{-1} is too restrictive for the routine clinical use of most radiotherapy equipment. The transitory nature of the dose rate at a point from a linear accelerator, primarily due to the movement of the gantry and from the modulation of a small beam, results in a person outside the bunker being exposed to the beam for only a few seconds. This supports the approach that it is more appropriate to use the annual dose constraint as the limiting factor for shielding design for this type of equipment, even in high dose rate (flattening-filter-free (FFF)) mode (see chapter 4). It is recommended that shielding calculations are carried out with the aim of achieving the annual dose constraint and that the IDRs are reviewed to ensure they are not too high. These reviews can indicate numerical values of some tens of μSv h^{-1} and are considered acceptable under current operational circumstances for FFF linear accelerators. Some RPAs experienced in bunker design will accept up to 100 μSv h^{-1}. It is important that the RPA understands how the equipment will be used, any weaknesses in shielding such as penetrations through barriers, and the critical points outside the bunker to enable appropriate advice to be offered.

Restricting this value to, for example, 7.5 μSv h^{-1} will lead to more shielding being installed than is required. Controlled areas are defined in IRR99 Regulation 16(1) (IRR 1999) as being areas where special procedures are required to restrict significant exposure to an individual in that area or to limit the probability of a

[1] In the USA a shielding design goal of 1 mSv per year is advocated for uncontrolled areas (NCRP 2005).

radiation accident and to limit its magnitude, or if it is likely that an individual in that area would receive an effective dose in excess of 6 mSv per year or three-tenths of any other dose limit for a radiation worker aged 18 years or over. Provided the dose in areas outside the bunker meet the constraint then there is no need to designate areas as controlled under the regulations. This aspect should be kept under review in risk assessments to ensure that the basis for the original design is still relevant.

This is in line with the views expressed in the British Institute of Radiology (BIR) report *Radiation Shielding for Diagnostic Radiology* (Sutton *et al* 2012a) which uses only a design constraint of 0.3 mSv per year (3/10 of 1 mSv per year), with no reference to TADRs over a minute. This view has been further clarified in a letter in the *Journal of Radiological Protection* (Sutton *et al* 2012b) that states that the 0.3 mSv per year constraint should be adhered to but that a 7.5 μSv h^{-1} IDR averaged over a minute constraint is not considered valid for diagnostic radiology. It is the view of the authors that using this constraint in shielding calculations for linear accelerator bunkers using FFF beams is also neither valid nor appropriate.

3.7.6 Other dose constraints/time averaging

It might be appropriate in some circumstances to apply a dose constraint over a shorter period to ensure doses are as low as reasonably achievable. A weekly dose or daily dose might be reasonable for some circumstances; for example if patterns of treatment were not constant. The dose constraint should not be lower than 1/50 of the annual dose constraint for a weekly constraint or 1/250 for a daily constraint, but could be much higher to take account of the distribution of radiation exposures over time.

The recommendations of this section are summarised in table 3.7.

3.8 Engineering controls

A hierarchy of control measures are used to restrict exposure of persons. Shielding is foremost, but medical applications require access to treatment rooms, so it is expected that there will be interlocks, warning devices and safety features built in

Table 3.7. Parameters used for optimising exposure in the design process.

Parameter	Recommended values
A year	2000 h
Annual dose constraint	Maximum of 0.3 to 1 mSv
IDR	No numerical limit provided the annual constraint is met.[a]
Other dose constraints	Weekly greater than or equal to 1/50 of the annual dose constraint. Daily greater than or equal to 1/250 of the annual dose constraint.[b]
TADR2000	<0.15–0.5 μSv h^{-1}
Occupancy factors	See table 3.5

[a] Provided the use of the equipment is well understood and applied in the design as described in section 3.7.
[b] Could be much higher than the fraction quoted.

at the design stage. Only then should written systems of work be used to restrict exposure.

Interlocks are generally required at the entrance to radiotherapy treatment rooms. These may be incorporated into a door closing mechanism, a physical barrier or a light curtain at the maze entrance. The interlock terminates the radiation beam if the door or barrier is opened or the light path is broken. The interlock circuitry should require the treatment unit to be reset before the radiation exposure continues; the exposure should not continue if a door or barrier is simply closed.

A 'last person out' (LPO) button is generally incorporated within the treatment room. Its position is sited such that the whole room should be visible from its position. Whilst industrial practice is to sweep an area and place the LPO button in the far side of a room, this could be disconcerting for the patient. The local risk assessment will consider the location of the button. Common practice is for it to be sited close to the inner maze entrance but where the operator has clear sight of the whole room. Some installations may have areas which are not visible, e.g. areas behind linear accelerators or room furniture. The latter is not desirable and may therefore require an audible warning of imminent radiation exposure to be installed. This again is disconcerting for the patient who may already be anxious. Interlocked doors are recommended for equipment areas behind linear accelerators which are incorporated into a fascia. If a light curtain is used a final closure of the interlock should be made with a second button outside the room to confirm no one other than the patient is inside.

There should be a visible indication of radiation present in the treatment room such as a red panel light indicating its presence, visible to anyone in the room or the maze.

Warning lights are normally fitted at the entrance to the controlled area to cover the regulatory requirement to demarcate the controlled area. These are ideally positioned at eye level either side of the entrance to the treatment room, but the design of many entrances means the exact positioning is sometimes above or to one side of the entrance. The wording needs to include a description of the hazard which may include x-rays, electrons and neutrons. Care is needed in the specification of any legend. A two stage warning light is commonly used (see figure 7.16). The upper yellow section is illuminated when the equipment is powered and can provide radiation. The red section is illuminated when radiation is being generated. Some centres use a three stage warning light with one section confirming to those outside the bunker when the LPO circuit has been closed.

When a radioactive source is part of the equipment, an independent radiation monitor to measure the presence of ionising radiation should also be installed in the treatment room with an audible indication of dose rate to indicate whether or not the source has returned to the safe position after treatment.

The equipment itself contains many engineering controls, fail safe devices and warning devices to restrict exposure and to fail safely should fault conditions develop. International standards exist for the specification of these (IEC 2009) and their operation should be understood, in particular by those carrying out the critical examination of the installation so that their operation can be checked.

Wherever there are engineering controls, their operation should be checked regularly to ensure they are operating correctly. The frequency of those checks will be decided as part of the risk assessment and will depend on their criticality and their potential for failure. Some will be checks before use or daily, others will be less frequent. They will be incorporated into the quality assurance regime for the equipment concerned (e.g. *Technical Quality Control Guidelines* of the Canadian Partnership for Quality Radiotherapy (CPQR 2016)).

3.9 Prior risk assessment

An assessment is required of the risk to employees and members of the public from the use of the ionising radiation. This is required to identify the measures required to restrict the exposure of those persons to the radiation. Consideration must also be made of any potential accidents and the nature and magnitude of any potential exposure. There are many sources providing advice on risk assessment, for example on the Health and Safety Executive website (www.hse.gov.uk/risk) or in the Medical and Dental Guidance Notes (IPEM 2002). All findings from the assessment should be recorded.

The assessment should include the following:

- The nature of the sources, e.g. x-rays, electrons, sealed sources, other radiation (e.g. neutrons), or unsealed material including radon gas. This shows the type of hazard—external dose, internal radiation or contamination.
- The likely doses that individuals might receive in normal circumstances and in potential accidents. It is common for separate assessments to be completed during commissioning and in routine clinical use. The design criteria for the installation can be used for this assessment and consideration of where individuals might be in the event of an incident, e.g. accidental exposure to the source or a requirement to enter the treatment room during an exposure. Consideration needs to be given to possible exposure in the event of failure of any of the engineering controls and design features planned for the installation.
- The results of the shielding survey will almost always form part of the assessment. Long term assessment of doses around the site is often carried out but the siting of dosimeters, but their lack of sensitivity may limit the actual value of such measurements. If the room was used for a similar purpose previously, previous monitoring results may help in this assessment. These can be updated with data from the actual facility once results are available.
- Additional consideration is required for equipment using radioactive material where potential exposures and accidents will need considering and also whether contamination needs to be considered and what levels might be encountered. Consideration is also required of source movement, loss and theft.
- Safe systems of work. These should be considered as part of the design stage and are likely to include a requirement for persons to be outside the controlled area during any exposure.

The outcome of the assessment will result in the following:

- Confirmation that the dose constraints will be met.
- Specification of the shielding required.
- The engineering controls required such as interlocks, etc.
- Local rules including systems of work.
- The contingency plans required.
- The requirements for personal dose monitoring.
- Designation of controlled areas.
- The methods required to restrict access to controlled areas.
- The training needs of staff who need access to controlled areas.
  Consideration needs to be given to all groups of staff who may need to gain access including cleaners and hospital maintenance staff.
- Any restrictions for pregnant staff so that the foetus is not exposed to significant levels.
- If unsealed radionuclides are used, the restrictions (if any) for breast feeding staff so that the child is not exposed to significant levels.

The risk assessment can also be used to record the requirements for decommissioning of the facility. All these findings may impact on the content of the local rules. An example for a linear accelerator is given in figure 3.1 and an example for HDR brachytherapy in figure 3.2.

The local rules may be different during the installation and commissioning phases of new equipment. The controlled area is generally under the control of the equipment manufacturer or supplier during the installation phase. This is often handed over to the user after joint acceptance testing, which will include the critical examination, has been completed. Access arrangements and modes of operation may differ from normal clinical operation during these phases and particular care is required to ensure all hazards have been considered and the risks minimised.

3.10 Additional regulatory requirements

A number of other requirements are identified in the regulations. These are applicable to radiotherapy and other areas. Specific additional requirements are described in individual chapters.

3.10.1 Investigation level and personal dose monitoring

Doses received by employees and members of the public will be much lower than the dose limit. An investigation level is set as an aid to optimisation to demonstrate doses are as low as reasonably achievable. For staff who are unlikely to get significant doses these can be set quite low. The doses recorded on personal dosimeters can also be used to carry out investigations of unexpected high readings. It should be noted that personal doses in radiotherapy can be very low. In some centres staff are not monitored routinely. In others the dosimeter results are used to

RISK ASSESSMENT	Hospital Anytown Room LA1 Date 2014
Radiation equipment/sources involved	Linear accelerator make/model/serial no. Room is a purpose built bunker on the ground floor designed for 15 MV and 10 MV x-rays. Adjacent to staff room on one side. All other sides—low occupancy. Two walls external walls—car park and roadway. No routine access required to area above bunker.
Clinical procedures & anticipated workload	Radiotherapy treatments are standard isocentric treatments with x MV x-rays, y patients per day and z Gy per patient.
Staff involved	Radiographers, physicists, engineers, porters, other maintenance staff.
Other persons involved	Patients being treated. Visitors.
Exposed groups & dose constraints	Members of the public 0.3 mSv. Staff x mSv whole body (and fingers if appropriate). Pregnant staff 1 mSv to abdomen (consider emergency situation). Comforters and carers 5 mSv.
Diagram 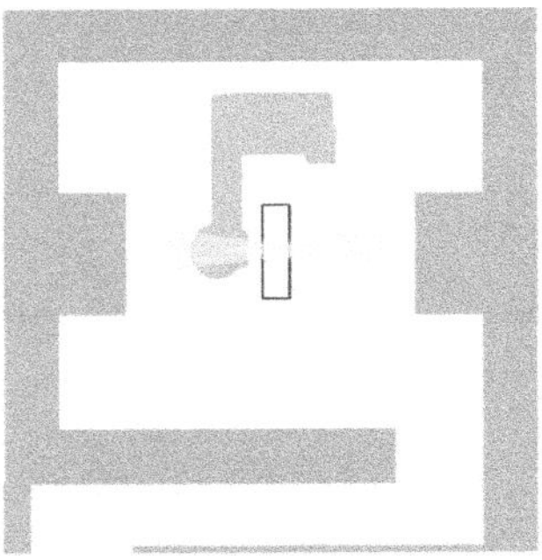	Room layout. Surrounding areas occupancy (including above and below). Monitoring devices location. Warning lights location. Engineering controls location, especially emergency off position. LPO button, other interlocks. Operator(s) positions(s). Equipment/source location.
Potential emergency situations	Fire. Medical emergency. Security. Damage.
Assessment of likely doses: routine operation	Average body doses for 2013 were less than 0.1 mSv in 3 months for radiographers, physicists and engineers.

Emergency situations	In an emergency situation dose limits could be approached in a few seconds.
Control measures	Shielding. LPO button. In-room monitor/light. Door interlock. Operation of equipment. Emergency off switches. Records. Engineering controls. Other warning devices. Monitoring arrangements. Access restrictions to roof.
Action to be taken	Training-equipment and radiation protection. Local rules. Checking of interlocks and warning devices. Review monitoring results. Contingency plan.

Signature ________________ **Date**__________

Title ______________________

Review date_________

Figure 3.1 Sample risk assessment for a linear accelerator in standard operation.

confirm that environmental doses are not approaching levels of concern and to reassure staff.

3.10.2 Critical examination

The installer of equipment producing radiation, including medical equipment such as linear accelerators and CT scanners, is responsible for ensuring a critical examination of the equipment is carried out under IRR99 Regulation 31 (IRR 1999). An RPA is required to be involved in the UK, although not necessarily present during this examination. IPEM has published guidance on critical examinations in diagnostic radiology (IPEM 2012). An example of the points that might be covered in a critical examination in radiotherapy is set out in table 3.8. If the installer of the equipment is not responsible for the bunker design or is installing into an existing bunker, they cannot be responsible for the shielding or its integrity.

3.10.3 Warning signs

Radiation installations must have warning signs to demarcate the controlled area (IRR 1999). Their format is documented in the Medical and Dental Guidance Notes

RISK ASSESSMENT	Hospital Anytown Room HDR Date 2016
Radiation equipment/sources involved	Afterloader make/model/serial no. Activity and radionuclide. Room details. External occupancy.
Clinical procedures & anticipated workload	Brachytherapy treatment procedures. Patients/procedure. Dose/procedure.
Staff involved	Doctors, nurses, radiographers, physicists, engineers, porters, other maintenance staff.
Other persons involved	Patient being treated.
Hazards	External irradiation. Loss or damage to the source.
Exposed groups & dose constraints	Members of the public 0.3 mSv. Staff x mSv whole body (and fingers if appropriate). Pregnant staff 1 mSv to abdomen (consider emergency situation). (Comforters and carers 5 mSv.)
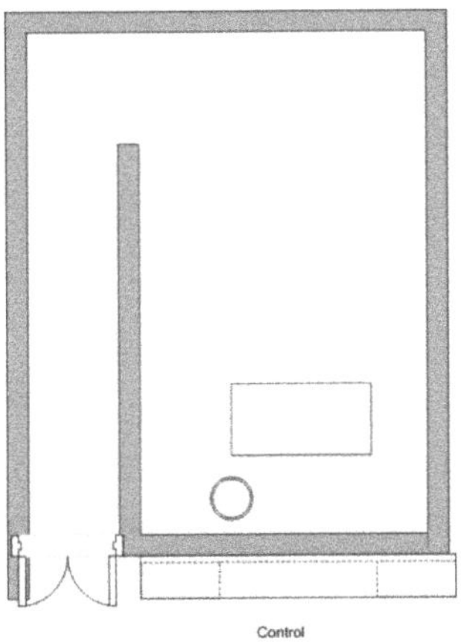	Room size/door/protective screens. Surrounding areas occupancy (including above and below). Monitoring devices location. Warning lights/sign location. Engineering controls location (if applicable). Patient orientation. Operator(s) positions(s). Distance to source. Equipment/source location. Lead pot, etc.
Potential emergency situations	Fire. Medical emergency. Security. Damage. Source stick.
Assessment of likely doses: Routine operation	<0.3 mSv routine operation.
Emergency situations	In an emergency situation dose limits to fingers could be approached in a few seconds.

Control measures	Shielding/protective screens. Handling of radioactive sources/operation of equipment. Records. Engineering controls especially emergency off switches. Warning devices. Personal protective equipment (PPE). Monitoring arrangements. Measures to minimise spread of contamination. Access arrangements.
Action to be taken	Training-equipment and radiation protection. Local rules. Checking of interlocks and warning devices. Review monitoring results. Contingency plan rehearsals.

Signature ________________ **Date**__________

Title ______________________

Review date__________

Figure 3.2. Sample risk assessment for HDR brachytherapy.

(IPEM 2002) and is enshrined in law in the Safety Signs Regulations (Safety Signs 1996). These are normally supplemented by warning lights (see section 3.8 above).

3.10.4 Quality assurance and maintenance

The life cycle of equipment is well documented with requirements for quality assurance, quality control checks and maintenance. This is particularly important for radiotherapy to ensure the correct dose is delivered to the planned location. Regular maintenance should be undertaken according to the equipment manufacturer's recommendations. Guidance about equipment, its life cycle and action to be taken when there is an equipment failure is the subject of specific guidance in PM77 (HSE 2006). Regular quality control checks are required and professional guidance is available (e.g. CPQR 2016).

Equipment handover before and after maintenance is of particular importance in radiotherapy and the availability/non-availability of equipment for clinical use should be clearly indicated at the control desk. Some centres keep a signed record of handovers. This forms part of the quality system (quality assurance in radiotherapy (QART)) within the radiotherapy department.

3.10.5 Incidents

Radiation incidents involving equipment failure in radiotherapy are rare. Because of the potentially fatal consequences in the event of equipment failure, equipment is

Table 3.8. Points to be considered in the critical examination of a linear accelerator.

Parameter
Room warning signs
Room warning lights: ready to emit radiation.
Room warning lights: 'do not enter'.
Audible exposure warning.
Visible exposure warning in maze.
Warning signals:
Mains on.
Exposure warning lights/indicators on the control panel.
Room protection:
General adequacy of protection.
Adequate shielding of walls and doors.
Surrounding dose rates meet design specification.
Engineering controls
LPO button.
Maze barrier interlock.
Emergency off buttons.
Labelling
Controlled area.
All controls clearly labelled.
Model and serial number.
CE mark.

carefully designed with fail safe mechanisms central to all control systems. There are also back-up systems which can be multi-layered. Changes to operational software, however, add a new vulnerability and upgrades must be subject to careful checks before patient exposure.

In the UK, notification to regulatory authorities is required when a dose much greater than intended is given to a patient (10% for a course of treatment or 20% for an individual fraction in radiotherapy) as defined in PM77 (HSE 2006). However, such notifications due to equipment failure are rare. Incidents involving a breakdown in procedures or human error are more likely, but are outside the scope of this report.

3.10.6 Contingency plans

Contingency plans are required to be developed to consider all the relatively foreseeable events around the use of radiotherapy equipment such as fire, theft, equipment failure or a medical emergency. These should examine the risks to both staff and patients.

A contingency plan for a linear accelerator might be relatively simple and involve turning the unit off.

However, for HDR brachytherapy, the contingency plan needs to consider a range of scenarios. The most critical is the radiation source becoming stuck outside the safe, resulting in unintended doses to the patient and staff. The plan must be rehearsed at regular intervals and with new staff so that all the necessary processes are second nature to the staff operating the unit.

References

CPQR (Canadian Partnership for Quality Radiotherapy) 2016 *Technical Quality Control Guidelines* www.cpqr.ca/programs/technical-quality-control/ (Accessed: 10 October 2016)

EPR 2010 *The Environmental Permitting (England and Wales) Regulations* SI 2010/675 (London: The Stationery Office)

EPR 2016 *The Environmental Permitting (England and Wales) Regulations* SI 2016/1154 (London: The Stationery Office)

European Commission 2013 Laying down basic safety standards for protection against the dangers arising from exposure to ionising radiation *Council Directive* 2013/59/Euratom (Brussels: European Commission)

European Commission 1996 Laying down basic safety standards for the protection of the health of workers and the general public against the dangers arising from ionising radiation *Council Directive* 96/29/Euratom (Brussels: European Commission)

HASS 2005 *High Activity Sealed Source Regulations* SI 2005/2686 (London: The Stationery Office)

HSE (Health and Safety Executive) 2000 *Work with Ionising Radiation: Approved Code of Practice and Practical Guidance on the Ionising Radiations Regulations 1999* L121 (London: HSE)

HSE (Health and Safety Executive) 2006 *Equipment used in Connection with Medical Exposure* Guidance note PM77, 3rd edn (London: HSE)

HSE (Health and Safety Executive) 2009 *The Carriage of Dangerous Goods and Transportable Pressure Equipment Regulations* SI 2009/1348 (London: HSE)

IAEA (International Atomic Energy Agency) 2014 Radiation protection and safety of radiation sources *International Basic Safety Standards* 1578 (Vienna: IAEA)

ICRP (International Commission on Radiological Protection) 1991 *1990 Recommendations of the International Commission on Radiological Protection* Report 60, Ann ICRP 21(1-3) (Ottawa: ICRP)

ICRP (International Commission on Radiological Protection) 1996 *Conversion Coefficients for use in Radiological Protection against External Radiation* Report 74, Ann ICRP 26: 3/4 (Ottawa: ICRP)

ICRP (International Commission on Radiological Protection) 2007 *2007 Recommendations of the International Commission on Radiological Protection* Report 103, Ann ICRP 37: 2-4 (Ottawa: ICRP)

ICRP (International Commission on Radiological Protection) 2009 *Preventing Accidental Exposures from New External Beam Radiation Therapy Techniques* Report 112, Ann ICRP 39: 4 (Ottawa: ICRP)

ICRP (International Commission on Radiological Protection) 2012 *ICRP Statement on Tissue Reactions/Early and Late Effects of Radiation in Normal Tissues and Organs—Threshold*

Doses for Tissue Reactions in a Radiation Protection Context Report 118, Ann ICRP 41: 1/2 (Ottawa: ICRP)

IEC (International Electrotechnical Commission) 2009 *Medical Electrical Equipment—Part 2-1: Particular Requirements for the Safety of Electron Accelerators in the Range 1 MeV to 50 MeV* 60601-2-1 (2nd edn) (Geneva: IEC)

IPEM (Institute of Physics and Engineering in Medicine) 2002 *Medical and Dental Guidance Notes: A Good Practice Guide to Implement Ionising Radiation Protection Legislation in the Clinical Environment* (York: IPEM)

IPEM (Institute of Physics and Engineering in Medicine) 2012 *The Critical Examination of x-ray Generating Equipment in Diagnostic Radiology* Report 107 (York: IPEM)

IRMER 2000 *The Ionising Radiations (Medical Exposure) Regulations* SI 2000/1059 (London: The Stationery Office)

IRR 1999 *The Ionising Radiations Regulations* SI 1999/3232 (London: The Stationery Office)

MARS 1978 *Medicines (Administration of Radioactive Substances) Regulations* SI 1978/1006 (London: The Stationery Office)

NCRP (National Council on Radiation Protection and Measurements) 2005 *Structural Shielding Design and Evaluation for Megavoltage X- and Gamma-Ray Radiotherapy Facilities* Report 151 (Bethesda, MD: NCRP)

RCR (Royal College of Radiologists), SCoR (Society and College of Radiographers), IPEM (Institute of Physics and Engineering in Medicine) 2008a *A Guide to Understanding the Implications of the Ionising Radiation (Medical Exposure) Regulations in Radiotherapy* (London: RCR)

RCR (Royal College of Radiologists), SCoR (Society and College of Radiographers), IPEM (Institute of Physics and Engineering in Medicine) 2008b National Patient Safety Agency, BIR (British Institute of Radiology) *Towards Safer Radiotherapy* (London: RCR)

REPPIR 2001 *Radiation (Emergency Preparedness and Public Information) Regulations* SI 2001/2975 (London: The Stationery Office)

RSA 1993 *Radioactive Substances Act* SI 1993/0012 (London: The Stationery Office)

Safety Signs 1996 *The Health and Safety (Safety Signs and Signals) Regulations* SI 1996/341 (London: The Stationery Office)

Sutton D G, Martin C J, Williams J R and Peet D J 2012a *Radiation Shielding for Diagnostic Radiology* 2nd edn (London: British Institute of Radiology)

Sutton D G, Williams J R, Peet D J and Martin C J 2012b Application of the constraint on instantaneous dose rate in the UK Approved Code of Practice 249 is inappropriate for radiology *J. Radiat. Prot.* **32** 101

UNECE 2017 *Accord Europeen relative au transport international des marchandises Dangereuses par Route (European Agreement concerning the International Carriage of Dangerous Goods by Road)* www.unece.org/trans/danger/publi/adr/adr2017/17contentse0.html (Accessed: 21 January 2017)

Zankl M 1999 Personal dose equivalent for photons and its variation with dosemeter position *Health Phys.* **76** 162–70

IOP Publishing

Design and Shielding of Radiotherapy Treatment Facilities
IPEM report 75, 2nd Edition
P W Horton and D J Eaton

Chapter 4

Clinical practice, treatment room and control room design

W P M Mayles and C Walker

4.1 Clinical practice

W P M Mayles

4.1.1 General

The layout of a radiotherapy facility is of prime importance for patient comfort and dignity and their movement through the rooms and spaces. A good layout is also important for efficient operation by the staff. The design must include consideration of the equipment to be installed and its planned use. There are likely to be some constraints on the space available, e.g. the limiting positions of external walls and the link to existing buildings.

It is important to get the appropriate people discussing these aspects at the earliest possible stage and to agree the limitations on some of these parameters to enable draft layouts and the thicknesses of radiation shielding to be proposed. This requires a good understanding of the modes of operation of the equipment, together with a knowledge of the proposed workload. At a minimum this should involve the architect, the users and a Radiation Protection Adviser (RPA) experienced in the design of such facilities (see chapter 2). The users and managers will need to provide a good specification of the workload and use of the equipment. Manufacturers will provide data specifying equipment dimensions and service and delivery requirements.

The easy approach is to specify provision for extremes of possible use, e.g. at the highest treatment energy. However, thicker shielding will increase the cost and space required and, if designing to a tight city centre footprint, may also limit the facilities that can be included. On the other hand it must be borne in mind that adding shielding after the completion of the building may be very much more expensive.

doi:10.1088/978-0-7503-1440-4ch4

Planning for possible additions to the shielding (e.g. by the use of concrete blocks or steel sheets) in areas of uncertainty could be a useful compromise.

The dose constraint(s) for the radiation protection for members of the public and employees need to be specified and agreed. The RPA will normally recommend value (s) which can be agreed by the users (see chapter 3). The basis of the design including details of equipment operation and patient workload must be clearly documented so that any changes in use of the equipment can be compared to the original specification to see if radiation protection and other measures need to be altered.

4.1.2 Treatment modalities

4.1.2.1 Linear accelerators

The majority of radiotherapy treatments are given using linear accelerators producing a number of x-ray beams with end-point energies in the range 6–18 MV and a number of electron beams with energies ranging from 6 to 18 MeV. Traditional linear accelerators are mounted within a gantry that allows the accelerating structure to rotate around the patient (see figure 4.1). They are so designed that the centre of the radiation beam always passes through a point in space called the isocentre. The isocentre is usually 1 m from the point of generation of the x-rays in the treatment head of the accelerator. If the tumour tissue is placed at the isocentre of the machine it is simple to enable radiation beams to enter the patient from a number of different coplanar directions with the beams overlapping within the target tissue. This reduces the radiation dose to normal tissue. The patient support system, or treatment couch, is also designed to rotate about the isocentre and this allows non-coplanar beam directions to be achieved. The position of the isocentre within the treatment room provides a reference point for the whole design.

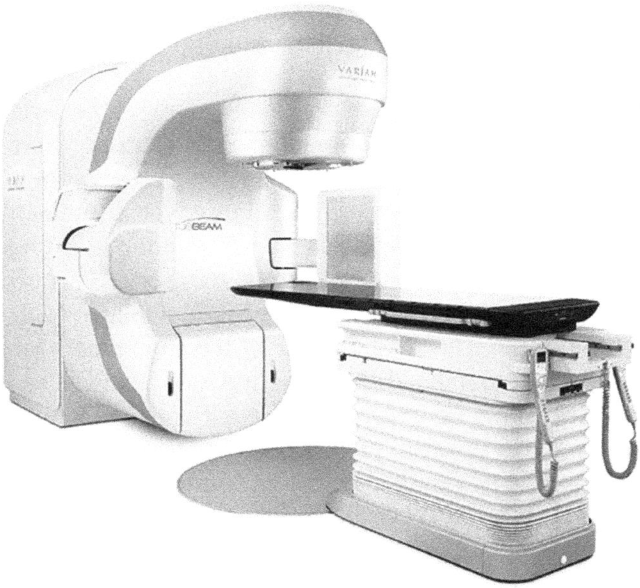

Figure 4.1. Linear accelerator with kilovoltage imaging equipment (courtesy of Varian Medical Systems).

The treatment beam from a linear accelerator is called the primary beam. This beam has an energy determined by the acceleration potential of the generator although its penetrative quality is also determined by any filtration that is incorporated into the beam. Areas of the walls, ceiling and floor that can be irradiated by the primary beam are called primary barriers. The primary beam is collimated (see below) with a maximum rectangular field size of 40 cm × 40 cm at the isocentre and the projection of this field rotated through 45° onto the barrier sets the width of the primary barrier in the walls and roof (see section 5.2). As well as the primary radiation there is some leakage radiation (limited by the International Electrotechnical Commission (IEC) specification (IEC 2009) to 0.1% of the primary beam intensity) which is emitted from the accelerator in an arbitrary direction. This is often of a similar energy to the primary beam. In addition the primary radiation is scattered from the patient and the walls of the treatment room. This scattered radiation has an energy spectrum considerably lower than that of the primary beam (except for very narrow angle scatter). Areas of the walls that are irradiated only by leakage and scattered radiation are called secondary barriers.

Conformal radiotherapy

To attenuate a megavoltage therapy beam requires a significant mass of material. The thick blocks of metal which confine the radiation to a specific area of the patient are called collimators. Traditional accelerators have a conical primary collimator which restricts the beam to a 50 cm diameter circle at the isocentre. Some accelerators then have two pairs of collimators that restrict the beam to a rectangular shape, usually up to 40 cm × 40 cm followed by a multi-leaf collimator (MLC) which enables irregular shaped fields to be produced (see figure 4.2). (In some recent designs the MLC is used without backup rectangular shaped collimation.) The MLC consists of a number of sheets of high density metal (called leaves) which cast a radiation shadow at the

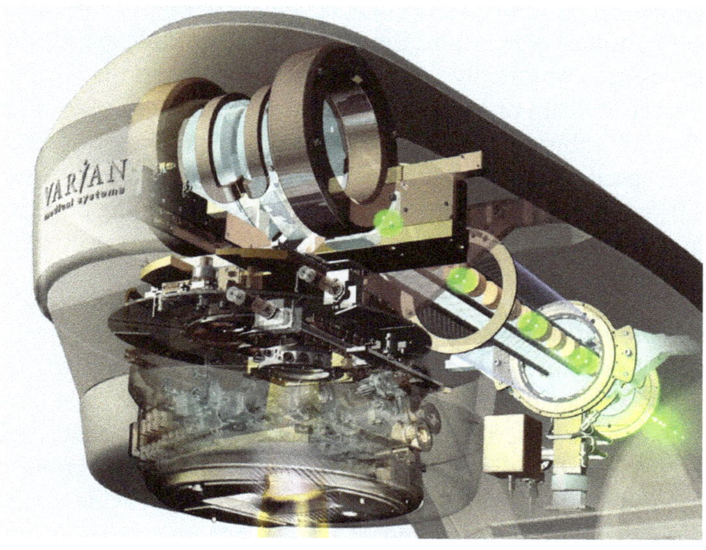

Figure 4.2. Linear accelerator treatment head (courtesy of Varian Medical Systems).

isocentre between 0.25 cm and 1 cm wide. The treatment field is thus normally much smaller than the maximum field size and is shaped to match the tumour volume. The use of such shaped fields is called conformal therapy.

Intensity modulated radiotherapy (IMRT)

Conformal therapy allows the beams to be shaped to the tumour volume but is unable to give different doses to different parts of the tumour volume to compensate for the outline of the entrance surface of the patient or to create concave dose distributions. By changing the field shape with the MLCs during the radiation exposure it is possible to achieve all these goals at the expense of having the beam on for longer. This increases the amount of leakage radiation, which is proportional to beam-on time, but not the contribution of the primary beam and the scattered radiation to the external dose. IMRT can be delivered in two ways: step-and-shoot and dynamic. In the step-and-shoot method each mini-field is irradiated and then the leaves are moved to the next mini-field position with the beam turned off. In the dynamic method the leaves are moved continuously with the beam on. In either case the beam-on time and hence the amount of leakage radiation is greater than for conformal therapy. Beam-on time is often quantified in terms of 'monitor units' (MU). These represent the beam-on time necessary to deliver a particular dose with a particular field size and position of the reference point of interest. The target dose is directly proportional to the number of MUs. To deliver a particular dose to the patient the number of MUs required compared to simple conformal treatment will be approximately 2.5 times greater for step-and-shoot IMRT and 5 times greater for dynamic IMRT. This multiplying factor is referred to as the IMRT factor and calculations of the shielding required in secondary barriers need to include this factor to allow for the increased treatment time.

Volumetric modulated arc therapy (VMAT)

This development of dynamic IMRT has been called VMAT. In this approach the gantry rotates continuously around the patient at a variable speed, the positions of the MLC leaves are continually adjusted and the dose rate is varied. The greatly increased number of beam orientations facilitates the delivery of even more precisely conformed dose distributions than IMRT. The efficiency in terms of the number of MUs to give a specified dose to the patient is roughly equivalent to step-and-shoot, i.e. the IMRT factor is 2.5. In addition the dose exiting from the patient is distributed more uniformly over the primary barrier leading to less radiation escaping the bunker in any given direction.

Stereotactic treatment techniques

With the advent of more accurate imaging and setup techniques it has become possible to treat smaller treatment volumes to a higher dose. The term *stereotactic radiotherapy* is used to described treatment of field sizes less that about 4 cm. The term *stereotactic* actually refers to a technique developed for neurosurgery in which a metal frame affixed to the patient's head was used to provide a rigid coordinate system to allow accurate introduction of probes into the patient's brain. In radiotherapy the term was first used to describe treatment of small lesions in the brain, but it has now been extended to cover the use of small precise fields in any part of the body, whether or not a frame is used. This is termed *stereotactic body radiotherapy* (SBRT) or more recently *stereotactic ablative body radiotherapy* (SABR). Because the volumes being treated are small it is less necessary to deliver treatments in small fractions to spare normal tissue so the dose delivered on each patient visit is likely to be higher. The term *stereotactic radiosurgery* is also used to describe very high doses given in a single fraction where the intention is to destroy tissue or tumour cells in the manner of surgery. A linear accelerator capable of stereotactic treatments is illustrated in figure 4.3.

Motion management techniques

When the tumour is moving, as is the case in particular with lung and liver tumours, it has been necessary to increase the field size to always encompass the tumour volume in the presence of such movements. Motion management techniques have been introduced to avoid the need for this increase in field size and reduce the volume of normal tissue irradiated. One such approach is to turn the treatment machine on only when the tumour is within the planned treatment volume; this is referred to as 'gating' the treatment. Another approach is to seek to limit the movement due to respiration by breath hold techniques or by limiting the movement of the diaphragm with a mechanical diaphragm clamp.

Flattening-filter free (FFF) treatments

In a linear accelerator, high energy electrons are converted into a photon beam by generating bremsstrahlung (braking radiation) x-rays when they hit a high atomic number target. The x-radiation is emitted preferentially in the forward direction. The extent to which the resulting beam is forward peaked is dependent on the energy of the incident electrons, with the effect being greater the higher the energy. In order to produce a uniform distribution of radiation over a 40 cm × 40 cm field a so-called flattening filter is introduced. This consists of an approximately conical piece of metal place beneath the x-ray target. The filter has three effects; it increases the penetrative quality of the beam in the centre of the field and produces the desired uniform dose across the beam while reducing the beam intensity on the central axis.

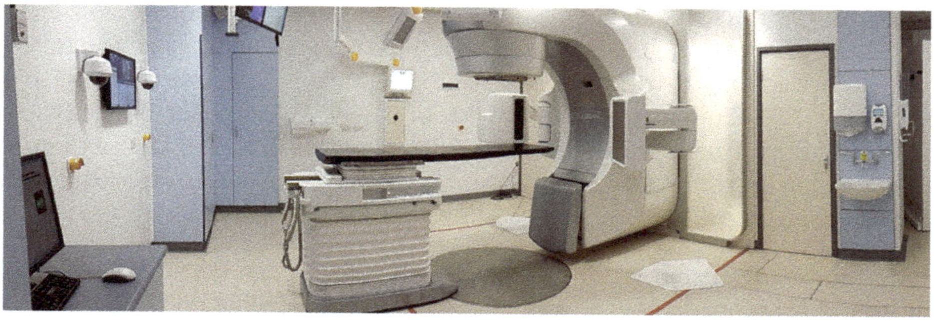

Figure 4.3. A bunker at the Northern Centre for Cancer Care, Newcastle, housing a stereotactic enabled linear accelerator with peripheral imaging equipment and a six degrees of freedom treatment couch.

With IMRT and stereotactic treatments the mini-fields are small and the need for a uniform dose distribution across a large field is much reduced. Consequently the flattening filter is not necessary and can be removed to produce FFF (or triple F) beams. These beams differ from the flattened beams in having a higher dose rate. More details on FFF beam characteristics are given in Budgell *et al* (2016). If the energy of the electrons striking the target is kept constant, the beam will be less penetrating at its centre and less primary beam shielding will be required to achieve the same primary beam dose per MU outside the bunker (Kry *et al* 2009). With this approach taken by one linear accelerator manufacturer the dose at a given depth in the patient will be less in FFF mode than in the conventional mode with a flattening filter. An alternative approach offered by another linear accelerator manufacturer is to increase the electron energy so that the dose at a depth in the patient compared to the dose at the surface is kept the same in FFF and conventional modes. In this case the thickness of material required to achieve the same attenuation depends on the energy of the beam (Paynter *et al* 2014). The absence of the flattening filter also removes a major contributor to the magnitude of the head leakage radiation, which is reduced by 50%. While it would appear unnecessary to increase the wall thickness to account for the higher dose rate (unless a substantial increase in dose delivered to the isocentre is intended), it would nevertheless be unwise to use less shielding, as alluded to by Kry *et al* (2009).

Total body irradiation (TBI)

TBI is used in conjunction with bone marrow transplants in the treatment of leukaemia and lymphomas. The patient is usually treated at an increased distance from the radiation source, which may be three or more times the standard treatment distance with the collimators opened as wide as possible. This requires the accelerator to be offset from the centre line of the treatment room to give the longer treatment distance required, with the patient placed close to one of the primary barriers in a horizontal position (see figure 2.2). Consequently the beam will be pointing in this one particular direction throughout the treatment and this beam orientation may occur more frequently than occurs with other treatments. This and the offset isocentre will need to be taken into account when calculating the necessary barrier thickness (see section 4.3.1).

Treatment with electrons

In a linear accelerator, it is possible to remove the x-ray target and allow the accelerated electrons to be used directly for treatment. Electrons are much less penetrating than photons. In addition the conversion of electrons to bremsstrahlung photons is an inefficient process and the electron beam current in the accelerator is much less than for the production of photons. Consequently any protection designed for x-ray photons will also be adequate for electrons.

Neutron production

An undesirable property of x-ray beams with end point energies above 8.5 MV is the production of neutrons. The ratio of neutrons to x-ray photons increases with the energy of the beam. At 10 MV the neutron dose is about 40 μSv per photon Gy, whereas at 15 MV it is about 1 mSv per photon Gy (McGinley 2002) quoted in NCRP Report 151 (NCRP 2005). The exact proportion is dependent on the material used for the flattening filter—a machine with a steel flattening filter will produce fewer neutrons for the same nominal beam energy than one with a tungsten filter (related to the amount of pair production). The neutrons in the beam are an issue for the dose delivered to the patient as well as being a radiation protection issue. The primary barrier penetration of neutrons will not be a problem because a barrier designed for the photon beam will be adequate for neutrons, provided it contains no high Z materials, but neutron transport down a maze and along ducts requires special design considerations, as discussed in chapters 5, 6 and 7.

Linear accelerators with magnetic resonance (MR) imaging

A linear accelerator with MR imaging is a hybrid of a MR scanner and a linear accelerator on a CT scanner style gantry. They have some room design features additional to those required for standard linear accelerators. As these features may vary by manufacturer it is important to understand the specific equipment and design requirements provided by the manufacturer prior to the design process. An MR safety expert should also be involved in the design process. Provision is required for screening patients and staff before they enter the scanner to cover such issues as pacemakers, metal implants and other sensitive materials. Metal detectors in the vicinity of the entrance are likely to be required.

There are MR requirements which affect the design of the bunker. Magnetic shielding may be necessary to contain the 0.5 mT (5 Gauss) line and a Faraday cage is essential to protect the machine from radio frequency (RF) interference. While not strictly an x-ray protection issue, maintaining the integrity of the Faraday cage means that power and signal cables may need to enter the room through new conduits created in the existing barriers; this may be easier to achieve in a new bunker. It is important that cable runs are positioned as far from the isocentre as possible and their channels should incorporate a maze rather than a direct line of sight for radiation. There will also need to be a quench pipe to take helium gas out of the room in the event of a failure of the superconducting system (quenching). This must have a significant diameter in order to carry the large volume of helium gas in a quench. Again, this should be positioned as far away from the isocentre as possible and is usually vertical, which prevents any direct line of sight for radiation. The area around the quench pipe exit must have restricted access for the eventuality of it being used, and restricting access near the quench pipe may be straightforward if these are also high dose rate areas. Standard maze calculations (see section 5.7) can be used for assessment of dose rates through these structures.

The energy spectrum of the linear accelerator may be different from a standard accelerator and it is important to understand the attenuation properties of the radiation produced. This difference is due to the specialised technology which may include shortened wave guides and FFF delivery. It is also important to note that field sizes can be smaller than for standard accelerators, and the source to isocentre distance may be greater than 1 m. Currently MR linear accelerators are closed gantry based, and offer some self-attenuation due to material directly opposite the accelerator head. The initial dose rate required for calculations may therefore be defined at the outer surface of the gantry housing using values provided by the manufacturer.

TomoTherapy® units

All modern high energy accelerators are mounted isocentrically. A special case of such a design is the TomoTherapy[1] unit in which a 6 MV linear accelerator is mounted on a CT scanner style gantry. This normally rotates constantly about the patient in a single plane and a permanently mounted beam stopper is incorporated into the gantry opposite the accelerator, thus reducing the need for a primary barrier. The unit has an MLC across the width of the primary beam, in which the leaves are either open or closed when they completely block the beam. The collimator varies the intensity distribution of the primary beam on the patient as the gantry rotates and the patient moves at constant speed through the gantry aperture. All patient treatments are therefore IMRT treatments. More details on the shielding required are given in section 8.2.

CyberKnife® units

A departure from the isocentric linear accelerator design is the CyberKnife[2] unit. In this a 6 MV linear accelerator is mounted on a robotic arm which allows the beam to be pointed at any point within the patient under robotic control. Because the beam can be pointed in any direction, with some restriction in the upward direction, all of the walls become primary barriers, although each direction will only be irradiated for a small proportion of the time. Usually the roof can be considered as a secondary barrier. More details on the shielding required are given in section 8.3.

4.1.2.2 Kilovoltage treatment and electronic brachytherapy

Most radiotherapy is delivered with megavoltage beams, but there are still a number of applications for which kilovoltage beams in the range 50–300 kV are appropriate and cost effective. Whereas kilovoltage x-rays were often regarded as a cheaper alternative for palliation, in recent years a number of specific areas of use have been developed for which there are significant advantages with the lower energy.

X-ray units working in the range 50 kV to about 140 kV are often termed *superficial units*. These are used mainly to treat skin cancers with applicators defining the treatment area and distance from the x-ray target. The unit is generally supported on a mounting that restricts the orientation of the radiation beam so that not all surfaces of the room can be irradiated with the primary beam. Scatter doses do need to be considered but will generally be of sufficiently low energy not to present a significant radiation protection challenge. *Orthovoltage units* operate up to 300 kV and apart from the increased energy have similar constraints to superficial machines. More information on the radiation protection measures needed for kilovoltage therapy units is given in chapter 9.

---

[1] TomoTherapy is a registered trademark of Accuray.

[2] CyberKnife is a registered trademark of Accuray.

The term *electronic brachytherapy* has been used to describe devices that use a treatment applicator with a very short distance between an x-ray source and the end of the applicator, and operate at around 50 kV. The applicator can be placed on the skin or inside a body cavity. These devices can sometimes be hand-held, but it is preferable for the applicator to be fixed independently of the operator. These devices are used for rectal, breast and skin treatments, and the intraoperative treatment of breast lesions. Treatment may take place in a conventional operating theatre and not in a radiotherapy centre. The term is also used to describe mobile accelerators producing electrons in the energy range 4–12 MeV and used in similar clinical applications. More information on the radiation protection measures needed with these devices is included in chapter 9.

4.1.2.3 Brachytherapy

Brachytherapy uses a sealed radioactive source which is inserted into the patient usually by a process of remote afterloading. The activity of the source depends on whether the equipment is rated as high dose rate (HDR), pulsed dose-rate (PDR) or low dose-rate (LDR). LDR afterloading equipment that used caesium-137 sources has been phased out largely in favour of HDR installations and a lower number of PDR installations. The penetration of the radiation will depend on the radionuclide source used; the most common is iridium-192, but cobalt-60 is also used. For a HDR installation a shielded room is required together with a control room and appropriate interlock systems, and treatment times are relatively short (minutes). PDR treatments are intended to have the same radiobiological effect as LDR treatments, and treatment times are longer—up to two days. This will require a shielded single room, control unit and appropriate interlocks. Since the radiation emerging from the patient is essentially isotropic, the walls, floor and ceiling of the shielded rooms will all be primary barriers (see chapter 10).

4.1.2.4 Gamma Knife® units

Cobalt-60 sources are no longer used for radiation therapy in the UK with the exception of the Gamma Knife[3]. This uses 192 cobalt-60 sources mounted in a helmet shaped array. Because the sources are close to the patient and contained within the helmet, relatively little shielding is required when compared to an isocentric cobalt-60 unit. More information on the shielding of Gamma Knife units is given in section 8.1.

Isocentric cobalt-60 units are usually sited in a bunker like a linear accelerator. Shielding calculations for such a bunker are the same as those for a linear accelerator bunker described in chapter 5. The source to isocentre distance is usually 80 cm and not 100 cm as in accelerators. Data for cobalt-60 radiation are included in tables 5.1–5.7.

Recently the GammaPod™ has been introduced in the USA, designed specifically for SBRT of the breast[4]. The GammaPod consists of 36 collimated cobalt-60 sources

[3] Gamma Knife is a registered trademark of Elekta.

[4] GammaPod is a trademark of Xcision Medical Systems.

with a total activity of 160 TBq in a hemispherical source carrier. Shielding calculations are not straightforward due to the beam geometry, but early studies suggest that it meets US regulatory requirements if sited in a linear accelerator bunker.

4.1.3 Information required for shielding calculations

4.1.3.1 Geometric considerations

The size of the treatment room will be determined by the requirements of the treatment unit manufacturer to allow for flexible and ergonomic use of the unit. It is normal for the room to be slightly larger than the minimum specified, but too large a room will be less ergonomically efficient because of the increased distances that the staff will need to walk. It is also essential to consider the requirements for patient access on trolleys and the installation of the unit. The primary barrier can either protrude into the treatment room or into the space outside, and the necessary clearance to the isocentre will define the position of the inside of the barrier. The further the primary barrier is from the isocentre the wider it will need to be (see section 5.2). Consideration also needs to be given to whether the room will be used for TBI, as in that case it will be necessary to offset the isocentre towards one of the walls so that an extended treatment distance becomes possible in the opposite horizontal direction (see above and section 2.2). A decision will also need to be made about the roof of the treatment room—whether this needs to be a primary barrier when the areas above are occupied, or whether a thinner barrier is sufficient if the area above is not occupied and access can be restricted during operation of the unit.

4.1.3.2 Dose and dose rate constraints

In order to determine the thickness of each barrier it will be necessary to know what dose rate will be acceptable on the outside of the barrier. For this purpose dose constraints are used (see also section 3.7.3). These may be specified in terms of the annual radiation dose that would be acceptable, and this will allow the maximum instantaneous dose rate (IDR) to be calculated. A typical constraint might be 0.3 mSv per annum for a member of the public with a higher constraint (1 mSv is sometimes used) being adopted for staff. A higher dose rate may be acceptable for the exterior of the roof if there is nothing above. In these circumstances skyshine is a deciding factor and an upper limit of 2 mSv h^{-1} is commonly used. This is discussed further in section 5.4.

To derive the acceptable IDR from the dose constraint it is necessary to know the duty cycle of the machine (i.e. what proportion of the time the beam is on), what proportion of time the beam will be pointing in the relevant direction and the occupancy of the area being considered. For areas with low occupancy, or for FFF beams where the dose rate at the isocentre is high, the calculation of the shielding based on TADR2000 (see the glossary) may lead to dose rates of several tens of μSv h^{-1}. Over-specification of the shielding to obtain low IDRs which will reduce the dose per annum to levels well below 0.3 mSv per annum is not necessary and is difficult to justify on a cost benefit basis (see also section 3.7.5). However, a risk assessment which evaluates possible unusual scenarios that might lead to staff or members of the public receiving high doses should always be carried out.

For FFF beams, the dose rate can increase from 6 Gy min^{-1} to 24 Gy min^{-1} at the isocentre. However, unless the throughput of patients increases significantly, the annual dose received outside the bunker may actually decrease. Kry *et al* (2009) examined this question for Varian linear accelerators. They found that because the penetrative quality of the beam was reduced in the absence of the flattening filter, the value of the tenth value layer (TVL) in concrete was reduced by about 12%. This is because the flattening filter hardens the beam and also because the dose rate at the centre of the beam is higher than that at the edges. Jank *et al* (2014) looked at this from the point of view of Elekta accelerators. Elekta increase the electron energy of the beam so that the TPR20/10 for the beam is unchanged. In spite of this Jank *et al* found that the dose rate outside the barrier was 30% lower for the same isocentre dose rate at 6 MV, although they did not consider matched 10 MV beams. However, Paynter *et al* (2014) found that for a matched 10 MV beam the effect of shielding was very slightly reduced.

In addition to this effect on the penetration quality of the primary beam, the leakage radiation is reduced for both types of accelerator because of the lower beam current needed to produce the same dose rate at the isocentre. The impact of lower leakage on the thickness of the secondary barriers has been discussed by Vassiliev *et al* (2007) and Jank *et al* (2014). Since the annual dose outside the bunker is going to be less with an FFF machine it is not difficult to argue that not increasing the thickness of the barriers meets the as low as reasonable practicable (ALARP) criterion since additional shielding would bring no actual benefit in reducing the doses received. Kry *et al* (2009) suggest that if a machine is to be used exclusively without a flattening filter, there is even a justification for reducing the shielding. The risk assessment should, however, consider the possibility that the throughput of the machine may increase. Beam-on time is in practice a small proportion of the time taken to treat a patient so a significant increase in throughput is unlikely, but FFF may be used in the future to facilitate hypofractionated treatments. Such treatments will probably be associated with an increased setup and imaging time, so the increase in total weekly dose delivered is still likely to be marginal.

4.1.3.3 Workload assessment

To determine the radiation workload at the isocentre over a specified period, the following information is required:

- The number of patients to be treated.
- The beam energies to be used and the proportion of patients at each energy.
- The proportion of patients at each energy to be treated with IMRT or VMAT.
- The average dose per patient treatment.

A suitable pro-forma for specifying the expected workload for a linear accelerator is given in figure 4.4. A simpler version can be used for kilovoltage units.

SPECIFICATION OF X-RADIATION WORKLOAD AT ISOCENTRE/APPLICATOR FACE

Centre:

Room Name:

X-Ray Energy 1, Specify: …………..

Conformal			IMRT/VMAT			FFF		
Patients / month	Dose / fraction (Gy)	Dose rate (Gy/min)	Patients / month	Dose / fraction (Gy)	Dose rate (Gy/min)	Patients / month	Dose / fraction (Gy)	Dose rate (Gy/min)

X-Ray Energy 2, Specify: …………..

Conformal			IMRT/VMAT			FFF		
Patients / month	Dose / fraction (Gy)	Dose rate (Gy/min)	Patients / month	Dose / fraction (Gy)	Dose rate (Gy/min)	Patients / month	Dose / fraction (Gy)	Dose rate (Gy/min)

X-Ray Energy 3, Specify: …………..

Conformal			IMRT/VMAT			FFF		
Patients / month	Dose / fraction (Gy)	Dose rate (Gy/min)	Patients / month	Dose / fraction (Gy)	Dose rate (Gy/min)	Patients / month	Dose / fraction (Gy)	Dose rate (Gy/min)

TBI **X-Ray Energy, Specify:** …………..

Patients / month	Dose / fraction (Gy)	Fractions/patient	Dose rate (Gy/min)

SRS **X-Ray Energy, Specify:** …………..

Patients / month	Dose / fraction (Gy)	Fractions/patient	Dose rate (Gy/min)

SBRT **X-Ray Energy, Specify:** …………..

Patients / month	Dose / fraction (Gy)	Fractions/patient	Dose rate (Gy/min)

Figure 4.4. Sample pro-forma for the specification of the radiation workload for a linear accelerator.

Most linear accelerators have the possibility of a choice of several x-ray energies. The conservative assumption is that the highest beam energy will be used 100% of the time, but this is in practice unlikely and will lead to excessive shielding and larger bunker footprints. Data from record and verify systems (or radiotherapy management systems) should be available to confirm the proportions of energies used.

As mentioned earlier IMRT in whatever form it is used will potentially affect the thickness of secondary barriers. The extent of IMRT use and the method of delivery should be considered when deciding what factor to use for IMRT. Similar considerations apply to TBI. Examples of TBI orientation factor calculations can be found in Rodgers (2001).

Regarding patient throughput, while it is just possible to treat six patients per hour, five is a more reasonable assumption.

Regarding patient dose, experience at the Clatterbridge Cancer Centre indicates that the average dose is 2.4 Gy per fraction, but it may be appropriate to allow for increased hypofractionation and assume 3 Gy per fraction. If one assumes that the average depth dose is 75% (12 cm deep at 6 MV), this implies that 4 Gy will be delivered to the isocentre, giving a dose per hour of 20 Gy and a weekly dose of 800 Gy (based on an eight hour day and five working days/week). For a linear accelerator operating with a dose rate of 6 Gy min^{-1} this is a duty cycle of 5.6% beam-on time. It will be seen that this is a conservative estimate. Some conservative factors for patient workload are suggested in table 4.1.

Dose fractionation is a particular area of uncertainty. There is a trend towards hypofractionation, which may lead to increased patient dose being delivered at each fraction. Some increase in setup and imaging time can be expected for such treatments because more accurate treatment is required for higher doses per fraction, reducing patient throughput, but it is still likely that the total number of MUs delivered per day will increase. Whereas with IMRT only the secondary barriers would be affected, hypofractionation will also affect the requirements for the primary barrier.

During commissioning it may be necessary to run the machine continuously for long periods which might affect the workload. Another approach is to separate this phase of the life of the bunker and manage the radiation implications separately by creating temporary controlled areas. The design of the bunker is unlikely to be affected by this relatively short phase.

4.1.3.4 Equipment use or orientation factor

The use or orientation factor is the proportion of the beam-on time that a unit spends pointing at a specified direction. In order to calculate this factor a detailed

Table 4.1. Conservative values for the calculation of radiation workloads.

Parameter	Conservative value	
Dose/patient fraction @ isocentre	4 Gy	
Patients treated	5 per hour	
Working day	8 hours	
Working week	5 days	
Working year	50 weeks	
Head leakage	0.001	
IMRT factor	IMRT	5
	VMAT	3
Orientation/use factor	0.3[a]	

[a] For general use; more accurate values are needed for specific applications, e.g. TBI.

knowledge of the planned use of the machine is required. For linear accelerators where the primary beam is confined to a vertical plane through the isocentre, the simple approximation that the accelerator spends equal amounts of time pointing down, up and in both lateral directions leads to a factor of 0.25 for the primary barriers, floor and ceiling when calculating TADRs. This is clearly a simplification when some gantry angles are used more frequently and, for example, will not reflect the increased use of lateral fields employed as part of pelvic irradiations with conventional radiotherapy or for TBIs. Almost all accelerators are now fitted with a record and verification system (or radiotherapy management system) and it is therefore possible to obtain an accurate record of the number of MUs delivered in any particular direction during the course of the day. Records such as this can be used as a guide to see if a more complex range of factors needs to be employed. This can be a risky strategy because of changes in practice that may be expected over the life of the bunker and suitable margins for uncertainty should be included. While it is desirable to plan for reasonably foreseeable changes, it can become excessively expensive to try to allow for all possible changes in the future. While it is generally more expensive to add shielding after the building is completed, it may be even more expensive to plan for a possible change in practice that is not expected for many years. While this may lead to a significant reduction in the shielding required, a system of risk assessments needs to be in place to ensure that future changes in practice do not invalidate the calculated doses. It is recommended that a factor of 0.3 is used for gantry angle 0° and 0.25 used for gantry angles 90°, 180° and 270° for standard clinical practice.

4.1.3.5 Occupancy factors

The occupancy factor is the time spent by an individual at the location in question. This has been discussed in section 3.7.2 and suggested factors in the report *Radiation Shielding for Diagnostic Radiology* (Sutton *et al* 2012) are reproduced in table 3.5 and the factors in NCRP151 (NCRP 2005) in table 3.6.

4.1.3.6 TomoTherapy units

In TomoTherapy units the linear accelerator is continuously rotating and the orientation factor can be taken as 0.1 (Baechler *et al* 2007). The primary beam stopper on the far side of the patient has a transmission factor of 0.004 (Balog *et al* 2005). The IMRT factor has been given as 8 (Balog *et al* 2005). Because of this increased beam-on time, Baechler *et al* (2007) have found that the principal requirement for shielding is from leakage radiation. They also describe an approach for calculating the additional shielding required. The shielding requirements for a room with a TomoTherapy unit are described in greater detail in section 8.2.

4.1.3.7 CyberKnife units

Due to its complete freedom of movement (except usually above an angle of 22°) the linear accelerator does not point in a particular direction for any length of time. NCRP151 (NCRP 2005) and the Accuray shielding guidelines suggest a value for the orientation factor of 0.05. This is based on the publication by Rodgers (2007).

Yang and Feng (2014) have re-examined these assumptions and found an orientation factor of 0.01 over a number of years of clinical practice. However, they suggest using their data to justify a conservative orientation factor of 0.05. NCRP151 (NCRP 2005) suggests that the IMRT factor may be as high as 15, which implies that the contribution of leakage radiation may be significant even in calculating the primary barrier thickness. Yang and Feng (2014) also examined this factor and found an IMRT factor of 7.4. The unit uses small treatment fields defined by cylindrical collimators or a micro-MLC and the contribution from patient scatter is small. The shielding requirements for a room with a CyberKnife unit are discussed in greater detail in section 8.3.

4.2 Treatment room design

C Walker

4.2.1 Introduction

The majority of this report is focused on providing methodologies for experienced hospital physicists to design radiotherapy facilities in terms of radiation protection. However, it is also important to consider those design requirements that affect the 'fitness for purpose' of the finished product and provide at least a measure of future-proofing for bunkers that will stand for a number of decades. Whilst the positioning of services such as heating and ventilation ducts remains the responsibility of the architect, the effects of a misconceived plan can be crucial for routine working.

4.2.2 Internal dimensions

Given the relative longevity of the built environment of 30 years or more compared to the life time of a linear accelerator of approximately 10 years, it is vital that bunkers are built with sufficiently large internal dimensions to allow for the installation of any manufacturers' upcoming equipment offerings as well as that for which they were initially designed. All manufacturers provide equipment specific site planning guides that provide guidance on all services required, as well as minimum sub-optimal room dimensions and minimum optimal room dimensions. The difference between optimal and sub-optimal is usually the ability to completely rotate the fully extended treatment couch. Further caution is required for sub-optimal installations in that they generally result in limited access to the machine to perform servicing functions which can in turn affect clinical uptime.

If minimal room dimensions are adopted, future-proofing will be difficult and the ability to provide appropriate 'in-room' storage will be compromised. If room dimensions are to be chosen to accommodate equipment from all manufacturers, then careful consideration must be given to the 'back wall to isocentre' distance. If this crucial distance is not considered explicitly, it may result in the isocentre of the machine being displaced from the centre of the primary barrier. If the minimal back wall to isocentre distances are being considered, displacement of the isocentre is likely to be of the order of 0.2 m. If the primary barrier has not been constructed of a sufficient width to accommodate this displacement, more width will need to be added to ensure the primary barrier encompasses the widest possible beam for the replacement accelerator. From the author's experience rooms that are of the order of 8 m long (gantry axis) and 7 m wide should be adequate for most installations, including currently available robotically mounted linear accelerators. More generous dimensions than this would allow for better storage solutions and mitigate against any space reduction caused by any maze construction. Finished ceiling heights of 2.8 m will generally suffice, but the robotically mounted accelerators require a greater head room of 3.05 m.

Whilst these suggested dimensions are suitable for present day equipment, advances in image guidance with MR imaging technology may necessitate the inclusion of RF and magnetic shielding in future bunker builds. Indicative dimensions would suggest that the width and length requirements given above would be suitable, but a greater ceiling height of 3.25 m coupled with a 1.05 m deep pit would also need to be provided.

4.2.3 Site access

Traditionally radiotherapy departments have been built on the periphery of hospitals in an attempt to mitigate radiation protection problems through low or zero occupancy adjacencies. The advantage of such a location is that it provides short access routes for the egress of obsolete equipment and installation of new equipment. Irrespective of the radiotherapy department position, space must be available for the safe unloading of the equipment from the delivery vehicle. Consideration must also be given, at this stage, to ancillary devices such as close coupled chiller units which may be installed in physically remote or in roof top plant rooms. In such cases safe crane lifting operations require space, short spans and unoccupied areas below the path of the jib.

The intended route that any equipment is to take into the treatment room must provide space for the equipment's movements in all planes, particularly if doorways are to be traversed. Consideration must also be given to the turning circle or minimum radius of curvature that the equipment can achieve, especially in treatment rooms with maze entrances. In addition to the floor of the treatment room, the floor of the access route must be strong enough to take the typical 2 kN m^{-2} equipment load. Special measures for floor ducts and inspection covers should be considered, possibly requiring steel plates during the installation process. Temporary floor coverings, e.g. plywood sheets, may also be necessary to avoid damage to floor coverings. Mitigation against complex access routes for future replacements can be made by the use of demountable blocks for the construction of all, or a single wall or a section of wall of the treatment room. Historically this was achieved through the use of barytes blocks, but alternative materials such as high density concrete or Verishield™ blocks are now readily available[5] (see chapter 7).

[5] Verishield is a trademark of Veritas Medical Solutions.

The future employment of MR imaging guidance will bring specific access requirements for the associated magnet which will need to be delivered intact. The magnet is likely to require a direct access route into the treatment room that is at least 2.75 m by 2.5 m, provided either through the roof or one of the shielding walls.

The problems identified above are significantly increased if the treatment rooms are not on the ground floor level and any lifts installed must be capable of taking the equipment weight.

4.2.4 Lintels, baffles and nibs

Lintels may be placed above the maze either for structural or neutron scatter reduction purposes. In the latter case this tends to have minimal impact except in the reduction of neutron streaming in high energy installations. However, placement of such a lintel, particularly if for structural purposes, can pose a challenge to the removal of and installation of new equipment via this route. This can cause a major problem if it is not appropriately penetrated for the installation of services and ductwork has to be fitted below it with a commensurate reduction in ceiling height. Ideally services should pass through lintels with suitable protection measures (see chapter 7). The inclusion of baffles or nibs in the maze design to prevent single reflection incident photons leaving the maze can also reduce the total useable maze width for equipment replacement processes and even make it impossible to access the room with a hospital bed. In such cases where the design calls for the inclusion of these scatter reducing features, consideration should be given to installing them in a demountable manner.

If a maze is designed in such a way that it relies on baffles to prevent scatter, caution should be applied to the dead spaces created by their inclusion. There may be a future temptation to use such spaces for storage, which would inadvertently introduce a further scatter source which would negate the effect of the original baffles.

4.2.5 Room access arrangement—last person out (search button)

Over recent years the use of motorised protective treatment room doors in conjunction with short mazes has grown in popularity over the traditional door-less but longer maze design. Whilst such doors will be necessarily heavy and will require motorised movements for general use, auxiliary means for opening the doors in the event of electrical or mechanical failure must also be provided. Provision of a single appropriately shielded and interlocked door removes the need for an additional neutron door for high energy x-ray beams, and the associated complexity of interlock arrangements required when switching between low or high energy modes.

As these large and heavy doors move relatively slowly, treatment efficiency can be gained through the use of a 'half open/closed' functionality, as well as judicious positioning of an additional door control switch at the linear accelerator control console. In addition to increasing efficiency, this measure allows rapid access to the treatment room in the event of patient distress or emergency. 'Crush' protection should be provided for the door in terms of infrared movement detectors and also, preferably, a physical proximity detection mechanism. These doors may also be used to provide security of access to the bunker and further act as fire doors.

Restriction of exposure (IRR99 Regulation 8 (IRR 1999)) is achieved through the judicious selection and placement of door interlock mechanisms. Such systems are discussed in the *Approved Code of Practice* (HSE 2000) and the *Medical and Dental Guidance Notes* (IPEM 2002). The door interlocks must be intrinsically 'fail safe' and it must not be possible to reset these interlocks by merely closing the opened barrier. The door interlocks, when reset, should not allow the equipment to resume emitting radiation without further positive confirmation from the operator at the control console. The door interlock mechanism should be achieved by the use of a two stage 'search and lock' system where the 'search' switch must be located at a position within the treatment room, such that the operator operating this switch when leaving the room has a clear view of the entire room. The operation of the 'search' switch should start a timing mechanism with enough of a delay to allow the operator to leave the room without delay and close the door interlock through operating the 'lock' switch. In the case of a room with a door the interlock switch will only be completed when the door is fully closed, but in the case of an open maze then a second physical interlock switch is required. A prior risk assessment will determine the location of the search button, but a room design that provides interrupted views with possible 'hiding' places may require additional search switch locations and an audible warning of radiation exposure.

When there is no door, half door or other physical barrier such as an interlocked bar, the room entrance must be protected by photo-electric beams or infrared movement detectors. Care should be taken to site such detectors to ensure that they will be activated by small children crawling or walking into the maze entrance. Appropriate interlock switching must also be provided to any equipment room doors that reside within the bunker itself, including gantry facia doors. These doors should have fail safe interlock switches that only 'make' with the door closed with a mechanism provided to hold them open if an engineer requires access. If the door is closed and it then becomes possible to initiate an exposure, then a suitable audible/visible warning should be provided to anybody who could still be inside the equipment area.

4.2.6 Emergency stops

Prior risk assessment will inform the location of emergency stops within the treatment and control rooms as well as in any 'in-bunker' equipment rooms (e.g. behind a gantry facia). These should be clearly identified as emergency stop switches and should be physically separated from 'search' or other interlock switches to avoid inadvertent activation. Whilst the main purpose of these switches, from the manufacturer's perspective, is to stop movement of the unit and therefore protect patients and operating/maintenance personnel from potential crush injuries, once activated they will also prevent the initiation of or terminate a radiation exposure. Their number and positioning in the treatment and equipment room should also be such as to allow for radiation exposure termination without the need for the operator to directly cross the beam path. These stop switches must be intrinsically 'fail safe' and must latch the machine in the 'stop' mode, requiring positive action from the operator to fully restore motion and/or the initiation of a radiation exposure.

In addition to the above emergency stops, a power shut down or 'fireman's' switch should be provided in an accessible position in the linear accelerator control room. Whilst it is important for this switch or switches to be accessible, they should be protected from inadvertent operation.

4.2.7 Lighting arrangements (including alignment lasers)

There are a number of conflicting considerations for room lighting, including the need for bright lighting to allow for maintenance personnel to carry out small and intricate maintenance operations, whilst treatment radiographers require dim lighting to enable them to see the patient positioning with respect to optical projection systems. It should be possible to switch between these two modes directly from the unit's control pendant, as well as from the room wall switches. Care should be taken to ensure that complex combinations of switching operations are not required to provide the required lighting levels.

Patient alignment is carried out through the use of specially mounted lasers that indicate the accelerator's isocentre position. Usually they comprise two sidewall lasers and at least one sagittal laser mounted at ceiling height to project along the full length of the couch. There may also be the requirement for a ceiling laser mounted directly above the isocentre. In all cases the lasers should be switched from the machine control pendant. Rigid thick steel mounting plates should be supplied for the lasers to ensure that they do not move with changes in room temperature. They should also be protected from inadvertent knocking by personnel or patient trolleys. There will be a temptation to mount the sidewall lasers in cut-outs or alcoves in the room sidewalls. As these cut-outs will necessarily be in the primary barrier, consideration must be given to the protection implications of potentially removing 10–20 cm of this barrier. It is also easier to cast these cut-outs in place during the pouring of the concrete walls as opposed to cutting them out later. If this approach is taken then the cut-outs should be wide enough to accommodate any anticipated move in isocentre position associated with equipment refresh.

4.2.8 Services

Electrical supply

An adequate supply of switched power sockets should be placed around the room including any plant room. It should be noted that a power supply is required in reasonable proximity to the isocentre to allow test phantoms and patient monitoring instruments to be powered. As all walls of the treatment room are radiation barriers it is best practice to surface-mount all junction boxes on the protective barrier walls with stud walls used to hide them behind a decorative finish. If the protective barrier is to be compromised by the installation of flush mounted junction boxes, they should be backed with a 3.8 cm thick steel plate extending to a 2.5 cm margin around the box.

Water

Whilst a wash hand basin may be required to ensure compliance with infection control requirements, other water supplies are not necessary as all linear accelerator manufacturers now provide close coupled chillers for equipment cooling purposes. Infection control requirements are also likely to require the mounting of an appropriate hand gel dispensing station.

Heating/cooling and ventilation ducts

With regard to the heating, ventilation and air-conditioning, consideration needs to be given to the semi-naked patient who will be expected to lie in a still and reproducible position on the treatment couch for a reasonable period of time. The architect will indicate the required number of air changes per hour for the room for this purpose. However it should be noted that some equipment will require ambient cooling, without recourse to chilled water mechanisms, and will therefore require increased ventilation. Advice on the requirements for this will be given in the manufacturer's site planning guide, as will the heat output from conventional water cooled equipment. It may be necessary to provide additional air changes for equipment that is going to be used for high dose rate electron treatments to dissipate ozone formed from the irradiation of oxygen in air. In all cases the ozone level should be kept below the maximum permissible concentration of 0.1 parts per million (ppm) (NCRP 2005).

Care needs to be taken over the siting of penetrations to carry the air input and extract ducts, as any penetration of a radiation barrier brings protection problems. Ideally installations should involve running duct work above a false ceiling along the route of the maze or under the radiation barriers through the floor slab in the case of the Forster-sandwich construction. More details are given in chapter 7.

IT connectivity (including linear accelerator control cabling)

The treatment unit will require the provision of significant amounts of ductwork for the interconnecting cables between it and the treatment control console in the treatment control room. In addition to this cabling, provision should also be made for IT cables and suitable sockets/connections to allow for the increasing data requirements of, for example, motion management systems and medical physics quality control systems. These cable runs can be cut into the floor as covered ducts or penetrate the concrete floor slab as described above.

Dosimetry cables

As well as the more permanent cabling described above, the medical physicists will require a dedicated duct through which they can pass dosimeter and water phantom signal and control cables. This will provide a fall-back solution in case of a permanent installation failure and will allow for the quick introduction of additional dosimetry equipment. The duct should have an opening of at least 120 mm to allow the passage of large 'D' type connectors. The duct should open at a suitable location in the control room to allow placement of the connected electrometers either on a desk or shelf. Similarly the opening in the treatment room should be readily accessible, not for example behind a cupboard, unless this is intended for storage of the cabled items and adequate access has been provided. The duct will present a radiation leakage pathway, which can be minimised if it is both sloped vertically downwards into the treatment room and angled away from the normal to the penetrated wall (see chapter 7).

Smoke detectors

These should be mounted away from any area which can be struck by the primary beam and should not rely on ionisation as the detection mechanism.

CCTV system

A closed circuit television (CCTV) system is required to monitor the patient during treatment delivery. However, the increased adoption of auto-sequencing techniques for treatment delivery, in particular VMAT, necessitates the careful observation of the relationship between the treatment unit and the patient through the full 360 degrees of possible gantry rotation. To facilitate this three camera installations are required: one in a sagittal line with the gantry/patient axis but avoiding impediment of the sagittal patient positioning laser and one on each sidewall of the room. These two sidewall cameras should be mounted such that they can be used to view the alignment laser isocentre marks on the patient skin to enable the implementation of deep inspiration breath hold (DIBH) treatment techniques. The cameras should be provided with remote control of motorised zoom and pan functionality, as well as focus and iris controls to allow adaption to the various light levels employed in the treatment room. The zoom and pan functionality will also greatly help in viewing any monitoring equipment required for the patient, such as cardiac monitoring in patients with pacemakers or the monitoring required for anaesthetised paediatric patients.

Intercom

There should be a two way intercom system between the control and treatment rooms. Whilst the primary use for this system is to monitor the patient, it is also increasingly required for the delivery of verbal coaching, particularly in breath hold delivery techniques. Communication with the patient should require positive operation of the intercom system so that the patient cannot inadvertently overhear control room conversations.

4.2.9 Gating interfaces

Whilst most modern radiotherapy gating interfaces rely on an optical projection onto the patient's surface, the projection system usually requires mounting just below ceiling height in line with the sagittal axis of the linear accelerator. In addition to the physical mounting, consideration needs to be given to the power and data requirement of the projector along with any associated 'in-room' display or computer control systems.

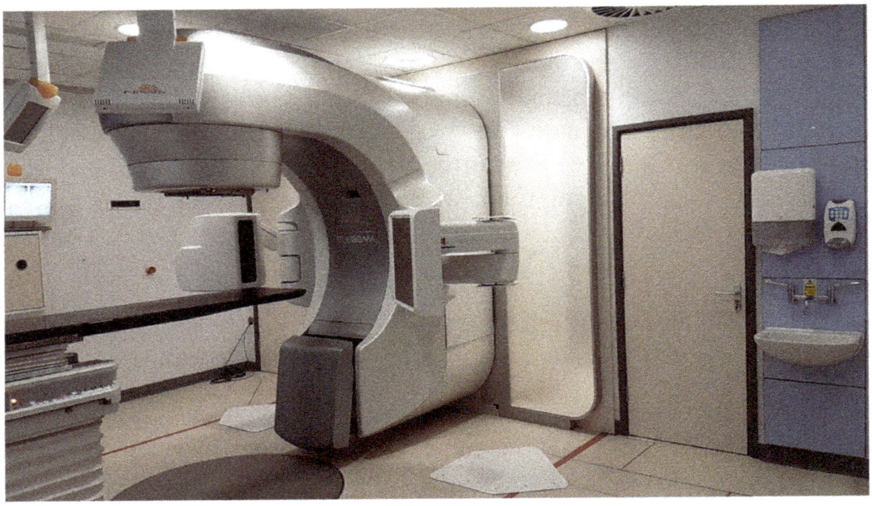

Figure 4.5. A bunker at the Northern Centre for Cancer Care, Newcastle, showing the Exac Trac X-Ray monitoring equipment.

4.2.10 Motion management systems

Motion management technology comes in many forms ranging from 4D capable integrated kilovoltage cone beam CT facilities to ceiling mounted x-ray tubes and detection panels on the floor (e.g. Exac Trac® X-Ray Monitoring[6]—see figure 4.5). Optical systems which use a stereoscopic multi-camera system (such as Align-RT®)[7] are also available. Careful planning is required to ensure appropriate physical installation along with the requisite power and data connections (see figure 4.6).

4.2.11 Storage solutions

Storage space is required for a large range of individual items ranging considerably in physical dimensions and weight. The best storage solution is a bespoke cupboard arrangement with integrated shelves and racks designed to take the individual pieces of equipment (see figure 4.7). The cupboards should have doors to obscure the items in storage to alleviate patient anxiety. The cupboard doors will also have to comply with local infection control policy. Likely storage requirements are listed below, but this list cannot be regarded as comprehensive given the present rate of technological development.

- Immobilisation equipment:
  - Head immobilisation shells.
  - Generic breast boards.
  - Generic pelvis boards.
  - Generic thorax boards.
  - Belly boards.
  - Customised vac-bags.

---

[6] Exac Trac is a registered trademark of Brainlab AG.

[7] Align-RT is a registered trademark of Vision RT.

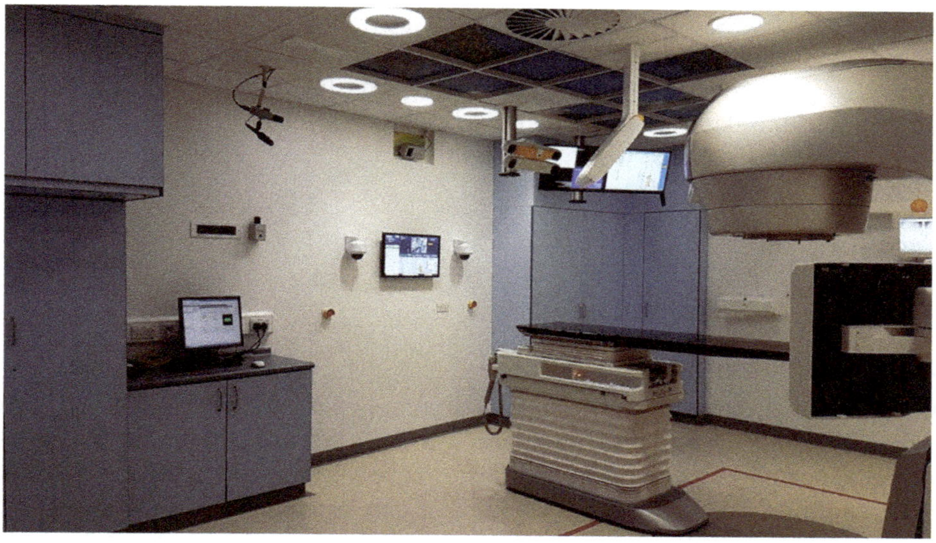

Figure 4.6. A bunker at the Northern Centre for Cancer Care, Newcastle, showing a range of motion management equipment installations.

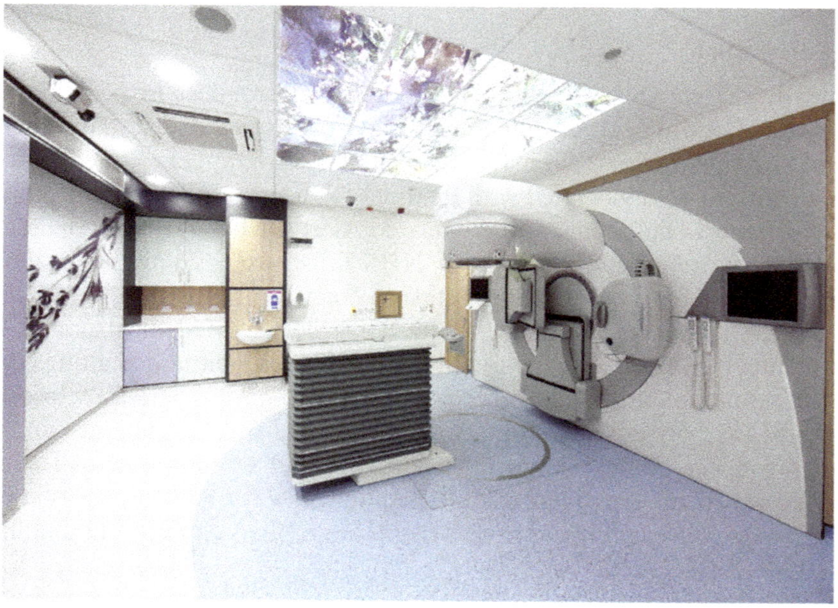

Figure 4.7. An adequately sized bunker with an Elekta linear accelerator at the James Cook University Hospital, Middlesbrough, with 'built-in' storage solutions.

- Couch panels.
- Patient mobility items such as 'pat-slides'.
- Dosimetry equipment, including phantoms (at a location convenient for power and data requirements).
- Imaging phantoms.
- Electron applicators.
- Electron inserts (cut-outs).
- Bolus.
- General storage.

4.2.12 Finishes and fittings

Whilst the room finishes and fittings must comply with the appropriate standards, it should be noted that such facilities will have a considerable impact on the anxious patient. Therefore, every effort should be taken to soften the hard technical appearance of the room and equipment. This can be achieved in a number of ways from the exact orientation of the linear accelerator in the room or by having illuminated 'sky ceilings' and innovative decorative room finishes.

4.3 Control room design

C Walker

4.3.1 Introduction

Historically control areas were little more than a control desk in a corridor outside the treatment room. More enlightened departments extended the benching to provide additional workspace for treatment radiographers to carry out the administrative duties associated with treatment delivery. Following the publication of the Toft report (Toft 2005) and the related Alert 4181 (DH 2004) concerning the safe delivery of radiotherapy treatment 'NHS Trusts were required to ensure that a suitable environment is provided for staff to concentrate fully on the task of data manipulation'. This has resulted in the construction of dedicated and private rooms from which control of the treatment machine is maintained alongside safety critical data manipulation and other administrative duties. These enclosed rooms also ensure that privacy and dignity is maintained for the patients undergoing radiotherapy. The control room must also be sited so that staff can effectively control access to the treatment room. It should always have a clear view of the entrance to the treatment room so that the radiographers can prevent unauthorised access.

4.3.2 Control room dimensions

The control room dimensions should be considered explicitly in the design in order to accommodate all the necessary equipment as well as the operating personnel and any professional visitors. Space needs to be available for the linear accelerator's treatment control cabinet/system, which can be as large as 0.8 m^2 and up to a height of 1.3 m. Vendor specific site planning guides will provide specific dimensions. However, it will be up to the architect to incorporate this large cabinet with its associated cabling into the general control room furnishing. Desk space needs to be provided for the operating console including its monitors, additional associated imaging monitors and computers (see figure 4.8). The monitors for the CCTV system, intercom and gating and or motion management systems will again need to be installed into this space (see figure 4.9). It is crucial that all of this equipment is accommodated ergonomically within the room to allow the radiographers to safely and efficiently treat patients. Away from the control console itself, provision will need to be made for additional computer and monitor workstations to allow for appointment scheduling and off-line image review. The move to paperless or at least paper-light workflows reduces the need for dockets and drawers, but places an increasing emphasis on computer workstation provision.

From the author's experience control rooms that are of the order of 7 m long and 3.5 m wide, excluding door and changing facilities, should be adequate for most installations. More generous dimensions than this could allow for better storage solutions, but care should be taken not to make this essentially private control room too big or busy for its intended purpose.

4.3.3 Patient access arrangements

Workflow efficiency can be maximised through the provision of two 'trap type' changing cubicles, at least one of which should be large enough for disabled patient

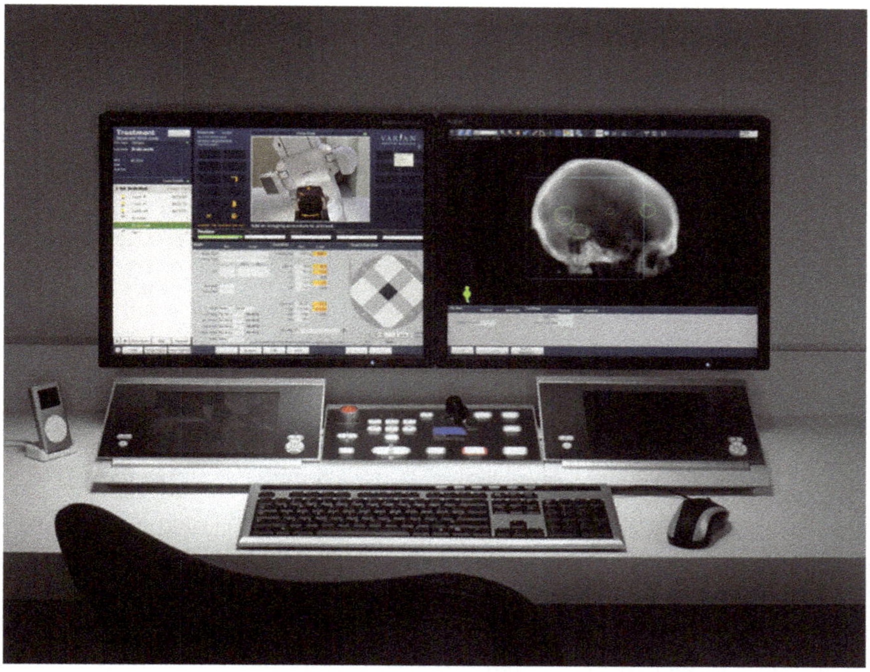

Figure 4.8. Linear accelerator control area (courtesy of Varian Medical Systems).

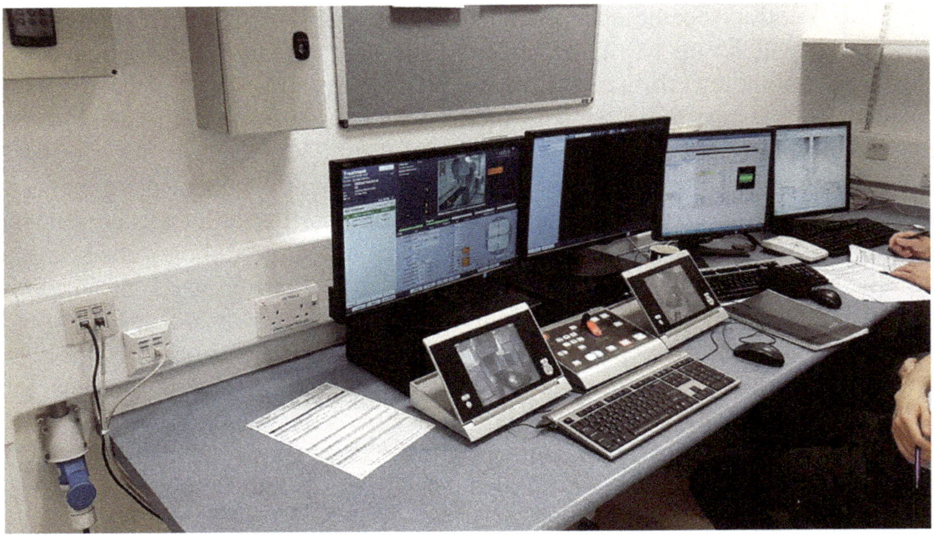

Figure 4.9. A typical control console configuration at the Northern Centre for Cancer Care, Newcastle, illustrating the space required for monitors.

changing. These will have external doors to the waiting or sub-waiting area and internal doors leading to the maze/treatment room entrance. Access to and through these cubicles will be controlled by the treating radiographers, ensuring patient privacy and dignity is maintained.

4.3.4 Treatment room door operation

If the treatment room has a heavy protected door, switching mechanisms should be provided to give a half-open functionality to reduce its closing/opening time and therefore maximise treatment efficiency. An additional opening switch located at the control console will allow the radiographers to start the door opening as soon as treatment has been completed. In addition to speeding up the workflow this will also ensure that the door can be opened as quickly as possible if a patient experiences difficulties inside the treatment room.

4.3.5 Warning lights/signs

As the treatment room will inevitably be a controlled area, physical demarcation could be provided by its physical walls and any protected door if installed. Additional consideration will have to be given to the demarcation of an 'open' maze entrance.

Illuminated warning signs (see figure 7.16) should be installed at the entrance to the treatment room. These signs should be energised by the radiation equipment itself such that when power is supplied to the equipment and it is in the preparatory state a radiation trefoil and 'Controlled Area' legend are illuminated. Once the beam-on state is reached and radiation is being emitted a red 'Radiation On' or 'X-rays On' legend must be illuminated. To avoid delay in illumination of the

'Radiation On' sign following beam initiation, florescent bulbs must not be used in this sign and in all cases the legend on such a sign should not be visible when the equipment and the lamps are off. Similar warning signs should be installed within the treatment room and any internal equipment rooms operating in conjunction with those at the room entrance. In all cases the signs should be mounted so that they are immediately obvious to any visitor, this necessitates mounting at eye level rather than above any door.

4.3.6 Equipment status notification

The *Medical and Dental Guidance Notes* (IPEM 2002) recommend that a clear indication should be available at the control panel when equipment is being serviced or repaired. As this is always necessary it is sensible to build in equipment status notification signage at the design stage. This should clearly indicate whether the unit is available or is not available for clinical use.

4.3.7 Lighting arrangements

As with the treatment room itself there are a number of conflicting considerations for the control room lighting. The best results will be achieved by the provision of dimmable lighting to allow radiographers to select the most appropriate ambient lighting for each task. This is particularly relevant to CT image review for image guided radiotherapy.

Ideally it should also be possible to switch off the lights in the treatment room from the control room, but the mechanism for this should be clear and transparent in use to avoid unnecessary complexity. Alternatively a switch to switch off all lights in the treatment room can be positioned at the entrance to the maze or the door to the treatment room.

4.3.8 Electrical services and IT connectivity

Dado trunking should be provided around the full extent of the benching in the control room with a significant number of power and data points. It should be possible to break into the trunking at any time in the future to install additional points.

References

Baechler S, Bochud F, Verellen D and Moeckli R 2007 Shielding requirements in helical tomotherapy *Phys. Med. Biol.* **52** 5057–67

Balog J, Lucas D, DeSouza C and Crilly R 2005 Helical TomoTherapy radiation leakage and shielding considerations *Med. Phys.* **32** 710–9

Budgell G, Brown K, Cashmore J, Duane S, Frame J, Hardy M, Paynter D and Thomas R 2016 IPEM topical report 1: guidance on implementing flattening filter free (FFF) radiotherapy *Phys. Med. Biol.* **61** 8360–94

DH (Department of Health) 2004 Safe Delivery of Radiotherapy Treatment *Safety Alert 4181* (London: Department of Health)

HSE (Health and Safety Executive) 2000 *Work with Ionising Radiation: Approved Code of Practice and Practical Guidance on the Ionising Radiations Regulations 1999* L121 (London: HSE)

IEC (International Electrotechnical Commission) 2009 *Medical Electrical Equipment—Part 2-1: Particular Requirements for the Safety of Electron Accelerators in the Range 1 MeV to 50 MeV* 60601-2-1 2nd edn (Geneva: IEC)

IPEM (Institute of Physics and Engineering in Medicine) 2002 *Medical and Dental Guidance Notes: a Good Practice Guide to Implement Ionising Radiation Protection Legislation in the Clinical Environment* (York: IPEM)

IRR 1999 *The Ionising Radiations Regulations* SI 1999/3232 (London: The Stationery Office)

Jank J, Kragl G and Georg D 2014 Impact of a flattening filter free linear accelerator on structural shielding design *Med. Phys.* **24** 38–48

Kry S F, Howell R M, Polf J, Mohan R and Vassiliev O N 2009 Treatment vault shielding for a flattening filter-free medical linear accelerator *Phys. Med. Biol.* **54** 1265–74

McGinley P H 2002 *Shielding Techniques for Radiation Oncology Facilities* (Madison, WI: Medical Physics)

NCRP (National Council on Radiation Protection and Measurements) 2005 *Structural Shielding Design and Evaluation for Megavoltage X- and Gamma-Ray Radiotherapy Facilities* Report 151 (Bethesda, MD: NCRP)

Paynter D, Weston S J, Cosgrove V P, Evans J A and Thwaites D I 2014 Beam characteristics of energy-matched flattening filter free beams *Med. Phys.* **41** 052103

Rodgers J E 2001 Radiation therapy vault shielding calculational methods when IMRT and TBI procedures contribute *J. Appl. Clin. Med. Phys.* **2** 157–64

Rodgers J E 2007 Analysis of tenth-value-layers for common shielding materials for a robotically mounted stereotactic radiosurgery machine *Health Phys.* **92** 379–86

Sutton D G, Martin C J, Williams J R and Peet D J 2012 *Radiation Shielding for Diagnostic X-rays* 2nd edn (London: British Institute of Radiology)

Toft B 2005 *Independent Review of the Circumstances Surrounding a Serious Adverse Incident that Occurred in the—Redacted—* www.who.int/patientsafety/news/Radiotherapy_adverse_event_Toft_report.pdf (Accessed: 8 November 2016)

Vassiliev O N, Titt U, Kry S F, Mohan R and Gillin M T 2007 Radiation safety survey on a flattening filter-free medical accelerator *Radiat. Prot. Dosim.* **124** 187–90

Yang J and Feng J 2014 Radiation shielding evaluation based on five years of data from a busy CyberKnife center *J. Appl. Clin. Med. Phys.* **15** 313–22

Chapter 5

Empirical shielding calculations for treatment rooms with linear accelerators

P W Horton, D J Peet and R M Harrison

5.1 General principles

The purpose of radiation shielding is to attenuate the radiation from the treatment unit, its surroundings and the patient, to areas outside the room and its entrance to a level less than a dose and/or a dose rate constraint adopted by the hospital and based on requirements and recommendations set in national legislation or international guidance. Walls at which the beam can be pointed directly are called primary barriers. Other walls in the treatment room need to provide protection from radiation leakage from the head of the treatment unit and scatter from the patient, and are called secondary barriers. Generally secondary barriers are thinner than primary barriers due to the lower energy of the scattered radiation and lower dose rates. For primary and secondary barriers, the dose rate at an external point of interest will be reduced by the inverse square law and the attenuation provided by the intervening shielding, the latter diminishing with increasing x-ray or gamma ray energy.

The entrance to the treatment room may be through a door or along a corridor with a number of bends, termed a 'maze'. Doors need to be substantial, especially for megavoltage treatment units, to provide the necessary shielding to attenuate the radiation, and are power operated. With maze entrances, multiple scattering and absorption along the length of the maze reduce the dose rate to an acceptable level at the entrance. The dose rate at the maze entrance during operation will diminish with increasing maze length due to the inverse square law and with the number of bends, which increase the number of scatter interactions with the walls of the maze. When space is limited, a combination of a short maze and a lighter door may be used to achieve acceptable dose rates. For linear accelerators operating at 8.5 MV and higher energies, neutrons will be produced in the treatment head of the accelerator and scattered by the walls down the maze. Again the inverse square law plays a part

doi:10.1088/978-0-7503-1440-4ch5

but special measures such as neutron absorber sheets on the walls of the maze and a door may be required to achieve the dose and/or dose rate constraint. These processes and the calculation of the external annual dose and instantaneous dose rate using empirical methods are considered in greater detail below. Typical arrangements for a shielded room containing a linear accelerator, often termed a bunker or a vault, and having a maze are shown in plan and elevation in figure 5.1.

5.2 Primary barriers

5.2.1 General

Radiation falling directly on a primary barrier originates from the target of the treatment unit and all distances for the inverse square law component of shielding calculations should have this as their origin.

The attenuating power of shielding materials can be empirically specified in terms of tenth value layers (TVLs), i.e. the thickness of the material, to reduce the intensity at normal incidence to one tenth of its incident intensity for megavoltage radiation, and in terms of the half value layer (HVL), i.e. the thickness to reduce the incident

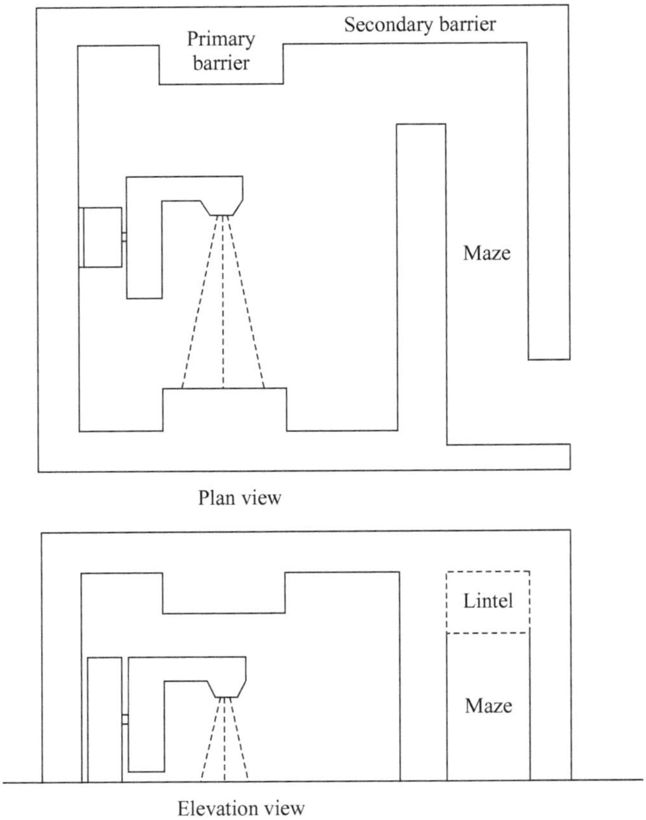

Figure 5.1. A typical linear accelerator bunker.

intensity by half, for kilovoltage radiation. The barrier transmission factor, B, is then given by

$$B = 10^{-n} \text{ or } 2^{-n},$$

where n is the number of TVLs or HVLs, respectively. To achieve a specific transmission factor, the number of TVLs or HVLs can be calculated using the expressions

$$n_{\mathrm{TVL}} = -\log_{10} B \quad \text{or} \quad n_{\mathrm{HVL}} = -\log_2 B.$$

The required thickness of the shielding can then be calculated by multiplying n by the relevant TVL or HVL value, i.e.

$$\text{thickness}\ (t) = n \times \text{TVL or } n \times \text{HVL}. \tag{5.1}$$

The TVL and HVL will decrease with increasing x-ray energy and n will need to be increased to achieve a specific dose rate on the exterior of the shielding for a given incident dose rate.

IPEM (1997) tabulates TVLs for standard concrete (2350 kg m^{-3}) for x-ray end-point energies ranging from 4 to 24 MV, and also has a graphical presentation of the TVL variation in concrete, steel and lead over the energy range 50 kV–10 MV. However, these are average TVL values. In practice the x-ray beam will be hardened as it penetrates the shielding and the TVL will increase, especially after the first TVL. NCRP (2005) adopts this more scientific approach and gives values for the first TVL (TVL_1) and the subsequent equilibrium TVL (TVL_e). These are reproduced in table 5.1. The barrier thickness, t, is then given by

$$t = \mathrm{TVL}_1 + (n - 1)\mathrm{TVL}_e. \tag{5.2}$$

Table 5.1. Primary beam TVLs for concrete, steel and lead for a range of endpoint energies (adapted from NCRP (2005) table B2).

	Concrete		Steel		Lead	
Density (kg m^{-3})	2350		7870		11 350	
Endpoint energy (MeV)	TVL_1 (mm)	TVL_e (mm)	TVL_1 (mm)	TVL_e (mm)	TVL_1 (mm)	TVL_e (mm)
4	350	300	99	99	57	57
6	370	330	100	100	57	57
10	410	370	110	110	57	57
15	440	410	110	110	57	57
18	450	430	110	110	57	57
20	460	440	110	110	57	57
25	490	460	110	110	57	57
30	510	490	110	110	57	57
Co-60	210	210	700	700	40	40

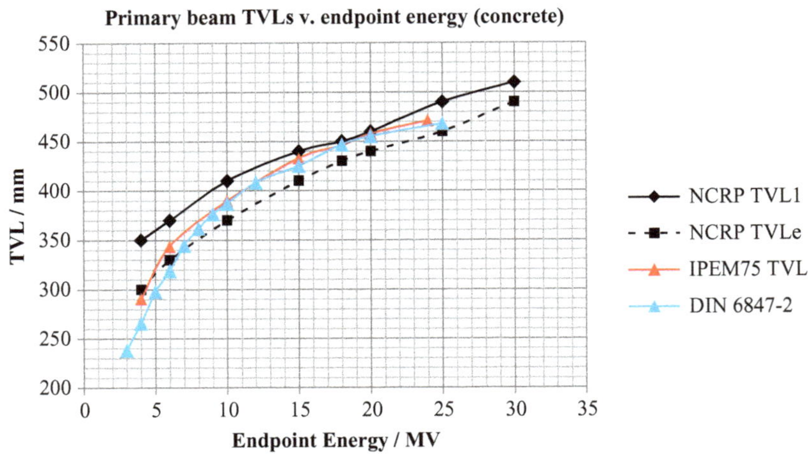

Figure 5.2. Variation of concrete TVLs with endpoint energy (density of concrete = 2350 kg m^{-3}). Data are taken from table 5.1, IPEM (1997) and DIN (2008).

Comparison of the two sets of TVL data shows that the IPEM (1997) values are closer to the equilibrium TVLs in the range 4–8 MV, and lie between the first and equilibrium TVLs at higher end point energies. This is illustrated in figure 5.2. It is recommended that the NCRP (2005) TVL values reproduced in table 5.1 are used in calculations.

5.2.2 Annual dose

The unattenuated annual dose (D_p) at a position outside the primary shielding around a treatment unit can be calculated from the annual radiation workload delivered to the isocentre (D_i) (see chapter 4) and the fraction of the treatment time (orientation or use factor) for which the beam is pointed at the barrier concerned (see section 4.1.3.4), i.e.

$$D_p = D_i \times U \times d_i^2/(d_i + d_p)^2,$$

where U is the orientation factor, d_i is the target to isocentre distance and d_p is the distance from the isocentre to a point 0.3 m from the barrier on the far side of the barrier.

This point, 0.3 m beyond the barrier, is chosen as it is representative for the whole-body exposure of a person standing next to the external surface of the barrier at the calculation point selected.

The annual workload can be calculated from the number (N) of patient treatments per day, the average dose per patient (D_f) and the number of treatment days per year; the last is taken as 250 days for 5 days per week and 50 weeks per year, i.e.

$$D_i = D_f \times N \times 250.$$

The attenuated annual dose (D_a) to a person outside the primary shielding is then given by

$$D_a = \left(D_f \times N \times 250 \times U \times T \times B \times d_i^2\right)/(d_i + d_p)^2 \qquad (5.3)$$

where T is the occupancy factor for the area concerned, i.e. the fraction of time the area is occupied by an individual (see section 3.7.2).

Re-arranging expression 5.3, the barrier transmission to achieve an annual dose constraint (D_{acc}) is given by

$$B = D_{acc} \times (d_i + d_p)^2 / \left(D_f \times N \times 250 \times U \times T \times d_i^2\right). \quad (5.4)$$

This will only be the case if a single energy is used for treatment. Commonly two energies are used, e.g. 6 MV and 10 MV or 6 MV and 15 MV, and for a given barrier thickness, the annual dose will be the sum of the annual doses at each of the energies taking into account the proportion of treatments at each energy. Calculation of the barrier thickness assuming all treatments take place at the higher energy will result in a safe situation, but will overestimate the thickness required in practice and calculation at the lower energy will result in an underestimate. A number of trial calculations between these two thicknesses taking into account the proportion of treatments at each energy may be required to arrive at an optimal thickness that meets the dose constraint. Some centres adopt the highest energy approach as a means of future-proofing the bunker for future developments but this adds to the costs. Worked example 1 below shows the thicknesses of concrete required to achieve 0.3 mSv per year at 6, 10 and 15 MV for a typical radiation workload at a single energy for a fully occupied area outside the barrier. As stated above, more complex situations are met in practice.

Worked example 1

Suppose

$D_{acc} = 0.3$ mSv per year
$d_i + d_p = 5.0$ m and $d_i = 1.0$ m
$D_f = 2$ Gy
$N = 50$ patients per day
$U = 0.25$
$T = 1$

then

$B = 1.2 \times 10^{-6}$
$n = -\log_{10} B = 5.92$
$t = \mathrm{TVL}_1 + 4.92 \times \mathrm{TVL}_e$.

The required barrier thicknesses in standard concrete (2350 kg m^{-3}) at 6, 10 and 15 MV using the TVL_1 and TVL_e values in table 5.1 are as follows:

Energy (MV)	Thickness (m)
6	1.99
10	2.23
15	2.46

5.2.3 Dose rate measures and verification of shielding

Whilst the annual dose constraint is the principal criterion for shielding design, it is recommended that external dose rates for each barrier are calculated to check that they are not excessive (see chapter 3). The external dose rate may also be a constraint in national legislation, usually expressed in μSv h^{-1}. In the UK, the term 'instantaneous dose rate' is used to describe the dose rate averaged over one minute to take account of the response time of the measuring instrument and the pulse repetition rate if a linear accelerator is the radiation source. To check the adequacy of the shielding, the dose rate on the exterior of the barrier when the radiation beam is pointing directly at the barrier at normal incidence can be measured and compared with these predicted values.

For an existing barrier with a transmission factor B, the external dose rate, DR in μSv $\min^{-1}$, will be given by

$$\mathrm{DR} = \left(\mathrm{DR_i} \times 10^6 \times B \times d_i^2\right)/(d_i + d_p)^2, \tag{5.5}$$

where $\mathrm{DR_i}$ is the dose rate at the isocentre (Gy $\min^{-1}$) and d_i and d_p have the meaning given above.

This value can be compared with a measured value at the same position to assess the adequacy of the shielding.

To calculate the barrier thickness to meet a dose rate constraint, $\mathrm{DR_{act}}$ in μSv h^{-1}, equation (5.5) can be re-arranged to calculate the transmission factor required as follows:

$$B = (\mathrm{DR_{act}} \times (d_i + d_p)^2)/(\mathrm{DR_i} \times 60 \times 10^6 \times d_i^2). \tag{5.6}$$

The required thickness can then be calculated from B in TVLs as above and be converted to actual thickness using the relevant TVL values. In general a dose constraint based on dose rate over a short period of time will lead to thicker barriers as this does not take account of the absence of radiation between patient fields and between patients. This is illustrated in worked example 2A, where an actual dose rate of 7.5 μSv h^{-1} has been specified for 6 Gy $\min^{-1}$ operation. As can be seen, the thickness of concrete at each energy is slightly greater than in worked example 1. Worked example 2B shows the thickness of concrete required for an actual dose rate of 20 μSv h^{-1} with flattening-filter-free (FFF) mode operation at 24 Gy $\min^{-1}$. The thickness of concrete at each energy is slightly greater than in worked example 2A. US practice (NCRP 2005) has shielding design goals for controlled and uncontrolled areas based on equivalent dose limits per week.

Worked example 2A: Standard mode operation

Suppose

$\mathrm{DR_{act}} = 7.5$ μSv h^{-1}

$d_i + d_p = 5.0$ m and $d_i = 1.0$ m (as before)

$\mathrm{DR_i} = 6$ Gy $\min^{-1}$

then

$B = 5.21 \times 10^{-7}$

$n = -\log_{10}B = 6.28$

$t = \text{TVL}_1 + 5.28 \times \text{TVL}_e$.

The required barrier thicknesses in standard concrete (2350 kg m^{-3}) at 6, 10 and 15 MV using the TVL_1 and TVL_e values in table 5.1 are as follows:

Energy (MV)	Thickness (m)
6	2.11
10	2.36
15	2.60

Worked example 2B: FFF mode operation

Suppose

$\text{DR}_{act} = 20\ \mu\text{Sv h}^{-1}$

$d_i + d_p = 5.0$ m and $d_i = 1.0$ m (as before)

$\text{DR}_i = 24\ \text{Gy min}^{-1}$

then

$B = 3.47 \times 10^{-7}$

$n = -\log_{10}B = 6.46$

$t = \text{TVL}_1 + 5.46 \times \text{TVL}_e$.

The required barrier thicknesses in standard concrete (2350 kg m^{-3}) at 6, 10 and 15 MV using the TVL_1 and TVL_e values in table 5.1 are as follows:

Energy (MV)	Thickness (m)
6	2.17
10	2.43
15	2.68

5.2.4 Primary barrier width

For bunkers containing linear accelerators where the radiation beam is confined to a rotational plane through the isocentre (sometimes termed 'C-arm accelerators'), the primary barriers will be limited in width to reduce concrete volume and cost (see figure 5.1). The width of the barrier will primarily be set by the extent of the beam at the barrier distance using the diagonal of largest field size, commonly 400 mm $\times \sqrt{2} = 570$ mm at the isocentre distance. Whilst at the end point energies of linear accelerator beams, 6 MV and higher, the radiation scatter within the barrier will be predominantly in the forward direction, there will still be some lateral scatter, sometimes termed the 'plume effect'. To absorb this scattered radiation and to allow for building tolerances, it is good practice to add 300 mm to each side of the projected maximum beam width at the barrier to give the barrier width for

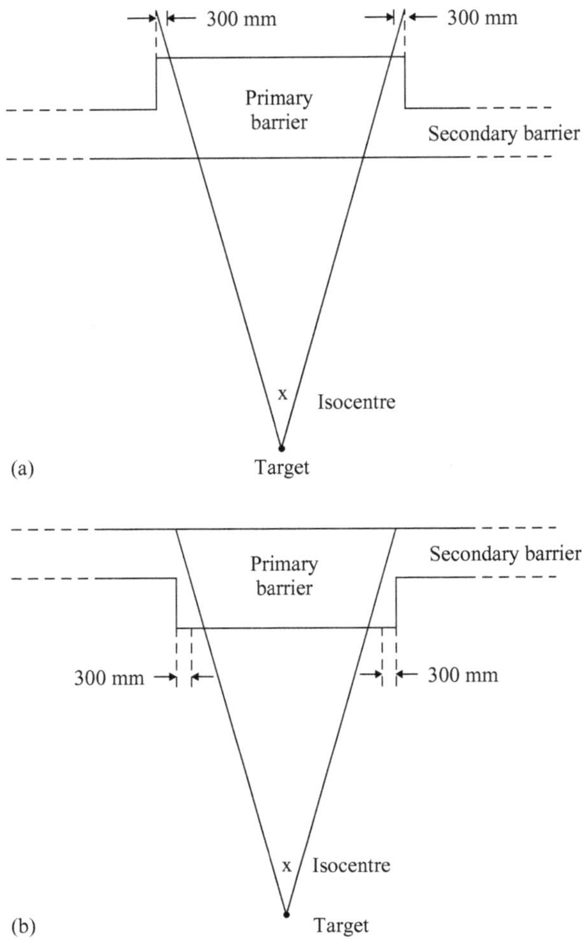

Figure 5.3. (a) Primary barrier external to treatment room. (b) Primary barrier intruding into treatment room.

construction. This is illustrated in figure 5.3 for barriers intruding into the treatment room, where 300 mm is added at the distance of inner wall provided by the secondary shielding, and extending outside the room, where 300 mm is added at the external wall. The width of the primary wall barrier will need to be maintained for the primary barrier in the roof of the bunker (figure 5.1) if the exterior is accessible.

5.3 Secondary barriers

5.3.1 General

Radiation falling on the secondary barriers originates from leakage radiation from the head of the treatment unit, scattered radiation from the patient and to a lesser extent scattered radiation from the walls. At large scatter angles, the intensity and energy of the radiation scattered from the patient is less than the leakage from the treatment head, especially with small field sizes, and the latter is used alone in calculations of adequate secondary shielding. This practice is followed in the examples below. When the scatter angle is small, patient scatter should not be ignored. Scatter fractions from a human-size phantom are given in NCRP (2005, table B4); these are reproduced in table 5.8. When calculating the secondary barrier thicknesses for leakage and patient scattered radiation, the larger thickness should be used if the two thicknesses differ by more than a TVL. If the two thicknesses differ by less than a TVL, use the larger thickness and add an HVL of the shielding material to give the total thickness required (IAEA 2006).

International standards (IEC 2009) limit the leakage dose rate to 0.1% of the dose rate in the primary beam at the isocentre to restrict the patient's body dose in comparison with the tumour dose. Linear accelerator manufacturers achieve a lower leakage rate in practice and the rate is typically halved when the accelerator is in FFF mode due to the absence of the flattening filter as a source of scattered radiation.

All distances for the inverse square law component of secondary shielding calculations have the isocentre as their origin. This is assumed to be the mean position of the treatment head over a large number of treatments at different gantry angles for leakage radiation and is also the origin of the patient scatter.

The scattered radiation is also assumed to be isotropic in its distribution around the isocentre, when averaged over all gantry angles. The orientation factor, U, is therefore taken as unity in all directions in dose calculations.

The end point energy of the leakage radiation will be degraded by the scatter interactions with components in the treatment head, and the mean energy of the scattered radiation will be less than the primary radiation. Consequently the TVL values for scattered radiation will be lower than those for the primary beam and generally secondary shielding will be thinner than primary shielding. Again, IPEM (1997) tabulates secondary TVLs for standard concrete (2350 kg m^{-3}) for x-ray end point energies ranging from 4 to 24 MV. These are an average value as the scattered x-ray beam will be hardened as it penetrates the shielding and the TVL will increase, especially after the first TVL. Again NCRP (2005) adopts a more scientific approach and gives values for the first TVL (TVL_1) and the subsequent equilibrium TVL (TVL_e) for leakage Co-60 radiation and x-radiation with end point energies in the range 4–30 MV. These are reproduced in table 5.2. Comparison of the two sets of TVL data shows that the IPEM (1997) values are broadly in agreement with the NCRP (2005) equilibrium TVLs although the IPEM (1997) values are lower at 4–6 MV. This is illustrated in figure 5.4. NCRP (2005, tables B.5a and B.5b) also gives mean TVL values for patient scattered radiation in concrete for Co-60 radiation and x-radiation with end point energies in the range 4–24 MV and in lead for 4, 6 and 10 MV for a range of scatter angles; these are reproduced in tables 5.3 and 5.4, respectively, for completeness. IPEM (1997) has extensive data for kilovoltage end point energies and limited data at 4 and 6 MV only in the megavoltage range; the latter data are typically 25% higher than the corresponding NCRP (2005) values.

As described in section 4.1, many current radiotherapy treatments employ intensity modulated radiotherapy (IMRT) or volumetric intensity modulated arc

Table 5.2. Leakage TVLs for concrete at 90° for a range of endpoint energies (adapted from NCRP (2005) table B7).

Endpoint energy (MeV)	TVL_1 (mm)	TVL_e (mm)
4	330	280
6	340	290
10	350	310
15	360	330
18	360	340
20	360	340
25	370	350
30	370	360
Co-60	210	210

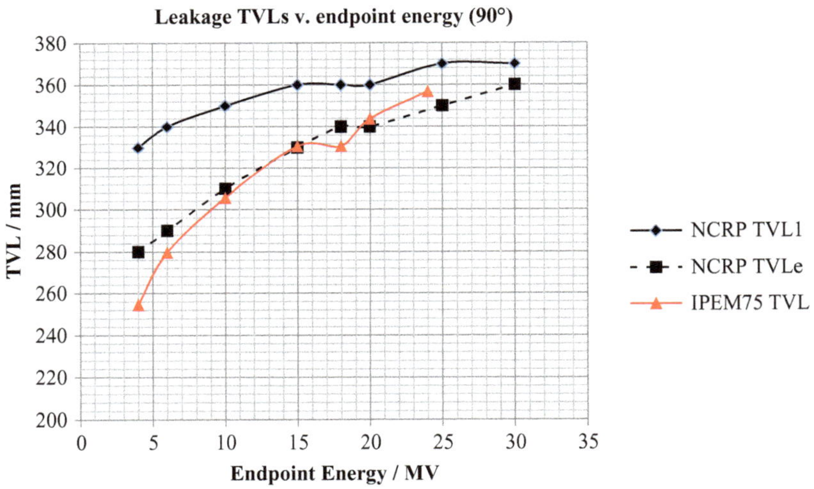

Figure 5.4. Variation of concrete leakage TVLs (90°) with endpoint energy (density of concrete = 2350 kg cm^{-3}). Data are taken from table 5.2 and IPEM (1997).

therapy (VMAT) to build up complex non-uniform dose distributions within the tumour treatment volume. This requires the application of many small shaped fields of different intensity. The total dose will generally be the same as that in a conventional single large field of uniform intensity, and primary shielding calculations are unchanged unless the total dose is increased for clinical reasons. However, the build-up using small fields will require a much longer period of irradiation (beam-on time) for the same prescribed dose, and this longer period of radiation increases the amount of leakage and scattered radiation per treatment. An

Table 5.3. TVL values in concrete for patient scattered radiation versus scatter angle (adapted from NCRP (2005) table B.5a).

Scatter angle °	TVL (mm)					
	Co-60	4 MV	6 MV	10 MV	15 MV	18 MV
15	220	300	340	390	420	440
30	210	250	260	280	310	320
45	200	220	230	250	260	270
60	190	210	210	220	230	230
90	150	170	170	180	180	190
135	130	140	150	150	150	150

Table 5.4. TVL_1 and TVL_e in lead for patient scattered radiation versus scatter angle (adapted from NCRP (2005) table B.5b).

Scatter angle °	4 MV		6 MV		10 MV	
	TVL_1 (mm)	TVL_e (mm)	TVL_1 (mm)	TVL_e (mm)	TVL_1 (mm)	TVL_e (mm)
30	33	37	38	44	43	45
45	24	31	28	34	31	36
60	18	25	19	26	21	27
75	13	19	14	19	15	19
90	9	13	10	15	12	16
105	7	12	7	12	9.5	14
120	5	8	5	8	8	14

IMRT factor is introduced into secondary shielding calculations to take account of this practice; it is defined as follows:

$$\text{IMRT factor (IF)} = \frac{\text{MU(IMRT)}}{\text{MU(conventional)}},$$

where MU(IMRT) is the number of monitor units (typically 1 MU~1 cGy) to give the prescribed dose using IMRT, and MU (conventional) is the number of monitor units to give the prescribed dose with a single uniform treatment field.

NCRP (2005) notes that the IMRT factor ranges from 2 to 10 for IMRT treatments and a factor of 5 is commonly used in calculations of secondary shielding. VMAT employs arc therapy to deliver similar doses to IMRT in a shorter treatment time and an IMRT factor of 2.5 has been determined for some treatments (see section 4.1.2.1). A value of 3 is considered conservative.

In planning adequate secondary shielding it is important that the proportion of patients having IMRT and VMAT is determined and the IMRT factor is derived from the range of existing or planned clinical procedures in the centre. For example if the fraction of patients having IMRT and/or VMAT is P and the IMRT factor is IF, then the fractional increase, f, in the 'beam-on time' will be given by

$$f = 1 - P + P \times \mathrm{IF}.$$

5.3.2 Annual dose

The unattenuated annual dose (D_p) at a position outside the secondary shielding around a treatment unit can be calculated from annual radiation workload delivered to the isocentre (D_i) and the fractional leakage dose rate (0.001) and the increase in beam-on time, i.e.

$$D_p = D_i \times 0.001 \times f / d_p^2,$$

where d_p is the distance from the isocentre to the far side of the barrier.

The annual radiation workload can be calculated from the number (N) of patient treatments per day, the average dose per patient (D_f) and the number of treatment days per year; the last is often taken as 250 days for 5 days per week and 50 weeks per year, i.e.

$$D_i = D_f \times N \times 250.$$

The attenuated annual dose (D_a) to a person outside the secondary shielding is then given by

$$D_a = (D_f \times N \times 250 \times 0.001 \times f \times T \times B)/d_p^2, \tag{5.7}$$

where T is the occupancy factor for the area concerned and B is the transmission factor.

Re-arranging equation (5.7), the barrier transmission to achieve an annual dose constraint (D_{acc}) is given by

$$B = D_{acc} \times d_p^2/(D_f \times N \times 250 \times 0.001 \times f \times T). \tag{5.8}$$

This will only be the case if a single energy is used for treatment. Commonly two energies are used, e.g. 6 and 10 MV or 6 and 15 MV, and for a given barrier thickness, the annual dose will be the sum of the annual doses at each of the energies taking into account the proportion of treatments at each energy. Calculation of the barrier thickness assuming all treatments take place at the higher energy will result in a safe situation, but will overestimate the thickness required in practice and calculation at the lower energy will result in an underestimate. A number of trial calculations between these two thicknesses taking into account the proportion of treatments at each energy may be required to arrive at an optimal thickness that meets the dose constraint. Worked example 3 below shows the thicknesses of concrete required to achieve 0.3 mSv per year at 6, 10 and 15 MV for a typical radiation workload at a single energy for a fully occupied area outside the barrier. As stated above, more complex situations are met in practice.

Worked example 3

Suppose

D_{acc} =0.3 mSv per year
$d_p = 4.0$ m
$D_f = 2$ Gy
$N = 50$ patients per day
$U = 1$
$T = 1$
IF = 5
fraction of patients having IMRT and/or VMAT = 0.4
$f = 0.6 + 0.4 \times 5 = 2.6$,

then

$B = 7.38 \times 10^{-5}$
$n = -\log_{10}B = 4.13$
$t = \mathrm{TVL}_1 + 3.13 \times \mathrm{TVL}_e$.

The required barrier thicknesses in standard concrete (2350 kg m^{-3}) at 6, 10 and 15 MV using the TVL_1 and TVL_e values in table 5.2 are as follows:

Energy (MV)	Thickness (m)
6	1.25
10	1.32
15	1.39

5.3.3 Dose rate measures and verification of shielding

Whilst the annual dose constraint is the principal criterion for shielding design, it is recommended that external dose rates for each barrier are calculated to check that they are not excessive (see chapter 3). The external dose rate may also be a constraint in national legislation, usually expressed in μSv h^{-1}. To check the adequacy of the shielding, the dose rate on the exterior of the barrier can be measured and compared with predicted values. This is normally done with a water phantom at the isocentre to mimic the patient scatter and is done at a number of gantry angles to cover all beam orientations.

For an existing barrier with a transmission factor *B*, the external dose rate, DR in μSv min^{-1}, will be given by

$$DR = (DR_i \times 10^6 \times 0.001 \times B)/d_p{}^2, \tag{5.9}$$

where $\mathrm{DR_i}$ is the dose rate at the isocentre (Gy min^{-1}) and d_p has the meaning given above.

This value can be compared with a measured value at the same position to assess the adequacy of the shielding.

To calculate the barrier thickness to meet a dose rate constraint, $\mathrm{DR_{acc}}$ in μSv h^{-1}, equation (5.9) can be re-arranged to calculate the transmission factor required as follows:

$$B = \left(\mathrm{DR}_{\mathrm{acc}} \times d_{\mathrm{p}}^{2}\right)/(\mathrm{DR}_{\mathrm{i}} \times 60 \times 10^{6} \times 0.001). \tag{5.10}$$

The required thickness can then be calculated from B in TVLs as above and converted to actual thickness using the relevant TVL values. This is illustrated in worked example 4, where a dose constraint of 7.5 μSv h^{-1} has been specified for 6 Gy min^{-1} operation and 20 μSv h^{-1} has been specified for 24 Gy min^{-1} operation. US practice (NCRP 2005) has shielding design goals for controlled and uncontrolled areas based on equivalent dose limits per week.

Worked example 4A: Standard mode operation

Suppose

$\mathrm{DR}_{\mathrm{acc}} = 7.5$ μSv h^{-1}

$d_{\mathrm{p}} = 4.0$ m

$\mathrm{DR}_{\mathrm{i}} = 6$ Gy min^{-1}

then

$B = 3.33 \times 10^{-4}$

$n = -\log_{10}B = 3.48$

$t = \mathrm{TVL}_{1} + 2.48 \times \mathrm{TVL}_{\mathrm{e}}$.

The required barrier thicknesses in standard concrete (2350 kg m^{-3}) at 6, 10 and 15 MV using the TVL_1 and $\mathrm{TVL}_{\mathrm{e}}$ values in table 5.2 are as follows:

Energy (MV)	Thickness (m)
6	1.06
10	1.12
15	1.18

Worked example 4B: FFF mode operation

Suppose

$\mathrm{DR}_{\mathrm{acc}} = 20$ μSv h^{-1}

$d_{\mathrm{p}} = 4.0$ m

$\mathrm{DR}_{\mathrm{i}} = 24$ Gy min^{-1}

then

$B = 2.22 \times 10^{-4}$

$n = -\log_{10}B = 3.65$

$t = \mathrm{TVL}_{1} + 2.65 \times \mathrm{TVL}_{\mathrm{e}}$.

The required barrier thicknesses in standard concrete (2350 kg m^{-3}) at 6, 10 and 15 MV using the TVL_1 and $\mathrm{TVL}_{\mathrm{e}}$ values in table 5.2 are as follows:

Energy (MV)	Thickness (m)
6	1.11
10	1.17
15	1.23

5.4 Roofs and skyshine

Where the space above the bunker(s) is routinely accessible or occupied, the same annual dose and possibly dose rate constraints for x-rays will apply to these areas as apply to areas outside the walls of the bunker(s). In this situation the thicknesses of the primary and secondary shielding in the roof of the bunker are calculated using the methodology in sections 5.2 and 5.3, respectively, taking into account the occupancy of the areas concerned and the orientation factor U in the direction of the roof for the primary beam.

When there are no rooms above the bunker, access to the area over the roof can be prohibited during operation of the treatment unit and an instantaneous dose rate of 2 mSv h^{-1} adopted for the primary and secondary shielding calculations. This dose rate is accepted (IPEM 1997) as the threshold for a significant dose from radiation transmitted through the roof and scattered from the air above the bunker to reach people on the ground nearby or in adjacent buildings, this is called 'skyshine' (NCRP 1977). This can be especially important if radiation sensitive equipment, e.g. gamma cameras, is located in adjacent buildings. For a linear accelerator operating at 6 Gy min^{-1} and a distance of 3.5 m from the isocentre to the upper surface of the roof, this requires 3.95 TVLs of primary shielding and 1.17 TVLs of secondary shielding (not taking obliquity into account). For 15 MV operation, this corresponds to 1.65 m of conventional concrete for the primary barrier and 0.42 m for the secondary barrier.

If an assessment of x-ray skyshine is required, the following expression (McGinley 2002) can be used to estimate the dose rate (Gy h^{-1}) at ground level using the configuration in figure 5.5:

$$\mathrm{DR_{sky}} = (2.5 \times 10^{-2} \times \mathrm{DR_0} \times \mathrm{B_{roof}} \times \Omega^{1.3})/\left((d_r + 2) \times d_c^{\,2}\right) \tag{5.11}$$

where $\mathrm{DR_0}$ is the dose rate at the isocentre (Gy h^{-1}), B_{roof} is the transmission factor of the roof with a vertical beam, Ω is the angle subtended by the primary beam at the

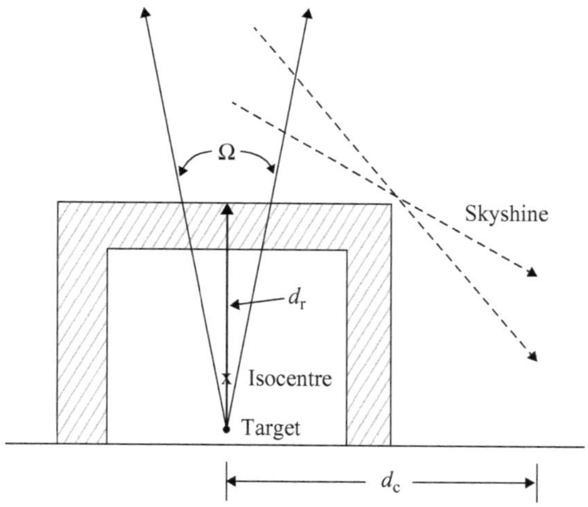

Figure 5.5. Elevation showing the position of the target and the position of the calculation point for the estimation of skyshine.

external surface of the roof, d_r is the distance from the radiation source to the external surface of the roof (m) and d_c is the horizontal distance from the radiation source to the point of interest (m).

McGinley (1993) has compared measurements of x-ray skyshine with calculated dose rates using the above methodology for an 18 MV accelerator with a roof having a transmission factor of 10^{-1}. The calculated dose rates are more than the measured dose rates close to the building because attenuation by the building is ignored but are lower farther away. The highest dose rates occur when d_c is similar to the height of the bunker wall. It is suggested that equation (5.11) should be used only to estimate an order of magnitude dose rate.

NCRP (2005) also considers the dose rate from x-rays scattered laterally from thin roof barriers and the skyshine dose rate from neutrons produced by linear accelerators operating at x-ray energies over 8.5 MV.

5.5 Groundshine

With a bunker built with conventional concrete the wall thickness will be at least 1 m and this will attenuate the radiation scattered upward when the beam is directed toward the floor at the bottom of a wall. However, with a thin wall made of high Z material, e.g. lead or steel, it is possible for scattered radiation to emerge on the far side of the wall when the primary beam is directed toward the bottom of the wall, e.g. in a CyberKnife® installation[1]. One solution to this problem is to place additional shielding of lead or steel on the floor at the foot of the wall (figure 5.6) or let into the floor. Alternatively the wall can be extended below floor level to ensure the primary beam passes through the same thickness of material. The obliquity of the beam in this situation (see below) reduces the thickness of lead or steel required.

5.6 Obliquity factor

Generally bunkers made of conventional concrete are built with primary and secondary barriers of constant thickness for simplicity and ease of construction; the thickness of the barrier being calculated for radiation at normal incidence to give the attenuation required. Away from radiation beams passing horizontally or vertically through the isocentre, the beam will strike the barrier at an oblique angle. This will increase both the distance to the barrier and the path length in the barrier, termed the slant thickness. The slant thickness t_s is given by

$$t_s = t / \cos\theta,$$

where t is the thickness of the barrier and θ is the angle of obliquity between the radiation and the normal to the surface of the barrier.

In practice, the use of t_s in transmission calculations will underestimate the barrier thickness required because scattered photons will originate inside the barrier and will have a path length less than t_s. This will vary with the angle of incidence and the

[1] CyberKnife is a registered mark of Accuray.

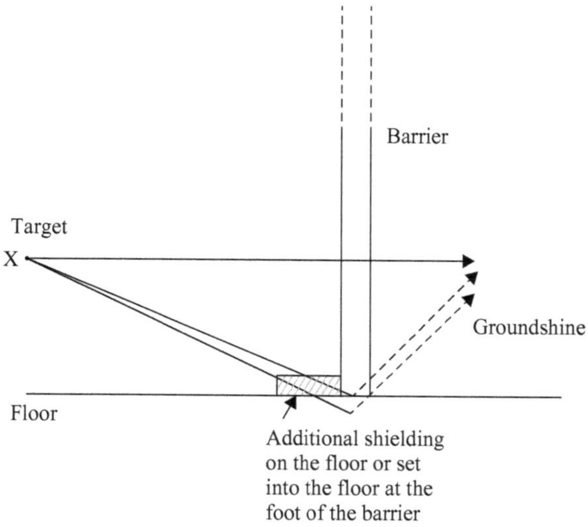

Figure 5.6. Groundshine at a physically thin barrier.

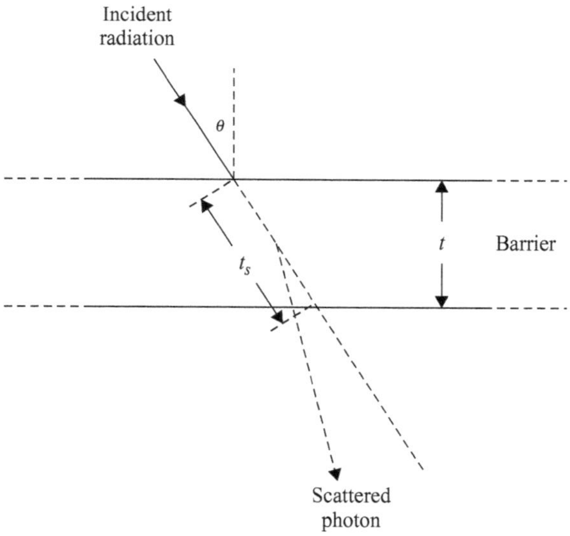

Figure 5.7. Calculation of slant thickness and origin of scattered radiation.

beam energy. This is illustrated in figure 5.7. The effective path length can be calculated by dividing the slant thickness by an obliquity factor (Biggs 1996). These are listed in table 5.5. As can be seen, the factors only become significant with incidence at 45° or greater. In practice obliquity is most often employed to reduce the wall thickness and cost when expensive high Z materials, e.g. lead, steel or high density concrete, are used when space is limited or when floor to floor height is limited and/or areas above are occupied.

Table 5.5. Obliquity factors for calculating effective slant thickness (Biggs 1996).

Angle	Concrete				Lead	Steel
	Co-60	4 MV	10 MV	18 MV	4–18 MV	4–18 MV
30	1.04	1.02	1.00	1.00	1.03	1.02
45	1.20	1.07	1.04	1.04	1.08	1.07
60	1.34	1.20	1.13	1.08	1.22	1.20
70	1.86	1.47	1.28	1.22	1.50	1.45

5.7 X-ray scatter down the maze

The dose rate due to x-rays at the external entrance to the bunker maze arises from four sources which need to be summed to give the total dose rate. These are:

- scatter of the primary beam from the bunker and maze walls,
- scatter from the patient,
- scatter of the head leakage radiation from the bunker walls and
- transmission of head leakage radiation through the inner maze wall.

These components will be considered individually. In general calculations assume that the intensity of the scattered radiation is linearly related to the irradiated wall area of the maze at each wall scatter and diminishes according to the inverse square law. This leads to multiple terms of the form $\alpha_n A_n / d_n^2$, where α_n is the reflection coefficient dependent upon the x-ray energy, wall material, and the angles of incidence and reflection, A_n is the area of wall irradiated and d_n is the distance to the next scatter or the exit in the case of the last scatter. It should be noted that barrier thicknesses calculated to adequately attenuate head leakage will also be adequate to satisfactorily attenuate all components of scattered radiation incident on a barrier and not reflected. The scattered radiation from the floor and roof of the bunker is not usually considered significant as both require an additional reflection at the floor or roof to reach the inner maze entrance. Typically this will add 0.1% to the intensity striking the inner maze walls in the examples in the following sections.

It is also generally assumed in these calculations that the radiation scattered by the patient and reflected at the walls after the first and subsequent scatters has an energy of 500 keV (NCRP 2005, IAEA 2006). However, Al-Affan (2000) using Monte Carlo modelling to simulate scatter down a two-leg maze from a 6 MV accelerator found that the scattered photon energy fell from about 350 keV at the inner maze entrance to about 100 keV at the outer maze entrance. McGinley and James (1997) also found that the average x-ray energy at the outer maze entrance of a similar maze was 150 keV for a 6 MV accelerator and 200 keV for a 10 MV accelerator. The lower energies will increase the reflection coefficients (see tables 5.6 and 5.7) for reflections close to the outer maze entrance. The lower energy from these calculations has been used to advocate less shielding in the door at the end of the maze if one is required. However, this suggestion should be treated with caution as higher energy x-rays from leakage radiation transmitted through the inner maze wall (see section 5.7.4) may also be present.

Table 5.6. Reflection coefficients for normal incidence on concrete as a function of angle of reflection for several endpoint energies (taken from NCRP (2005) table B8a). A table entry of 6.7 (e.g. for 4 MeV with normal reflection) means a reflection coefficient of 6.7×10^{-3}.

Endpoint energy (MeV)	Reflection coefficient $\times 10^3$ for normal incidence on concrete				
	Angle of reflection (degrees) Measured from the normal				
	0	30	45	60	75
4	6.7	6.4	5.8	4.9	3.1
6	5.3	5.2	4.7	4	2.7
10	4.3	4.1	3.8	3.1	2.1
18	3.4	3.4	3	2.5	1.6
24	3.2	3.2	2.8	2.3	1.5
30	3	2.7	2.6	2.2	1.5
Co-60	7	6.5	6	5.5	3.8
Effective energy (MeV)					
0.25	32	28	25	22	13
0.5	19	17	15	13	8

Table 5.7. Reflection coefficients for 45° incidence on concrete as a function of angle of reflection for several endpoint energies (taken from NCRP (2005) table B8b). A table entry of 7.6 means a reflection coefficient of 7.6×10^{-3}.

Endpoint energy (MeV)	Reflection coefficient $\times 10^3$ for 45° incidence on concrete				
	Angle of reflection (degrees) Measured from normal				
	0	30	45	60	75
4	7.6	8.5	9	9.2	9.5
6	6.4	7.1	7.3	7.7	8
10	5.1	5.7	5.8	6	6
18	4.5	4.6	4.6	4.3	4
24	3.7	3.9	3.9	3.7	3.4
30	4.8	5	4.9	4	3
Co-60	9	10.2	11	11.5	12
Effective energy (MeV)					
0.25	36	34.5	31	25	18
0.5	22	22.5	22	20	18

Table 5.8. Scatter fractions at 1 m from a human phantom for a reference field size of 400 cm^2 and target to phantom distance of 1 m (adapted from NCRP (2005) table B4). A table entry of 10.4 means a scatter fraction of 10.4×10^{-3}

	Scatter fraction $\times 10^3$			
Angle (degrees)	6 MV	10 MV	18 MV	24 MV
10	10.4	16.6	14.2	17.8
20	6.73	5.79	5.39	6.32
30	2.77	3.18	2.53	2.74
45	1.39	1.35	0.864	0.830
60	0.824	0.746	0.424	0.386
90	0.426	0.381	0.189	0.174
135	0.300	0.302	0.124	0.120
150	0.287	0.274	0.120	0.113

5.7.1 Scatter of the primary beam from the bunker walls

This is illustrated in figure 5.8(a) for a two-leg maze and in (b) for a three-leg maze, where the radiation beam is incident on the primary shielding and the plane of beam rotation is parallel to the inner maze wall in both cases.

In general, the dose rate at the maze entrance, S_1, will be given by:

$$S_1 = S^* \alpha_1 A_1 \alpha_2 A_2 \ldots \alpha_n A_n / (d_i d_1 d_2 \ldots d_n)^2, \tag{5.12}$$

where S^* is the dose rate at the isocentre; d_i is the distance from the target to the primary barrier (m); α_1 is the reflection coefficient at the first scatter dependent upon the x-ray energy, wall material, and the angles of incidence and reflection; A_1 is the beam area at the first scatter (m^2); d_1 is the distance from the first scatter to the second scatter (m); α_2 is the reflection coefficient at the second scatter dependent on the energy of the scattered radiation (generally assumed to be 0.5 MeV), and the angles of incidence and reflection; A_2 is the irradiated area at the second scatter (m^2); d_2 is the distance from the second to the third scatter (m); α_n is the reflection coefficient at the maze wall (nth scatter) dependent on the energy of the scattered radiation (generally assumed to be 0.5 MeV), and the angles of incidence and reflection; A_n is the area of the maze wall from which scatter is able to travel down the maze after the nth scatter; and d_n is the distance from the nth scatter to the maze entrance (m).

In figure 5.8(a) and (b), the first scatter takes place at the primary barrier and the distance d_i from the target to the primary barrier is 4.4 m and the area irradiated on the primary barrier is 1.8 m $\times$ 1.8 m = 3.2 m^2 for the largest field size. The second scatter takes place at the inner maze entrance and the distance d_1 from the primary barrier to the inner maze entrance is 6.3 m. Suppose we have a linear accelerator operating at 10 MV with a dose rate at the isocentre of 6 Gy min^{-1}. The reflection coefficient α_1 at the primary barrier will be 2.1×10^{-3} (table 5.6) assuming a typical scattering angle of 75°, and α_2 at the inner maze entrance will be 8×10^{-3} assuming a

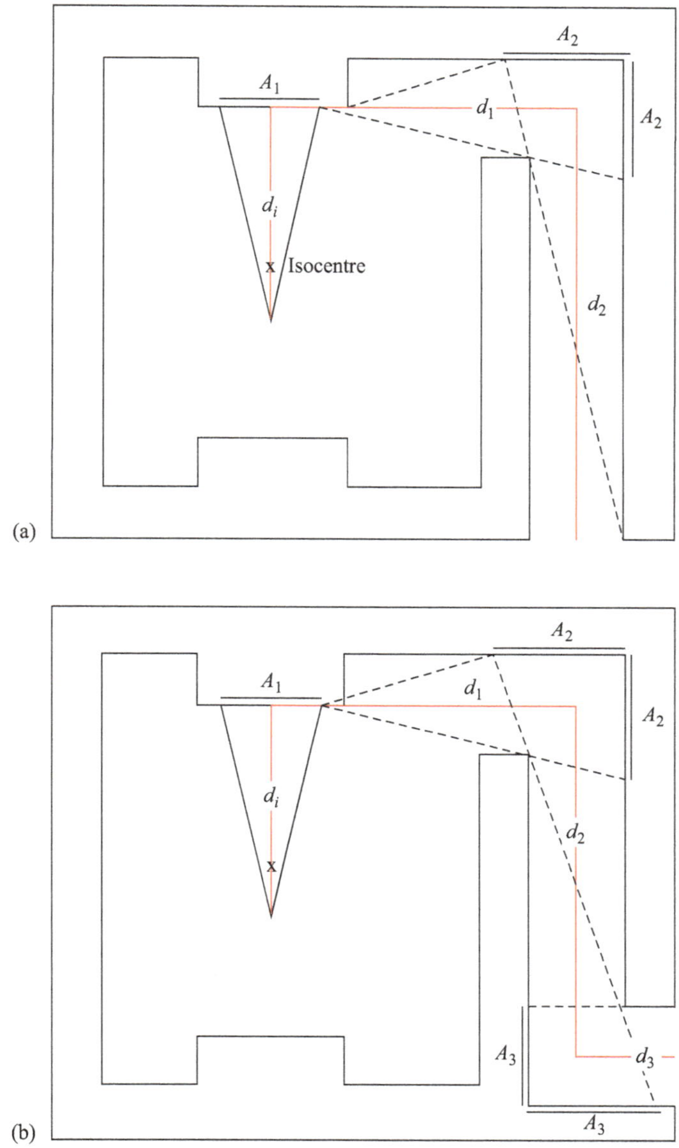

Figure 5.8. Bunker plans with the primary beam parallel to the maze showing the factors for calculating the x-ray scatter down the maze from the primary beam striking the bunker wall for a two leg maze (a) and three leg maze (b).

scattered energy of 0.5 MeV and a typical scattering angle of 75°. The bunker is assumed to be 3.7 m high.

In figure 5.8(a), the distance d_2 to the maze entrance is 8.8 m and the area A_2 of the inner maze walls irradiated by scattered radiation from the primary barrier and visible from the maze entrance is (2.6 + 2.4) m long by 3.7 m high, giving an irradiated area of 18.5 m^2. Inserting these values into equation (5.12) with two scatters gives a dose rate of 6.0 μSv h^{-1} at the maze entrance due to the scatter from the primary beam hitting the primary barrier.

For the three-leg maze in figure 5.8(b), the maze length d_2 is reduced to 7.2 m and the extra leg d_3 has a length of 2 m. The area A_2 of the inner maze walls irradiated by scattered radiation from the primary barrier and visible from the bend in the maze is (2.8 + 2.4) m long by 3.7 m high, giving an irradiated area of 19.2 m^2 and the area A_3 of the maze walls irradiated by scattered radiation from the inner maze entrance and visible from the maze entrance is (2.0 + 2.8) m long by 3.7 m high, giving an irradiated area of 17.8 m^2. The reflection coefficient α_3 is again assumed to be 8×10^{-3} with a scattered energy of 0.5 MeV and a typical scattering angle of 75°. Inserting these values into equation (5.12) with three scatters gives a dose rate of 0.3 μSv h^{-1} at the maze entrance due to the scatter of the primary beam hitting the primary barrier.

When the primary beam is pointing at the opposite primary barrier, further from the maze entrance, an additional reflection will be introduced into the path of the scattered radiation reaching the maze entrance. At 10 MV the scattered radiation will have a reflection coefficient of 4.1×10^{-3} (table 5.6) at normal incidence and a reflection angle of 30° and this factor combined with a distance of 8–9 m to the wall adjacent to the inner maze entrance will result in a negligible dose rate compared with the dose rates calculated for figure 5.8(a) and (b).

Inspection of tables 5.6 and 5.7 shows that the reflection coefficients increase with lower beam energy. A worse case calculation can be performed, assuming that all treatments take place at the lowest beam energy, e.g. 6 MV.

Some texts introduce a factor of 0.20 or 0.25 into equation (5.12) to allow for attenuation of the primary beam in the patient. Quite often this factor is omitted for a conservative result.

The situation when the plane of beam rotation is perpendicular to the inner maze wall is illustrated in figure 5.9(a) and (b) when the radiation beam strikes the primary shielding away from the maze entrance and for a two-leg and three-leg maze, respectively. In these figures, the distance d_i from the target to the primary barrier is 4.4 m, the distance d_1 from the primary barrier to the inner maze entrance is 9.3 m, and the area irradiated on the primary barrier is 1.8 m × 1.8 m = 3.2 m^2 for the largest field size. Suppose again we have a linear accelerator operating at 10 MV with a dose rate at the isocentre of 6 Gy min^{-1}. The reflection coefficient α_1 at the primary barrier will be 2.1×10^{-3} (table 5.6) assuming a typical scattering angle of 75° and α_2 at the inner maze entrance will be 8×10^{-3} assuming a scattered energy of 0.5 MeV and a typical scattering angle of 75°.

In figure 5.9(a), the distance d_2 to the maze entrance is 7.8 m and the area A_2 of the inner maze walls irradiated by scattered radiation from the primary barrier and visible from the maze entrance is (2.6 + 1.6) m long by 3.7 m high, giving an irradiated area of 15.5 m^2. Inserting these values into equation (5.12) with two scatters gives a dose rate of 2.9 μSv h^{-1} at the maze entrance due to the scatter of the primary beam hitting the primary barrier.

For the three-leg maze in figure 5.9(b), the maze length d_2 is reduced to 6.2 m and the extra leg d_3 has a length of 2 m. The area A_2 of the inner maze walls irradiated by

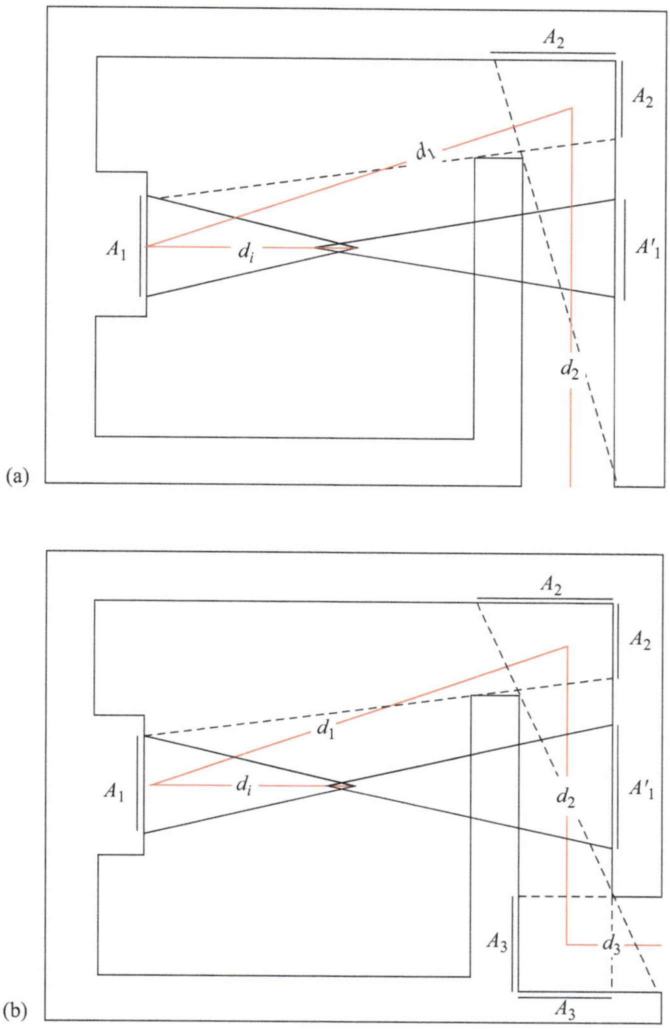

Figure 5.9. Bunker plans with the primary beam perpendicular to the maze showing the factors for calculating the x-ray scatter down the maze from the primary beam striking the bunker wall for a two leg maze (a) and a three leg maze (b).

scattered radiation from the primary barrier and visible from the bend in the maze is (2.8 + 1.6) m long by 3.7 m high, giving an irradiated area of 17.8 m^2, and the area A_3 of the maze walls irradiated by scattered radiation from the inner maze entrance and visible from the maze entrance is (2.0 + 2.8) m long by 3.7 m high, giving an irradiated area of 17.8 m^2. The refection coefficient α_3 is again assumed to be 8×10^{-3} with a scattered energy of 0.5 MeV and a typical scattering angle of 75°. Inserting these values into equation (5.12) with three scatters gives a dose rate of 0.2 μSv h^{-1} at the maze entrance due to the scatter of the primary beam hitting the primary barrier.

The annual maze entrance doses from this source can be estimated by multiplying the annual primary dose at the isocentre for each treatment energy by the factors in equation (5.12), taking into account the proportion of time the beam points at the primary barrier concerned (the orientation or use factor, U) and the occupancy factor (T) at the maze entrance, i.e.

$$D_a = D_f \times N \times 250 \times \alpha_1 A_1 \alpha_2 A_2 \cdots \alpha_n A_n/(d_i d_1 d_2 \ldots d_n)^2 \times U \times T.$$

The annual doses for each energy need to be summed to a give the total annual dose at the maze entrance contributed by this source.

In the situation shown in figure 5.9(a) and (b), the primary beam can also strike the inner maze wall. The beam will be attenuated by the inner maze wall before striking the inner face of the outer maze wall where it can be scattered toward the maze entrance.

In general, the dose rate at the maze entrance, S_1 will be given by

$$S_1 = S^* B_i \alpha_1 A_1 \alpha_2 A_2 \cdots \alpha_{n-1} A_{n-1}/(d_i d_1 d_2 \cdots d_n)^2, \quad (5.13)$$

where S^* is the dose rate at the isocentre; B_i is the transmission factor of the inner maze wall; d_i is the distance from the target to the outer maze wall (m); α_1 is the reflection coefficient at the first scatter (outer maze wall) dependent upon the x-ray energy, wall material, and the angles of incidence and reflection; A_1 is the beam area at the first scatter (outer maze wall) (m^2); d_1 is the distance from the first scatter to the second scatter (m); α_2 is the reflection coefficient at the second scatter dependent on the energy of the scattered radiation (generally assumed to be 0.5 MeV), and the angles of incidence and reflection; A_2 is the area of the inner maze wall from which scatter is able to travel towards the next scatter; d_2 is the distance from the second to the third scatter (m); α_n is the reflection coefficient at the maze wall (nth scatter) dependent on the energy of the scattered radiation (generally assumed to be 0.5 MeV), and the angles of incidence and reflection; A_n is the area of the maze wall from which scatter is able to travel down the maze after the nth scatter; and d_n is the distance from the nth scatter to the maze entrance (m).

For the two-leg maze in figure 5.9(a), the inner maze wall is 1 m thick and has a transmission factor of 2.54×10^{-3} at 10 MV, the distance d_i is 6.4 m, the maximum beam width on the far maze wall is 2.6 m, giving an irradiated area of 2.6 m × 2.6 m = 6.76 m^2 and the distance d_1 from the centre of the irradiated area to the maze entrance is 4.9 m. The scatter coefficient α_1 at 10 MV is 2.1×10^{-3} assuming normal incidence and a scatter angle of 75°. Inserting these values into equation (5.13) gives a dose rate at the maze entrance of 13.2 μSv h^{-1}.

For the three-leg maze in figure 5.9(b), the attenuation of the inner maze wall, the irradiated area of the outer maze wall A_1, d_i and α_1 are unchanged. The distance from the centre of the irradiated area to the corner of the maze is 4.7 m and the irradiated corner of the maze visible from the entrance is (2 + 2) m × 3.7 m = 14.8 m^2. The distance d_2 to the maze entrance from the centre point of the corner is 2 m and the scatter coefficient is 18×10^{-3} assuming 0.5 MeV scattered radiation with 45° incidence and a scatter angle of 75°. Inserting these values into equation (5.13) gives a dose rate at the maze entrance of 0.06 μSv h^{-1}.

The annual maze entrance doses from this source can be estimated by multiplying the annual primary dose at the isocentre for each treatment energy by the factors in equation (5.13), taking into account the proportion of the time the beam points at the inner maze wall (the orientation or use factor, U) and the occupancy factor (T) at the maze entrance, i.e.

$$D_a = D_f \times N \times 250 \times B_i\alpha_1 A_1 \alpha_2 A_2 \cdots \alpha_{n-1}A_{n-1}/(d_i d_1 d_2 \cdots d_n)^2 \times U \times T.$$

The annual doses for each energy need to be summed to a give the total annual dose at the maze entrance contributed by this source.

It should be noted that these are worst case calculations for the largest possible beam area incident on the primary barriers corresponding to a 40 cm × 40 cm field at the isocentre of the accelerator. In clinical practice, especially with IMRT and VMAT, the beam areas will be considerably smaller and the area of the beam A_1 striking a primary barrier or the outer maze wall will be considerably less than in the examples above.

5.7.2 Scatter of the primary beam by the patient

This is illustrated in figure 5.10(a) for a two-leg maze and in (b) for a three-leg maze, where the plane of beam rotation is parallel to the inner maze wall in both cases.

In general, the dose rate at the maze entrance, S_2, will be given by

$$S_2 = S^*\alpha\left(F/400\right)\alpha_1 A_1 \cdots \alpha_n A_n/\left(d_i d_1 \cdots d_n\right)^2, \quad (5.14)$$

where S^* is the dose rate at the isocentre; d_i is the distance from the target to the isocentre (m); α is the patient scatter factor (tabulated per 400 cm^2 incident field area on the patient, F is the field area incident on the patient (cm^2); d_1 is the distance from the isocentre (in the patient) to the second scatter (maze wall) (m); α_1 is the reflection coefficient at the second scatter (maze wall) dependent on the energy of the scattered radiation (generally assumed to be 0.5 MeV for patient scattered radiation), and the angles of incidence and reflection; A_1 is the area of the maze wall from which scatter is able to travel down the maze; α_n is the reflection coefficient at the maze wall (nth scatter) dependent on the energy of the scattered radiation (generally assumed to be 0.5 MeV), and the angles of incidence and reflection; A_n is the area of the maze wall from which scatter is able to travel down the maze after the nth scatter; and d_n is the distance from the nth scatter to the maze entrance (m).

In figure 5.10(a) and (b), the distance d_i from the target to the isocentre is 1 m, the distance d_1 from the isocentre to the inner maze entrance is 7.4 m, and the area A_1 of the inner maze walls irradiated by scattered radiation from the patient and visible from the maze entrance is (2.5 + 0.2) m long by 3.7 m high giving an irradiated area of 10.0 m^2. Suppose we have a linear accelerator operating at 10 MV with a dose rate at the isocentre of 6 Gy min^{-1} and a maximum field area of 400 cm^2. The patient scatter factor α will be 1.35 × 10^{-3} (table 5.8) assuming a typical scattering angle of 45° with a horizontal beam and α_1 at the inner maze entrance will be 22 × 10^{-3} assuming a scattered energy of 0.5 MeV, 45° incidence and a typical scattering angle of 45°.

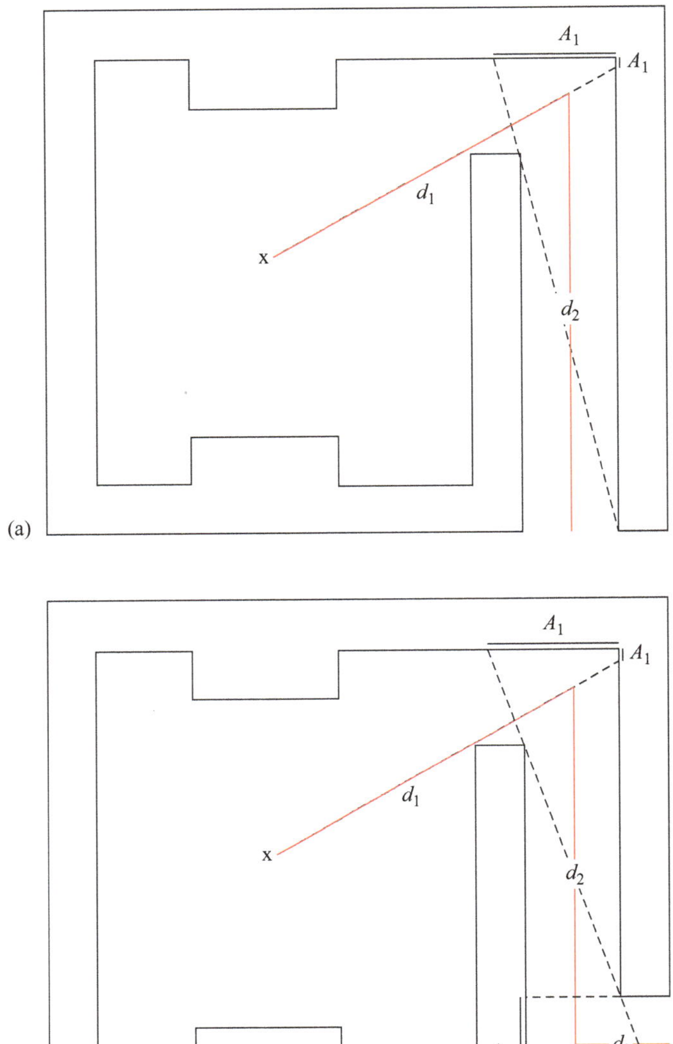

Figure 5.10. Bunker plans with the primary beam parallel to the maze showing the factors for calculating the x-ray scatter down the maze from the patient for a two leg maze (a) and three leg maze (b).

In figure 5.8(a), the distance d_2 to the maze entrance is 9.8 m. Inserting these values into equation (5.14) gives a dose rate of 20.3 μSv h^{-1} at the maze entrance due to scatter from the patient.

For the three-leg maze in figure 5.10(b), the maze length d_2 is reduced to 8.2 m and the extra leg d_3 has a length of 2 m. The area A_1 of the inner maze walls irradiated by scattered radiation from the patient and visible from the bend in the maze is (2.7 + 0.2) m long by 3.7 m high, giving an irradiated area of 10.7 m^2 and the area A_2 of the maze walls irradiated by scattered radiation from the inner maze entrance and visible from the maze entrance is (2.0 + 2.8) m long by 3.7 m high, giving an irradiated area of 17.8 m^2. The reflection coefficient α_1 is again taken to be 22×10^{-3} with a scattered energy of 0.5 MeV and a typical scattering angle of 45°. The reflection coefficient α_2 is taken as 8×10^{-3} with a scattered energy of 0.5 MeV at normal incidence and a scattering angle of 75°. Inserting these values into equation (5.14) with two wall scatters gives a dose rate of 1.1 μSv h^{-1} at the maze entrance due to the scatter from the patient.

Inspection of table 5.8 shows that the patient scatter coefficients at scatter angles of 45° or greater (which is normally the direction of the inner maze entrance) increase with lower beam energy. The scatter coefficients also decrease with increasing scatter angle, e.g. with a vertical beam when the scatter angle will be 90°. Coupled with a similar variation with wall scatter, a worse case calculation can be performed assuming that all treatments take place at the lowest beam energy, e.g. 6 MV.

The situation when the plane of beam rotation is perpendicular to the inner maze wall is illustrated in figure 5.11(a) and (b) for a two-leg and three-leg maze, respectively. This situation is very similar to the situation where the plane of the beam is parallel to the inner maze wall, because the patient scattering with a horizontal beam will again be at 45° in the direction of the inner maze entrance. The coefficients for patient scatter and the one or two wall scatters will be the same since the maze geometries are unchanged. Only the physical shape of the bunker and hence the distances are changed. In figure 5.11(a), the distance d_1 from the isocentre to the inner maze entrance is 6.4 m, the distance d_2 to the maze entrance is 8.8 m and the irradiated area A_1 of the inner maze walls visible from the entrance is (2.5 + 0.4) m long by 3.7 m high, giving an irradiated area of 10.7 m^2. Inserting these values into equation (5.14) gives a dose rate of 36.2 μSv h^{-1} at the maze entrance due to patient scatter of the primary beam. For the three-leg maze in figure 5.11(b), the maze length d_2 is reduced to 7.2 m and the extra leg d_3 has a length of 2 m. The area A_1 of the inner maze walls irradiated by scattered radiation from the patient and visible from the bend in the maze is (2.9 + 0.2) m long by 3.7 m high, giving an irradiated area of 11.5 m^2 and the area A_2 of the maze walls irradiated by scattered radiation from the inner maze entrance and visible from the maze entrance is (2.0 + 2.9) m long by 3.7 m high, giving an irradiated area of 18.1 m^2. Inserting these values into equation (5.14) gives a dose rate of 2.2 μSv h^{-1} at the maze entrance due to the scatter of the primary beam by the patient.

The annual maze entrance doses from this source can be estimated by multiplying the annual primary dose at the isocentre for each treatment energy by the factors in equation (5.14), taking into account the occupancy factor (T) at the maze entrance, i.e.

$$D_{\mathrm{a}} = D_{\mathrm{f}} \times N \times 250 \times \alpha(F/400)\alpha_1 A_1 \ldots \alpha_n A_n/(d_{\mathrm{i}} d_1 \ldots d_n)^2 \times T.$$

The annual doses for each energy need to be summed to a give the total annual dose at the maze entrance contributed by this source.

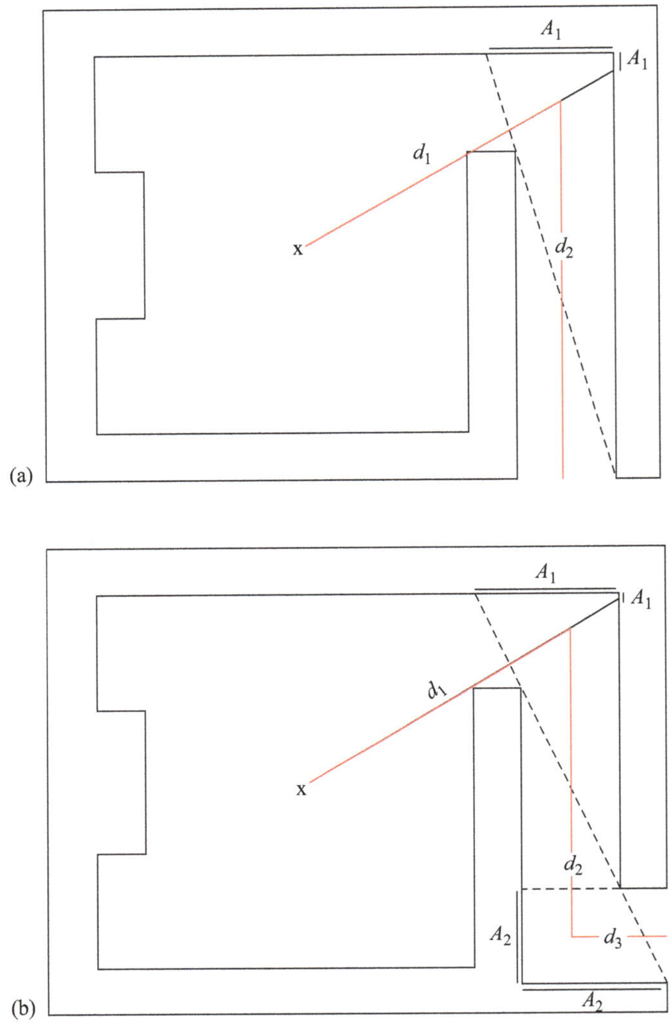

Figure 5.11. Bunker plans with the primary beam perpendicular to the maze showing the factors for calculating the x-ray scatter down the maze from the patient for a two leg maze (a) and three leg maze (b).

5.7.3 Scatter of head leakage radiation by the bunker walls

This is a similar geometrical situation to the scatter introduced by the patient, in that the source position is taken as the isocentre, this being considered the mean position of the treatment head during patient treatments. However, leakage radiation is considered to be isotropic whilst patient scatter has an angular dependence. Since the leakage radiation is considered to be isotropic this will be the same in principal whether the primary beam is parallel or perpendicular to the inner maze wall. The only difference may lie again in the size and shape of the bunker, and hence the distances between the source and the first scatter and the distances between subsequent scatters.

In general, the dose rate at the maze entrance, S_3, will be given by

$$S_3 = S^* \times 0.001 \times \alpha_1 A_1 \alpha_2 A_2 \ldots \alpha_{n-1} A_{n-1} / (d_i d_1 d_2 \ldots d_n)^2, \qquad (5.15)$$

where S^* is the dose rate at the isocentre; 0.001 is the fraction of the dose due to head leakage at 1 m from the target relative to the dose on the beam axis 1 m from the target; d_i is the distance from the isocentre to the first wall scatter (m); α_1 is the reflection coefficient at the first wall scatter dependent upon the x-ray energy (generally assumed to be 1.5 MeV (IAEA 2006, Nelson and Lariviere 1984)), wall material and the angles of incidence and reflection; A_1 is the irradiated area at the first scatter (inner maze wall); d_1 is the distance from the first to the second scatter (m); α_2 is the reflection coefficient at the second wall scatter dependent on the energy of the scattered radiation (generally assumed to be 0.5 MeV), and the angles of incidence and reflection; A_2 is the irradiated area at the second scatter (m^2); d_2 is the distance from the second to the third scatter (m); α_n is the reflection coefficient at the maze wall (nth scatter) dependent on the energy of the scattered radiation (generally assumed to be 0.5 MeV), and the angles of incidence and reflection; A_n is the area of the maze wall from which scatter is able to reach the maze entrance after the nth scatter; and d_n is the distance from the nth scatter to maze entrance (m).

Equation (5.15) can be numerated using figure 5.10(a) and (b) for the situation where the primary beam is parallel to the maze. For the two-leg maze in figure 5.10(a) $d_i = 7.4$ m, $A_1 = 10.0$ m^2 and $d_1 = 9.8$ m as before. The scatter coefficient α_1 at 1.5 MeV (using the Co-60 data in table 5.7) assuming 45° incidence and 45° reflection is 11×10^{-3}. Inserting these values into equation (5.15) gives a dose rate of 7.5 μSv h^{-1} at the maze entrance. For the three-leg maze d_i, A_1, d_1, A_2, α_2 and d_2 are unchanged from figure 5.10(b) and α_1 has the value above. Inserting these values into equation (5.15) gives a dose rate of 0.4 μSv h^{-1} at the maze entrance. Similarly it can be enumerated for figure 5.11(a) and (b) where the primary beam can strike the maze wall. The dose rate at the maze entrance is calculated as 13.4 μSv h^{-1} for the two-leg maze and 0.8 μSv h^{-1} for the three-leg maze.

The annual maze entrance doses from this source can be estimated by multiplying the annual secondary dose at the isocentre for each treatment energy by the factors in equation (5.15), taking into account the increase in beam on time (f) due to IMRT treatments and the occupancy factor (T) at the maze entrance, i.e.

$$D_a = D_f \times N \times 250 \times f \times 0.001 \times \alpha_1 A_1 \alpha_2 A_2 \ldots \alpha_{n-1} A_{n-1} / (d_i d_1 d_2 \ldots d_n)^2 \times T.$$

The annual doses for each energy need to be summed to a give the total annual dose at the maze entrance contributed by this source.

5.7.4 Transmission of head leakage radiation through the inner maze wall

This is illustrated in figure 5.12(a) for a two-leg maze and in (b) for a three-leg maze, where the plane of beam rotation is parallel to the inner maze wall in both cases. The dose rate at the maze entrance, S_4, will be given by

$$S_4 = S^* \times 0.001 \times B / d_m{}^2, \qquad (5.16)$$

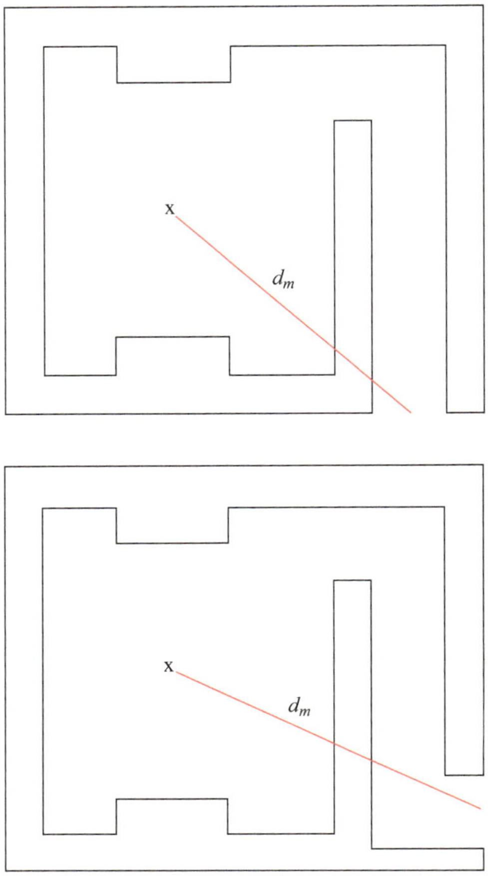

Figure 5.12. Bunker plans showing the path of head leakage radiation though the inner maze wall for a two leg maze (a) and a three leg maze (b).

where S^* is the dose rate at the isocentre; 0.001 is the fraction of the dose due to head leakage at 1 m from the target relative to the dose on the beam axis 1 m from the target; B is the transmission factor through the maze wall for 1.5 MeV x-rays; and d_m is the distance from the target to the maze entrance.

The transmission factor of the inner maze wall at 1.5 MeV (not taking obliquity into account) is 1.74×10^{-5}. The distance d_m in figure 5.12(a) is 8.3 m and 9.1 m in (b). Inserting these values into equation (5.16) gives dose rates at the maze entrance of 0.09 and 0.08 μSv h^{-1}, respectively. A similar situation exists when the beam strikes the inner maze wall and reference to figure 5.9(a) and (b) yields values of d_m of 7.2 m for the two-leg maze and 8.0 m for the three-leg maze. Inserting these values into equation (5.16) gives dose rates at the maze entrance of 0.12 and 0.10 μSv h^{-1}, respectively, due to the shorter distance with this geometry.

The annual maze entrance doses from this source can be estimated by multiplying the annual secondary dose at the isocentre for each treatment energy by the factors in equation (5.16), taking into account the increase in beam on time (f) due to IMRT treatments and the occupancy factor (T) at the maze entrance, i.e.

$$D_a = D_f \times N \times 250 \times f \times 0.001 \times B/d_m^2 \times T.$$

The annual doses for each energy need to be summed to give the total annual dose at the maze entrance contributed by this source.

5.7.5 Total x-ray dose rate and annual dose at the maze entrance

To confirm the design and shielding calculations, the maximum dose rate at the maze entrance can be calculated by summing the above four dose rate components and comparing the results with the measured dose rates at each treatment energy.

Table 5.9 shows the results of adding the four dose rate components using the example of 10 MV operation in the bunker configurations shown in figures 5.8–5.12. As can be seen, the additional scatter in a three-leg maze results in a considerable reduction in the total dose rate by comparison to a two-leg maze, especially for patient scatter which is the dominant component in this example. These examples also show that in general terms the total maze entrance dose rate is lower when the plane of the primary beam is parallel to the inner maze wall. For a two-leg maze with the beam able to point at the inner maze wall, the entrance component due to wall scatter (13.2 μSv h^{-1}) can be reduced by having a thicker inner maze wall than in this example; the outer wall can then be made thinner.

As shown in the sections above, the total annual dose at the maze entrance can be estimated for each of the four components, taking into account the primary or secondary annual doses at the isocentre at each energy, together with the use factor

Table 5.9. Total x-ray dose rates (μSv h^{-1}) at the maze entrance at 10 MV using the examples in figures 5.8–5.12.

Source	Two-leg maze			Three-leg maze		
	Beam parallel to maze wall	Beam perpendicular to maze wall		Beam parallel to maze wall	Beam perpendicular to maze wall	
		Directed away from maze	Directed toward maze		Directed away from maze	Directed toward maze
Walls/primary beam	6.0	2.9	13.2	0.3	0.2	0.1
Patient/primary beam	20.3	36.2		1.1	2.2	
Walls/head leakage	7.5	13.4		0.4	0.8	
Maze transmission of head leakage	0.1	0.1		0.1	0.1	
Total	33.9	52.6	62.9	1.9	3.3	3.2

and occupancy factor at the maze entrance where appropriate. The annual dose needs to be calculated separately for each energy and summed.

5.8 Neutron scatter down the maze

Neutron production occurs in linear accelerators operating with x-ray beams above 8.5 MV. Photoneutrons are produced when the x-ray beam interacts with the high atomic number components in the treatment head, e.g. lead and tungsten. Lead for example has a peak cross-section for neutron photoproduction at about 13 MeV. Production takes place at the target, flattening filter and collimators. The neutrons produced are moderated by the x-ray shielding in the treatment head and further moderated by scattering off the walls of the bunker. The total neutron fluence at any point in the room therefore comprises direct (fast) neutrons, scattered neutrons and thermal neutrons. IAEA (2006) states that for accelerators operating in the range 10–25 MV, the mean energy of direct neutrons from the treatment head is about 1 MeV and the mean energy of neutrons scattered by the walls of the room is about 0.24 MeV. This gives a mean neutron energy (excluding thermal neutrons) of 0.34 MeV (NCRP 1984). The TVL of 0.34 MeV neutrons in concrete is 210 mm (IAEA 2006). NCRP (2005) suggests a conservative TVL value of 250 mm. Comparison to tables 5.1 and 5.2, respectively, shows that this is about half of the TVL for 10 MV and 15 MV primary shielding (410 and 440 mm, respectively, for TVL_1) and around 60% of the secondary TVL at these energies (350 and 360 mm, respectively, for TVL_1). *Consequently if the primary or secondary shielding is adequate for x-rays it is adequate for neutrons, provided the x-ray TVL is greater than 210 mm for the density of the material concerned.* The neutron TVL is not altered by density and is the same in high density concrete. It is primarily related to hydrogen content and all concretes have a significant hydrogen content, being 4%–5% water by weight.

The ratio of neutrons to x-ray photons increases with beam energy. NCRP (2005) quotes values at 1.41 m from the target of 0.04 mSv Gy^{-1} at 10 MV, 0.17–1.3 mSv Gy^{-1} at 15 MV and 0.55–1.6 mSv Gy^{-1} at 18 MV for a variety of accelerator manufacturers. These are given in table 5.10 together with values

Table 5.10. Neutron dose equivalent at 1.41 m from the target and neutron production per Gy per absorbed dose of x-rays at the isocentre (taken from NCRP (2005) table B9).

End point energy	mSv Gy^{-1}	Neutrons/Gy × 10^{12}	Linear accelerator
10 MeV	0.04	0.06	Varian 1800
	–	0.08	Siemens MD2
	–	0.02	Siemens Primus
15 MeV	0.79–1.3	0.76	Varian 1800
	0.17	–	Siemens MD
	–	0.2	Siemens MD
	–	0.12	Siemens Primus
	–	0.21	Siemens Primus
	0.32	0.47	GE Saturne 41

for neutron production per gray. Barish (2009) has given more recent values (mSv Gy^{-1} @ 1 m) for neutron dose as a fraction of primary x-ray dose at the isocentre in Elekta and Varian accelerators. These are listed in table 5.11.

However the neutron fluence will be able to travel down the maze and, for accelerators operating above 8.5 MV, the dose rate at the maze entrance must include the neutron dose and the gamma ray dose from neutrons captured by the maze walls, as well as the doses to x-ray scatter and maze wall penetration considered in section 5.7. In general fast neutrons obey the inverse square law but scattered and thermal neutrons are isotropically distributed and consequently the neutron fluence down the maze does not fall off as fast as an inverse square law relationship.

McCall *et al* (1999) have shown that the total neutron fluence at the inner maze entrance (point A in figure 5.13) per unit x-ray absorbed dose at the isocentre is given by

$$\Phi_A = \beta Q/4\pi d_1^2 + 5.4\beta Q/2\pi S + 1.3Q/2\pi S. \tag{5.17}$$

Table 5.11. Neutron dose equivalent per unit absorbed dose of x-rays at the isocentre (mSv Gy^{-1}) (Barish 2009). Note: A radiation weighting factor (w_R) for neutrons of 10 has been used to convert to equivalent dose.

	Manufacturer	End point energy		
		10 MeV	15 MeV	18 MeV
Neutron dose equivalent (mSv Gy^{-1})	Elekta	0.1	0.7	1.5
	Varian	0.04	0.7	1.5

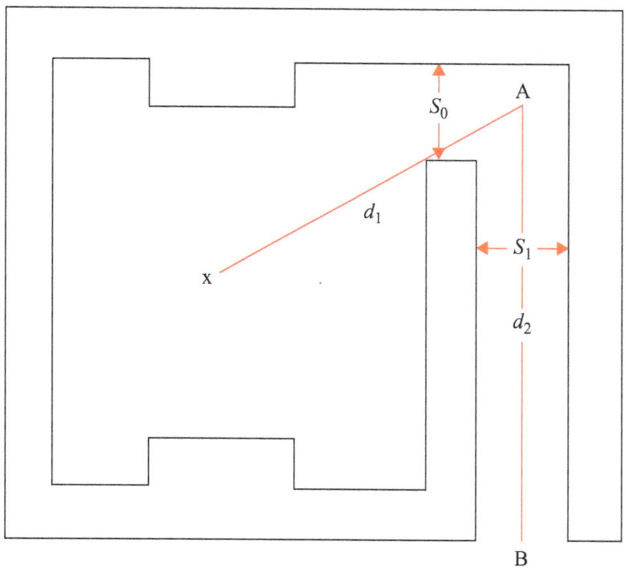

Figure 5.13. Bunker plan showing the factors for calculation of the neutron dose rate at the maze entrance.

These terms represent the direct, scattered and thermal neutron components respectively where β is the head shielding transmission factor for neutrons (1 for lead, 0.85 for tungsten); Q is the neutron source strength per gray of the x-ray absorbed dose at the isocentre (neutrons Gy^{-1}); d_1 is the distance from the isocentre to point A (m); and S is the total surface area of the treatment room (m^2).

For short mazes where the distance d_2 (AB in figure 5.13) in less than 2.5 m, NCRP (2005) states that x-ray fluence at the outer maze entrance (B) is dominated by neutron capture gamma rays and the contribution from scattered x-rays can be ignored. The dose equivalent H_γ from the neutron capture gamma rays at the outer maze entrance (McGinley *et al* 1995) is given by

$$H_\gamma = 6.9 \times 10^{-16} \times \Phi_A \times 10^{-(d_2/\mathrm{TVD})}, \tag{5.18}$$

where the factor 6.9×10^{-16} is the ratio of the neutron capture gamma ray dose equivalent (Sv) to the total neutron flux at point A and was determined experimentally (NCRP151); Φ_A is the total neutron fluence (equation (5.17)); d_2 is the distance from point A to the outer maze entrance (m); and TVD is the distance for the photon fluence to fall tenfold and is given as 3.9 m for 15 MV x-rays.

Evaluating equations (5.17) and (5.18) using figure 5.13, where $d_1 = 7.2$ m, $d_2 =$ 8.9 m, $S = 260$ m^2, $Q = 7.6 \times 10^{11}$ neutrons Gy^{-1} (taken from table 5.10), TVD = 3.9 m and $\beta = 1$ gives the following values:

$$\Phi_A = 1.167 \times 10^9 + 2.512 \times 10^9 + 6.048 \times 10^8 = 4.284 \times 10^9.$$

Substituting this value in equation (5.18) assuming a primary x-ray dose rate of 6 Gy min^{-1} gives

$$H_\gamma = 6 \times 60 \times 6.9 \times 10^{-16} \times 4.284 \times 10^9 \times 5.223 \times 10^{-3} = 5.6\ \mu\mathrm{Sv\ h^{-1}}.$$

The neutron dose equivalent at the outer maze entrance can be estimated in a number of ways. These use the finding by Maerker and Muckenthaler (1967) that the TVD for thermal neutrons is roughly given by the expression

$$\mathrm{TVD} = 3(h \times w)^{1/2},$$

where h is the height of the maze and w is the width of the maze.

They also found that the fluence of thermal neutrons is reduced threefold for each additional leg of the maze.

The earliest technique for estimating the neutron fluence at the outer maze entrance is due to Kersey (1979). The neutron dose equivalent H_n at the outer maze entrance is given by

$$H_n = H_A \times S_0 \times d_0^2 \times 10^{-(d_2/5)}/S_1 \times d_1^2, \tag{5.19}$$

where H_A is the total neutron dose equivalent at d_0 (1.41 m) from the target; S_0 is the cross-sectional area of the inner maze entrance; S_1 is the cross-sectional area of the maze; d_1 is the distance from the isocentre to the centre line of the maze just visible from the isocentre (point A); and d_2 is the distance from the point A to the outer maze entrance (point B) (see figure 5.13). When the maze has further legs, d_2 is the distance from point A to the outer maze entrance following the mid-line of the maze.

McGinley and Huffman (2000) modified equation (5.19) following measurements by McGinley and Butker (1991) who found the ratio of the calculated neutron dose equivalent to the measured dose equivalent ranged from 0.82 to 2.3 measured for 13 linear accelerator bunkers. McGinley and Butker introduced two exponential functions to better describe the variation of the neutron dose equivalent with distance d_2 down the maze. This was further developed by Wu and McGinley (2003) to cope with large treatment rooms or very long or very wide mazes. Wu and McGinley state that the neutron dose equivalent along the maze length is given by

$$H_n = 2.4 \times 10^{-15} \Phi_A \times (S_0/S_1)^{1/2} \times [1.64 \times 10^{-(d_2/1.9)} + 10^{-(d_2/\mathrm{TVD})}], \qquad (5.20)$$

where H_n is the neutron dose equivalent at the maze entrance (Sv) per unit absorbed dose of x-rays (Gy) at the isocentre; ΦA is the neutron flux per unit absorbed dose of x-rays (Gy) at the isocentre (equation (5.17)); S_0/S_1 is the ratio of the cross-sectional area of the inner maze entrance to the cross-sectional area of the maze; and TVD is the tenth value distance (m) for maze neutrons.

TVD varies with the cross-sectional area of the maze and is given by

$$\mathrm{TVD} = 2.06\, S_1^{1/2}. \qquad (5.21)$$

Again using figure 5.13, $d_1 = 7.2$ m, $d_2 = 8.9$ m and $S_0 = S_1 = (2\text{ m} \times 3.7\text{ m}) = 7.4\text{ m}^2$. Substituting for S_1 in equation (5.20) gives a TVD of 5.60 m. Substituting these values in equation (5.20) together with the value of Φ_A calculated above and assuming a dose rate of 6 Gy min^{-1} gives

$$H_n = 2.4 \times 10^{-5} \times 4.284 \times 10^9 \times 1 \times [1.64 \times 10^{-(8.9/1.9)} + 10^{-(8.9/5.6)}],$$

i.e.

$$H_n = 2.4 \times 10^{-5} \times 4.284 \times 10^9 \times 1 \times [1.64 \times 2.07 \times 10^{-5} + 0.026] = 96\ \mu\mathrm{Sv\ h}^{-1}.$$

For a three-leg maze, such as that shown in figure 5.12(b), the distance d_1 is unchanged but d_2 increases to 9.4 m and the additional bend reduces the neutron fluence by a factor of 3. This results in a dose rate $H_n = 26\ \mu$Sv h^{-1}.

5.9 Maze doors and lining

A shielded door will be necessary at the maze entrance if the constraints on annual dose or instantaneous dose rates cannot be achieved with a sufficiently long maze or a sufficient number of legs. For linear accelerators operating below 8.5 MV the dose rate at the maze entrance will arise from scattered x-radiation (see sections 5.7.1–5.7.3) and x-ray scatter from head leakage radiation through the inner maze wall (see section 5.7.4). The transmission factor necessary is given by

$$B = \mathrm{DR_{acc}}/\mathrm{DR_i}, \qquad (5.22)$$

where $\mathrm{DR_{acc}}$ is the dose rate constraint and $\mathrm{DR_i}$ is the total dose rate at the maze entrance incident upon the door.

In this situation maze doors usually contain lead in a supporting steel frame. NCRP (2005) states that door shielding should be based on broad beam transmission data for 0.2 MeV photons (Al-Affan 2000). For bunkers with a maze length longer than 5 m, Kersey (1979) has shown that lead has a TVL of 6 mm for the x-ray energies involved. For the situation described in table 5.9 for a linear accelerator operating at 10 MV in a bunker with a two-leg maze with the beam plane parallel to the inner maze wall, the total x-ray dose rate at the maze entrance is 33.9 μSv h^{-1}. If the dose rate constraint is 7.5 μSv h^{-1}, then $B = 7.5/33.9 = 0.22$ and the number of TVLs = $\log_{10} B^{-1} = 0.66$. The required thickness of lead in the door to achieve the given dose rate constraint is $0.66 \times 6 = 3.9$ mm.

For linear accelerators operating above 8.5 MV, the dose rate due to capture gamma rays and the neutron fluence often exceeds the scattered x-ray dose rates especially for short mazes. The mean energy of capture gamma radiation from concrete is 3.6 MeV (McGinley 2002) and with short mazes calculation of the thickness of the lead required for an acceptable dose rate needs to use a TVL of 61 mm (NCRP 1984). For longer mazes a TVL of 6 mm can be used (see above). IAEA (2006) states that the mean neutron energy at the maze entrance is 100 keV. Borated polyethylene (5% by weight) is normally used to absorb the neutron flux; the borating being particularly effective for thermal neutrons. Both NCRP (2005) and IAEA (2006) report that the TVL of 2 MeV neutrons is 38 mm and is 12 mm for thermal neutrons, but both recommend a conservative TVL of 45 mm for calculating the required thickness of borated polyethylene in a door. The usual door construction is to sandwich the borated polyethylene between two layers of lead within a steel door frame. The lead needs to be of sufficient thickness to attenuate the scattered x-rays and capture gamma rays. The lead on the incident side of the door reduces the neutron energy by scattering, which increases the effectiveness of the borated polyethylene. The lead on the outside of the door attenuates the capture gamma radiation from the borated polyethylene, which has an energy of 0.48 MeV. The external lead layer may not be necessary with a long maze that has substantially reduced the neutron fluence (McCall 1997).

IAEA (2006) has adopted a simple approach to calculating the required thicknesses of lead and borated polyethylene by supposing that each contributes half of the dose rate constraint, e.g. if the constraint is 7.5 μSv h^{-1} each results in 3.75 μSv h^{-1}. Suppose, using the example in figure 5.13, the scattered x-ray dose rate at the maze entrance is 27.7 μSv h^{-1}, the capture gamma dose rate is 5.6 μSv h^{-1} and the neutron dose rate is 96 μSv h^{-1}. The total dose rate due to scattered x-rays and capture gamma rays is $27.7 + 5.6 = 33.3$ μSv h^{-1}. The required lead transmission $B = 3.75/33.3 = 0.11$ and the number of TVLs = 0.95. The thickness required is 5.7 mm of lead (0.95×6). To reduce the neutron dose rate to 3.75 μSv h^{-1} requires a transmission $B = 3.75/96 = 0.04$ and 1.4 TVLs of borated polyethylene. This corresponds to a thickness of 63 mm (1.4×45). To meet the dose rate constraint the door can comprise two layers of lead with a total thickness of 6 mm with 65 mm of borated polyethylene between them.

Due to the uncertainty in neutron energies at the maze entrance, a radiation weighting factor of 10 is recommended for dose calculations.

Shielded doors are heavy, expensive and need to be motorised. This makes them slow to open and close and they require safety features to prevent the trapping of persons in the door opening. They also require a manual means of opening the door in the event of a power failure. Consideration should be given in the maze design to only needing the door to be shut when operating at 10 MV and above and to a partial open position allowing staff to enter and leave between treatment fields if required.

A number of measures can be taken to reduce the shielding in the door and its weight, primarily aimed at reducing the neutron fluence reaching the door. These include:

- reducing the cross-sectional area of the maze by having substantial lintels in the maze, especially at the inner maze entrance (see section 7.3.4) and
- lining the maze walls with borated polyethylene sheet.

McGinley and Miner (1995) describe how a reduced opening (1.22 m × 2.13 m) at the inner maze entrance reduced the dose rate due to capture gamma rays and neutrons at the outer maze entrance to one third for a bunker with an 18 MV accelerator. They also found that a door of 50 mm thick borated polyethylene placed at the inner maze entrance reduced the dose rate to 11%. IPEM (1997) describes a 50% reduction in neutron dose when 20 m^2 of the inner maze walls, especially the wall facing the treatment room, were covered in borated polyethylene sheet.

5.10 Direct doors

To save the space required for a maze, a direct shielded door can be used (see figure 2.1(b)). This must be sited in a secondary barrier and provide the same shielding as the secondary barrier. For accelerators operating below 8.5 V, the door is usually made of lead in a steel casing. In the absence of any TVL data for lead for leakage radiation, the primary barrier TVLs for lead in table 5.1 should be used, leading to a conservative result. For accelerators operating above 8.5 MV, the door will also need to shield for neutron capture gamma rays and neutrons. The door composition and construction will be similar to that described above for an indirect door with a substantial layer of lead on the radiation incident side followed by the layer of borated polyethylene and then a further layer of lead 20 mm thick to absorb the 0.48 MeV gamma rays from the boron. In some designs the central layer comprises a layer of polyethylene followed by a layer of borated polyethylene; the former being more effective for fast neutrons and the latter effective for thermal neutrons. McGinley and Miner (1995) suggest that 1 HVL is added to the thickness of the lead necessary to attenuate the scattered and leakage x-rays to an acceptable level to additionally shield against the capture gamma rays from the treatment room surfaces; there are no known measurements of capture gamma ray intensities inside a treatment room.

Such shielded doors are heavy. Hinged doors may be possible for the lesser shielding requirements for low energy accelerators but a sliding door running on a steel floor track is usually necessary for higher energy accelerators. This will need to be power operated and have the safety features mentioned in section 5.9. Leakage of the radiation around the edges and beneath the door can be unacceptable, and the special measures needed around the door opening to reduce the leakage are described in detail in section 7.3.6.

The weight of the door can be considerably reduced by introducing a short wall (sometimes called a 'nib') beside the door that prevents the head leakage radiation reaching the door directly. Barish (2005) states that this arrangement together with siting the gantry of the accelerator with its back to the wall containing the door reduces the door thickness by 50%. This is illustrated in figure 2.1(c). Such an arrangement reduces the complexity of the construction of the door and opening. It can also help with patient acceptability in that the short wall stops the patient seeing the door closing and perhaps feelingless claustrophobic at the start of treatment.

5.11 Laminated walls and roofs

The term 'laminated' is used to describe walls or roofs where steel plates or lead sheets have been introduced into the concrete walls or roof of the bunker to reduce the transmission when space is limited and there is not the depth or height to make the wall or roof completely of concrete. Normally this is only necessary in primary beam shielding and with higher energy linear accelerators. The total transmission is the product of the transmission factors for each of the constituents of the barrier. At energies above 8.5 MV, these materials will be a source of photoneutrons and there must be sufficient concrete on each side of the steel or lead to absorb the neutrons and capture gamma rays to reduce the internal and external surface dose rates to acceptable levels (see figure 5.14(a)). Lead (Pb-207) has a (γ,n) threshold of 6.7 MeV and steel (Fe-56) has a threshold of 11.2 MeV.

NCRP Report 144 (NCRP 2003) recommends that any steel sheeting should be backed by at least 0.6 m of concrete.

McGinley (1992) has developed an expression to estimate the neutron dose equivalent H_n (μSv per week) beyond the barrier when the beam collimation is opened to it maximum extent:

$$H_n = D_o \times R \times F_{max} \times 10^{-t_1/TVL_x} \times 10^{-t_2/TVL_n}/(t_m + t_2 + 0.3), \quad (5.23)$$

where D_o is the x-ray absorbed dose per week at the isocentre (cGy per week); R is the neutron production coefficient (neutron microsievert per x-ray centigray per beam area in m^2 ($\mu Sv\ cGy^{-1}\ m^{-2}$); F_{max} is the maximum field size at the isocentre (m^2); t_m is the thickness of the metal layer (m); t_1 is the thickness of the concrete on the side of the treatment room (m); t_2 is the thickness of the concrete beyond the metal layer (m); TVL_x is the TVL in concrete for the primary beam (m); TVL_n is the TVL in concrete for neutrons (m); and 0.3 is the distance from the external surface of the barrier to the point of calculation (m).

McGinley (1992) also gives values for the neutron production coefficient (R) of 3.5 and 19 $\mu Sv\ cGy^{-1}\ m^{-2}$ for lead at 15 and 18 MV, respectively, and 1.7 $\mu Sv\ cGy^{-1}\ m^{-2}$ for steel at 18 MV. NCRP (2005) suggests 0.25 m is a conservative value for TVL_n.

McGinley and Butker (1994) made measurements on the laminated ceilings of bunkers with accelerators operating at 15 and 18 MV. They found that a safe estimate of the photon dose equivalent from x-ray and capture gamma rays at the exterior

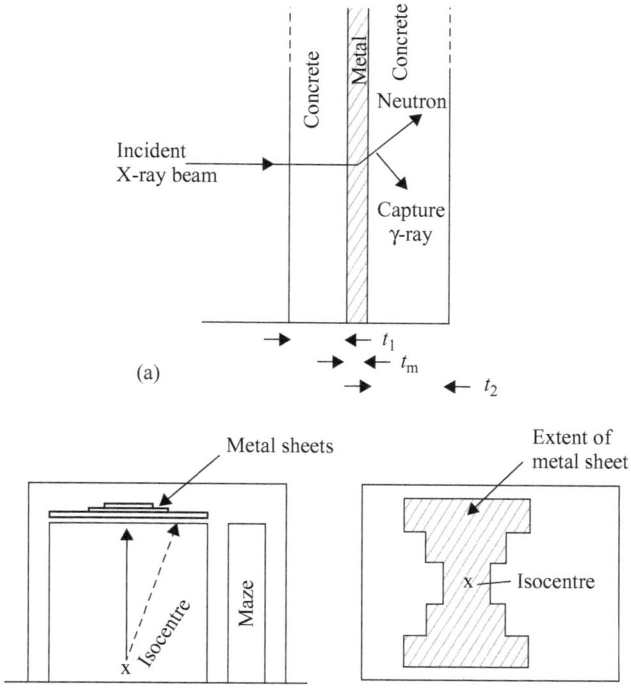

Figure 5.14. (a) Laminated wall section. (b) Shaping of metal sheet to minimise use.

surface can be obtained if the calculated transmitted x-ray dose equivalent (H_{tr}) is multiplied by 2.7. The total dose equivalent (H_{tot}) outside the barrier is then given by

$$H_{tot} = H_n + 2.7H_{tr}. \tag{5.24}$$

Rezende *et al* (2014) have used the Monte Carlo code MCNPX to check the validity of equation (5.23) using lead and steel layers in concrete at 15 and 18 MV. Calculations were performed with the metal layer one and/or two TVL thick with the layer on the incident surface, in the middle and on the external surface of the concrete barrier. This was done for each of total thicknesses of 4, 5 and 6 TVLs of concrete. In all cases the Monte Carlo calculated value exceeded the analytical value calculated using equation (5.23) by a factor ranging from 1.2 to 14.8. Selecting the simulations where the metal layer was two TVL thick and in the middle of the concrete yields the factors shown in table 5.12. The authors suggest that these multiplicative factors can be used to correct the values for neutron dose equivalent determined with equation (5.23) when the configuration of the barrier is similar to one of those used in the Monte Carlo simulation. They also found that equation (5.23) was very sensitive to the value of TVL_n and after determining this parameter for the different barrier configurations recommend that a value of 0.36 m is used in equation (5.23).

Because these materials are expensive, the number of the plates or sheets, i.e. the thickness, can be reduced away from the beam axis due to the increasing obliquity of

Table 5.12. Multiplication factors developed by Rezende *et al* (2014) to correct the neutron dose equivalents calculated with equation (5.23) at the exterior surface of laminated barriers.

End point energy (MeV)	Metal layer	Multiplying factor: Total thickness 4 TVL	5 TVL	6 TVL
15	Lead	7.3	8.5	[a]
18	Lead	3.4	3.1	1.9
18	Steel	2.1	4.4	[a]

[a] Values not considered because the uncertainties in MCNPX were greater than 20%.

the radiation path in the surrounding concrete. The width of the plates or sheets can also be matched to the width of the radiation beam at its greatest extent allowing for gantry rotation, being narrowest where the beam strikes the wall or roof perpendicularly (see figure 5.14(b)).

5.12 Spreadsheet approach for primary and secondary shielding

The required thickness of primary and secondary shielding can be calculated by incorporating the equations and factors described in sections 5.1 and 5.2 into a spreadsheet and is a good aid to optimising shielding design. It allows the ready recalculation of shielding thicknesses to achieve a particular dose constraint or the impact of altering the thickness on annual doses and instantaneous dose rates. It also enables the designer to examine the impact of different workloads.

References

Al-Affan I A M 2000 Estimation of the dose at the maze entrance for x-rays from radiotherapy linear accelerators *Med. Phys.* **27** 231–8

Barish R J 2005 Minimising entrance door thickness for direct-entry radiotherapy rooms *Health Phys.* **89** 168–71

Barish R J 2009 Neutron door design *Proc. Radiation Shielding in Medical Installations (Instituto Techologico e Nuclear, Unidade de Proteccao e Seguranca Radiologica, Ericeira, Portugal)*

Biggs P J 1996 Obliquity factors for Co-60 and 4, 10 and 18 MV x-rays for concrete, steel, and lead and angles of incidence between 0° and 70° *Health Phys.* **70** 527–36

DIN (Deutsches Institut für Normung) 2008 *Medical Electron Accelerators—Part 2: Rules for Construction of Structural Radiation Protection* DIN 6847-2 (Berlin: DIN)

IAEA (International Atomic Energy Authority) 2006 *Radiation Protection in the Design of Radiotherapy Facilities (Safety Report Series* No 47) (Vienna: IAEA)

IEC (International Electrotechnical Commission) 2009 *Medical Electrical Equipment—Part 2-1: Particular Requirements for the Safety of Electron Accelerators in the Range 1 MeV to 50 MeV* 60601-2-1, 2nd edn (Geneva: IEC)

IPEM (Institute of Physics and Engineering in Medicine) 1997 *The Design of Radiotherapy Treatment Room Facilities* Report 75 (York: IPEM)

Kersey R W 1979 Estimation of neutron and gamma radiation doses in the entrance mazes of SL75-20 linear accelerator treatment rooms *Medicamundi* **24** 151–5

Maerker R E and Muckenthaler F J 1967 Monte Carlo calculations, using the albedo concept, of the fast-neutron dose rates along the center lines of one-and two-legged square concrete open ducts and comparison with experiment *Nucl. Sci. Eng.* **27** 423–33

McCall R C 1997 Shielding for thermal neutrons *Med. Phys.* **24** 135–6

McCall R C, McGinley P H and Huffman K E 1999 Room scattered neutrons *Med. Phys.* **26** 206–7

McGinley P H 1992 Photoneutron production in the primary barriers of medical accelerator rooms *Health Phys.* **62** 359–62

McGinley P H 1993 Radiation skyshine produced by an 18 MeV medical accelerator *Radiat. Prot. Manag.* **10** 59

McGinley P H 2002 *Shielding Techniques for Radiation Oncology Facilities* (Madison, WI: Medical Physics)

McGinley P H and Butker E K 1991 Evaluation of neutron dose equivalent levels at the maze entrance of medical accelerator treatment rooms *Med. Phys.* **18** 279–81

McGinley P H and Butker E K 1994 Laminated primary ceiling barriers for medical accelerator rooms *Phys. Med. Biol.* **39** 1331–8

McGinley P H and Huffman K E 2000 Photon and neutron dose equivalent in the maze of a high-energy medical accelerator facility *Radiat. Prot. Manag.* **17** 43–7

McGinley P H and James J L 1997 Maze design methods for 6- and 10-MeV accelerators *Radiat. Prot. Manag.* **14** 59–64

McGinley P H and Miner M S 1995 A history of radiation shielding of x-ray therapy room *Health Phys.* **69** 759–65

McGinley P H, Miner M S and Mitchum M L 1995 A method of calculating the dose due to capture gamma rays in accelerator mazes *Phys. Med. Biol.* **40** 1467–73

NCRP (National Council on Radiation Protection and Measurements) 1977 *Radiation Protection Design Guidelines for 0.1–100 MeV Particle Accelerator Facilities* Report 51 (Bethesda, MD: NCRP)

NCRP (National Council on Radiation Protection and Measurements) 1984 *Neutron Contamination from Medical Electron Accelerators* Report 79 (Bethesda, MD: NCRP)

NCRP (National Council on Radiation Protection and Measurements) 2003 *Radiation Protection for Particle Accelerator Facilities* Report 144 (Bethesda, MD: NCRP)

NCRP (National Council on Radiation Protection and Measurements) 2005 *Structural Shielding Design and Evaluation for Megavoltage X- and Gamma-Ray Radiotherapy Facilities* Report 151 (Bethesda, MD: NCRP)

Nelson W R and Lariviere P D 1984 Primary and secondary leakage calculations at 6, 10 and 25 MeV *Health Phys.* **47** 811–8

Rezende G F S, Da Rosa L A R and Facure A 2014 Production of neutrons in laminated barriers of radiotherapy rooms: comparison between the analytical methodology and Monte Carlo simulations *J. Appl. Clin. Med. Phys.* **15** 247–55

Wu R K and McGinley P H 2003 Neutron and capture gamma along the mazes of linear accelerator vaults *J. Appl. Clin. Med. Phys.* **4** 162–71

Chapter 6

Monte Carlo methods

S Green, Z Ghani and F Fiorini

6.1 Introduction

The Monte Carlo technique offers the possibility of performing a complete simulation of a radiation shielding facility in all its geometrical complexity. In principle, the outcomes from such simulations are limited in accuracy only by the knowledge of the underlying cross-sections which govern the radiation interactions, the detail with which the shielding walls and other structures are modelled, the detailed representation of the radiation source and the available computing facilities. For radiotherapy treatment rooms where materials are generally quite standard and walls are constructed in large monolithic blocks, the main limitations in practice for calculation of the leakage radiation field intensity/dose rates are the accuracy with which the radiation source is modelled and the representation of the configuration and composition of shielding walls.

For calculation of other parameters, such as generated neutron spectrum and induced activity, there may be other limitations on accuracy which result from the chosen modelling code.

This chapter is a re-write and update of the Monte Carlo modelling chapter of IPEM Report 75 (1997). A slightly different approach is taken and the emphasis is changed to reflect the interest of the authors. It draws together the results of a number of research projects in Birmingham over the intervening period. These include O'Hara (2003) and Hall (2009) with additional input from the authors. Since the production of IPEM Report 75, the revolution in computer processing power has continued and this has changed the use to which Monte Carlo simulations for shielding can be put. In the mid-1990s, it was reasonable to perform Monte Carlo simulations to check a room design which had been arrived at by conventional approaches. It was reasonable to make a few minor changes to the room layout or the linear accelerator source characteristics and perform simulations which would each take many hours (in excess of around 24 h) on easily available computers. Now,

doi:10.1088/978-0-7503-1440-4ch6

20 years later, on modern high power parallel computers, results can be obtained in a few minutes, allowing in principle the opportunity to fully design and optimise the bunker layout based on Monte Carlo simulations.

6.2 Available Monte Carlo codes and deciding which one to use

One of the first decisions to be made by those wishing to embark on a programme of simulations is which of the available codes is most suitable. There is now a large list of candidates, which will be described only in general terms in this section. The major codes are included, but others which are not described may also have merit.

MCNP (in all its versions) is developed and supported by teams at Los Alamos Laboratory (https://mcnp.lanl.gov/). The code has its origins in the nuclear programme of the United States and is an excellent code for basic radiation shielding. The majority of the examples quoted in this chapter are of use of MCNPX, which is a version of MCNP initially developed to extend the capabilities of the code to charged particles. It is now merged into the main MCNP code in version 6. It is available in the UK, subject to security checks, to individual named users. In the past, access has been through the Nuclear Energy Agency (NEA) code data-bank[1] but now users must apply direct to the Radiation Safety Information Computational Centre (RISCC) in Oak Ridge. For linear accelerator bunker shielding it is greatly aided by the use of the visualisation and geometry editing package *Visual Editor* or *VISED* (http://www.mcnpvised.com/), which, amongst other functions, allows interactive viewing of transport calculations and particle tracks. For calculations to determine generated activity, there are companion codes such as FISPACT (now incorporated into the EASY-2010 (European Activation System) code) which provide valuable additional functionality. MCNP is now a coupled neutron, photon, electron and light-ion simulation package, and is capable of modelling the generation and transport of neutrons in higher energy linear accelerator bunkers (GEANT and FLUKA also have this capability).

GEANT is a general purpose physics modelling code developed at CERN for modelling of particle physics collisions, detector configurations and detailed interactions. It is a complex code which requires considerable investment to become proficient, but is very well capable of simulating all of the necessary components of a linear accelerator bunker. Geometry and particle track visualisation tools are well developed and available within the GEANT code package. All important particles are well modelled and there are a number of additional user codes which have been developed that can greatly help with generation of an accurate source model. As examples, GATE is an open source tool for imaging and radiotherapy simulation (http://www.opengatecollaboration.org/), TOPAS is a tool for modelling particle

[1] From the website of the NEA: 'The Nuclear Energy Agency (NEA) is a specialised agency within the Organisation for Economic Co-operation and Development (OECD), an intergovernmental organisation of industrialised countries based in Paris, France.... The Data Bank's primary role is to provide scientists in member countries with reliable nuclear data and computer programs for use in different nuclear applications.'

therapy beamlines (Perl *et al* 2012) and MULASSIS is a tool for simulation of layered shield-type geometries aimed at space applications (Lei *et al* 2002).

FLUKA (http://www.fluka.org, Ferrari *et al* 2005) is a general multi-purpose code developed by a world-wide collaboration headed by authors from CERN and the Italian Nuclear Physics Institute (INFN). Since the early phases of development, FLUKA has been focused on calorimetry, shielding calculations and radiation studies in high energy experimental physics and engineering, but it can currently be used for target and detector design, cosmic ray, space physics, radiation damage to electronics, dosimetry and medical physics studies.

It is underpinned by an accurate handling of a wide range of reaction channels, which are constantly corroborated with experimental data comparison in order to achieve better code performances. Of particular note for radiation protection are the tools to easily calculate induced activity and dose equivalents as well as its double capability to be used in a biased mode and as a fully analogue code. This means that while the code can be used to predict fluctuations, signal coincidences and other correlated events, a wide choice of statistical techniques are also available to investigate low statistics/rare events with the advantage of decreasing the simulation time.

McBend is developed and maintained by the ANSWERS group (now part of Amec Foster Wheeler). It is available on an annual licence and also via consultancy services from the ANSWERS team (http://www.answerssoftwareservice.com/mcbend/). The code has been through a high degree of quality assurance and implemented some leading features (such as adjoint calculations of importance maps to optimise calculation time) before they were available in other codes. It is able to transport neutrons, photons and electrons and has all the main elements for high quality linear accelerator bunker simulations.

The EGS codes (EGS4, EGSnrc, etc) were developed to accurately model coupled electron–photon problems in particle physics, with much work performed over the years to provide excellent modelling of electron condensed histories at lower energies such as those of interest to medical physics. EGSnrc is maintained by a team at the National Research Council of Canada (see http://www.nrc-cnrc.gc.ca/eng/solutions/advisory/egsnrc_index.html) and EGS by a team at the KEK the physics research facility (see http://rcwww.kek.jp/research/egs/egs5.html). The strength of EGS (and Penelope, see below) is in detailed studies of radiation dose to patients, detector modelling and other problems where a high degree of accuracy of electron transport models is required. It could in principle be used to model linear accelerator bunkers (and has been used for this purpose); this, however, is not the main strength of the code.

Penelope has been developed by the nuclear physics group at the University of Barcelona and is also available from the NEA data-bank (see http://www.oecd-nea.org/tools/abstract/detail/nea-1525). It provides excellent physics modelling of electron–photon physics and detailed transport, including transport of individual electrons. Such modelling accuracy comes at the expense of calculation time and since such detail is not generally necessary for a linear accelerator bunker, Penelope is little used for this purpose.

6.3 Using the MCNP code

To perform an MCNP simulation, users construct an input file where each line represents an instruction to configure all aspects of the problem to be simulated. The traditional method is to perform this task by hand, with a simple text editor, drawing from the knowledge and experience of the user and the detailed instructions of the code manual. While this section will focus on MCNP, the general approach of code-input specified through an edited text file is also followed by FLUKA and some of the other codes highlighted above.

6.3.1 Specification of the source characteristics

For linear accelerator shielding calculations this could be an approximated photon source defined to allow for a primary beam of a certain size plus the additional component of head-leakage. Alternatively, it is possible to directly simulate the linear accelerator head in some detail, modelling the key components that will influence the simulation results. This approach is required if induced neutron dose rates are to be considered. These neutrons are produced primarily by (γ, n) reactions in the tungsten alloy target, the primary collimation and flattening filter so their direct simulation is helpful. This was the approach taken by O'Hara (2003) for simulations of a 15 MV Elekta Precise accelerator and then more recently by the authors for simulation of a 10 MV Varian accelerator.

The final head geometry used for the Varian accelerator bunker design simulation is shown in figure 6.1 as displayed through VISED, where the head shielding is approximated by an iron shell surrounded by a lead shell.

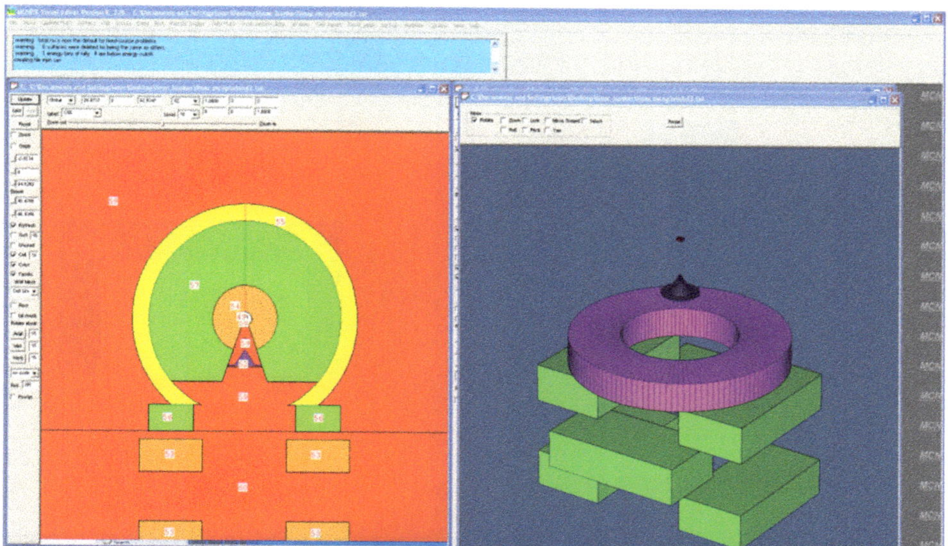

Figure 6.1. VISED screen shot of linear accelerator head model with gross shielding removed (right).

6.3.2 Specification of the room geometry and materials to be simulated

This is most likely where users will expend most effort; constructing and debugging the MCNP required definitions of surfaces and their intersections to form volumes (termed cells by MCNP). The user also specifies the materials of each cell through material cards which point MCNP directly to individual atomic cross-sections, which are part of the very large library of cross-sections distributed with MCNP. For linear accelerator shielding, all important materials are readily available from these libraries.

As an alternative to the traditional manual entry approach, it is possible using VISED to create a complete bunker model from architect's drawings using *Solid Works*. These drawings may require modification to remove 'complex' surfaces and superfluous details before the CAD files are converted into a format suitable for VISED. To create the room geometry shown in figure 6.2, VISED's native CAD conversion tool was used to create the cells and surfaces required by MCNP to define the problem geometry. Figure 6.2 shows a VISED plot of the final geometry model with the linear accelerator head in the room, the magnetite concrete primary barrier as blue cells and ordinary concrete as red cells. In figure 6.2, the beam is directed towards the primary barrier nearest the maze entrance and figure 6.3 shows a 30 cm × 30 cm × 30 cm water phantom positioned so that the isocentre lies at 5 cm deep in the phantom to reflect the calibration conditions for this machine.

As an alternative to VISED, Varian have developed the user-interface for the 3D discrete ordinates code ATTILA (Wareing *et al* 2001) to also allow geometry data import from a variety of CAD formats and specification of tally and other

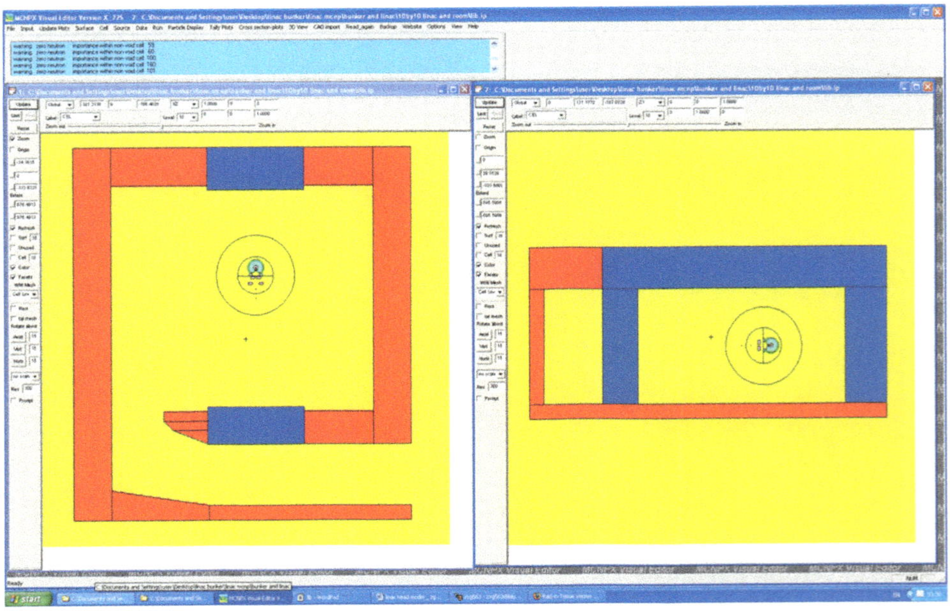

Figure 6.2. A basic room layout displayed in VISED as a horizontal section at isocentre height (on the left) and a vertical cut through the primary barrier, maze and linear accelerator treatment head (on the right).

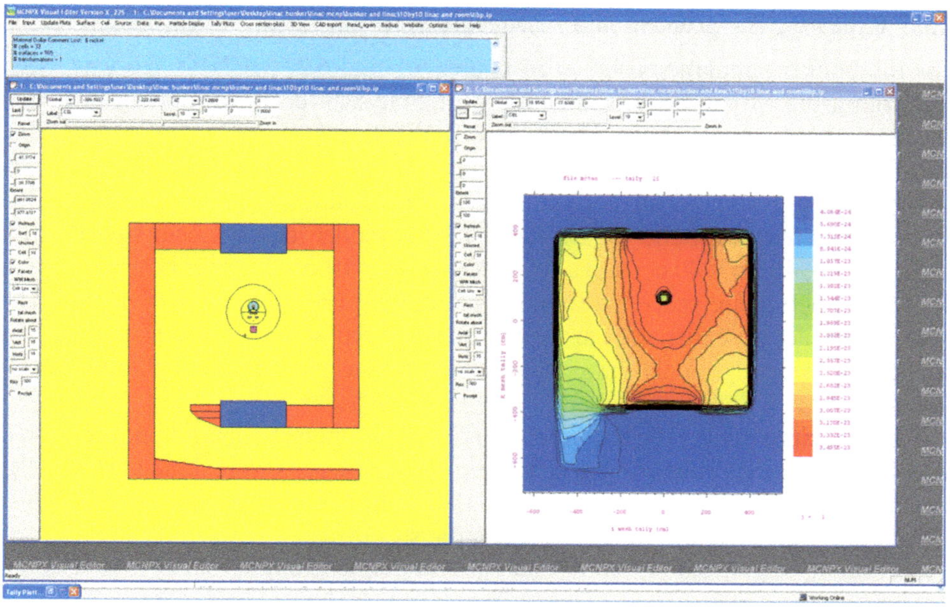

Figure 6.3. Linear accelerator bunker with treatment head (left) and photon ambient dose equivalent distribution (right). The colour scale is in units of Sv e^{-1}.

parameters to drive an MCNP calculation entirely from the user-interface (see Atilla4MC at http://www.varian.com/sites/default/files/Attila4MCOverview.pdf).

6.3.3 Description of the tally volumes and types

All Monte Carlo codes require the user to specify the locations within the simulated geometry at which the result (fluence, dose, etc) is required. Traditionally these so-called *tallies* take the form of volumes which are part of the simulated real-world geometry of the problem, and historically needed to be large volumes to maximise the efficiency of the simulation. Modern versions of codes such as MCNP make it possible to calculate the required result across a large mesh of tally volumes spread across the simulated geometry. This mesh is quite separate from the simulated real-world geometry. The quantity that MCNP will actually calculate is determined by the type of tally selected and any further conversion coefficient data which are specified by what are termed tally multipliers. MCNP includes tables for fluence-to-dose conversion factors, but users are also able to specify their own as required.

6.3.4 Other input cards

MCNP allows users to define a number of other aspects of the problem to be simulated. For problems which would otherwise be computationally inefficient, importance weighting can be used to preferentially increase the attention paid by MCNP to selected parts of the geometry, selected energy regions, etc. There are also basic controls of the number of simulated particles, computer run-time, etc.

6.3.5 Executing the problem in a reasonable time

For the bunker simulations shown in figures 6.1 and 6.2, MCNPX 2.6 was used to carry out a full Monte Carlo simulation of the physical problem running in electron, photon and neutron physics modes. ENDF/B-VII (http://www.nndc.bnl.gov/endf/b7.1) continuous energy, nuclear and atomic data were used, along with the current version of the LA150U photo-nuclear data libraries. To optimise run-time, separate phase spaces were created around the accelerator head model for each field size of interest (1 cm × 1 cm, 40 cm × 40 cm and a reference 10 cm × 10 cm field) for both photons and neutrons. Each phase space file took approximately 100 h of simulation time. These phase space files were then used in the complete simulations of the accelerator head and bunker and were repeatedly sampled, with simulations typically taking another 100 or so hours.

Thus the simulation time required to arrive at a total neutron and photon dose per field size was of the order of ~400 h. Fortunately these runs were done in parallel and concurrently on the University of Birmingham's high performance computer cluster (BlueBear) and took no more than a few days.

6.3.6 Validating the simulations

Before the results of any calculation are considered in detail, it is essential to take steps to validate the simulation model. In the case of the 10 MV Varian accelerator and bunker being modelled above, some data are available from published sources for benchmarking.

Photon leakage was evaluated in the accelerator head model using large spherical volumes to calculate track length estimates of fluence outside the head. These estimates of fluence were then used to calculate an absorbed dose to water or air. Data produced by Varian (Varian Medical Systems 2014) suggest that leakage 1 m from the target reaches a maximum of 0.0233% of the isocentre dose rate. On the assumption that the average level is lower than this, the thickness of the iron/lead layers shown in figure 6.1 was varied to achieve a leakage at 90 degrees of 0.01%.

Obtaining solid data for neutron head leakage dose rates from clinical accelerators is not easy. Varian themselves (Varian Medical Systems 2014) suggest that while neutrons can be measured at the isocentre in a 10 cm × 10 cm field (at 0.0013% of the isocentre dose rate), the leakage outside the patient plane is 0.0000% at 10 MV. This is an artefact of the suggested measurement approach for 10 MV which is intended to ensure that the IEC leakage criteria are met, rather than to accurately measure the actual (very low) neutron leakage.

The simulations performed here are outside the patient plane and give dose rates of approximately 25 μSv per photon Gy at 1 m from the target. A continuous-energy fluence-to-dose conversion function has been used to calculate ambient dose equivalent within the MCNP model. The value of 25 μSv per photon Gy is 0.0025% of the isocentre dose rate—which is not too different from the level quoted by Varian in the patient plane of 0.0013%. Of note here also is the work of the team from SLAC some years ago (Liu *et al* 1997) who used a complex model (necessary at the time) involving two other Monte Carlo codes (EGS for photon transport and

MORSE for neutron transport) plus an analytical step to link them together. Their results suggest that with jaws closed the neutron leakage rates at different positions around the head vary by less than a factor of 3, and they quote a neutron leakage figure of 20 μSv per photon Gy at 10 MV for Varian Clinac accelerators. This is in close agreement with the MCNP model described here, but of course also comes from a simulation.

Trends in the data should also be examined to ensure that they are sensible. It is regularly reported for Varian accelerators that larger field sizes are associated with reduced neutron dose rates surrounding the treatment head; this would be expected with the open jaws presenting less of a target for photo-neutron production.

6.3.7 Results and their interpretation

For the bunker simulations, results were tallied in such a way so as to show a dose 'everywhere' in the room, centred at the height of the isocentre. These results, known as mesh tallies in MCNPX, tally a track length estimate of neutron or photon fluence in a voxel mesh specified by the user. The results of these fluence calculations were multiplied by an ambient dose equivalent conversion function. All tallies are normalized per source particle with the source particle being an electron, therefore yielding results in terms of sieverts per electron. A sample photon ambient dose equivalent distribution is shown in figure 6.3 (right) for a 10 cm × 10 cm field, the colour scale is in units of Sv e^{-1}. A sample plot showing ambient dose equivalents for neutrons (left) and neutron induced photons (right) is shown in figure 6.4. As shown in figures 6.3 and 6.4, results are tallied separately for neutrons, photons and

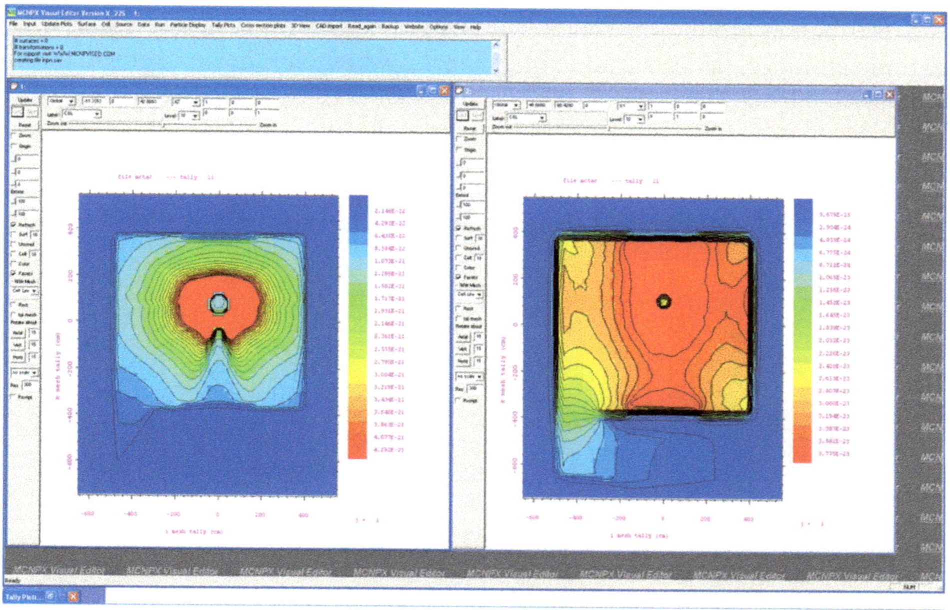

Figure 6.4. A mesh tally plot showing ambient dose equivalents for: neutrons (left) and neutron induced photons (right), i.e. prompt activation photons.

activation photons. Separate processing is then performed using utilities in codes such as *MatLab* to convert to more easily interpretable dose-rates and overlaying the knowledge that the linear accelerator will actually deliver a dose rate of (for example) 6 Gy min^{-1} at the isocentre.

6.3.8 Enhanced particle track visualisation capabilities

MCNP has always included a reasonable plotting package which helped to remove errors and inconsistencies in the specification of the simulated geometry. As noted above, in recent years this has been supplemented by VISED which provides vastly improved functionality for both geometry visualisation and alteration, and visualisation of particle tracks. It is possible to run MCNP within the environment provided by VISED and to select the nature of particle tracks to be displayed as the program executes. In this way, images such as the one in figure 6.5(a) have been generated. In figure 6.5 the bunker walls are shown in red and the air volume in yellow. A particular tally volume has been designated (in this case near to the maze entrance to the bunker) and the particle tracks which eventually reach this region are shown. It is clear from figure 6.5(a) that the majority of particles reaching the entrance are scattered from the phantom used to simulate the effect of the patient. These will be a small subset of the total particles simulated and if all were shown, the image would be impossible to interpret in this way.

It is also apparent to some extent from figure 6.5(a) that there is a variation in intensity in the radiation field reaching the door, which becomes more obvious when a full mesh tally simulation is performed. Figure 6.5(b) shows the bunker geometry superimposed with a colour-wash representation of a mesh tally calculation of the dose distribution around the room. The red primary beam is clearly visible and at the room entrance, the penetration of a higher dose region (shown in green) through the marked edge of the room door is clearly seen. The capability to see such detail in the dose-map is a function both of the mesh tally and a modern computer system to produce results in a short time (minutes rather than hours).

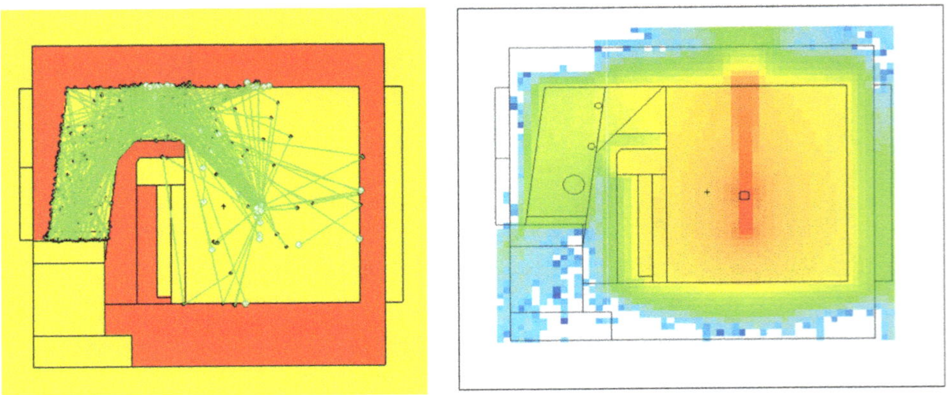

Figure 6.5. (a) A VISED plot of scattered photon tracks which ultimately reach the room door. (b) The MCNP mesh tally result for the same bunker geometry.

One situation which is commonly encountered in radiotherapy is the need to add shielding to an existing bunker where there are significant space constraints. This often leads to the use of high atomic number materials such as steel or lead. While this is very effective as a photon shield, adding such materials does have the potential to generate additional neutron (and prompt gamma) emissions, especially if they are placed in the arc of the primary beam. This issue is examined in terms of neutron production by Facure *et al* (2008) and Rezende *et al* (2014) with MCNP. In the paper from Facure *et al*, MCNP5 is used for a 10 MV linear accelerator bunker with consideration of steel or lead combined with concrete primary barriers. While steel has minimal impact, the use of lead significantly adds to neutron production and the location of the lead layer is critical. A lead layer outside the bunker increases neutron dose rates to staff outside, while a lead layer inside the bunker increases neutron dose rates for patients. This leads to a recommendation to surround the lead with a neutron absorbing layer (3 cm thick) of lithium or boron loaded polythene. The later paper from Rezende *et al* looks at linear accelerators energies of 15 and 18 MV and suggests that this kind of steel/lead/concrete laminated barrier geometry is not handled well by the analytical approach of McGinley (McGinley 1992a, 1992b) since MCNPX suggests neutron dose rates at least a factor of 2 higher than the analytical approach.

6.4 Using the FLUKA code

As noted in the introduction to this chapter, the difference between FLUKA and other Monte Carlo codes is mainly in the detailed modelling of a variety of partial reaction channels. This originates in improved modelling of hadronic–nuclear interactions and in nucleus–nucleus interactions. Since these are important in modelling the interactions of charged particles in the calculation of induced neutron spectra and induced activation, FLUKA is a good choice of code for these applications (Bohlen *et al* 2014). The examples which follow below are therefore calculations of this type, and are mainly drawn from the field of particle therapy (reflecting the interests of the authors).

The first FLUKA code, FLUKA86-87, was a specialised program to calculate shielding of high energy protons from accelerators. The current version has been adapted and developed for an extended range of applications and it is no longer limited to protons. Now the transport of more than 60 different particles can be simulated. However, its initial purpose is instructive and demonstrates that the activation calculation feature has always been one of the principal characteristics of the program (see http://www.fluka.org).

FLUKA can handle complex geometries using the Combinatorial Geometry (CG) package. The FLUKA CG code has been designed to track particles even in the presence of magnetic fields (but not yet electric fields). For most applications, no programming is required from the user, however, for more special requirements, such as peculiar source configurations or unusual scoring requirements, several user routines (written in Fortran77) are available for editing to the user needs. If scripting is not in the user capabilities, the program can now be entirely managed and run via an advanced graphical interface called Flair (Vlachoudis 2009) (http://www.fluka.org/flair/index.html), which has been appositely developed to edit FLUKA input files, execute the code and visualise the output files from a GUI environment without the need of command-line interactions. Flair is strictly connected to the development of FLUKA and with the Monte Carlo code improving with each release, Flair also grows in its capabilities. Another graphical interface mainly useful for 3D geometry visualisation that the users can find useful is SimpleGeo (Theis *et al* 2006); this program is an independent project developed at CERN to unify the various geometry modelling processes and syntaxes of radiation transport codes and it is not strictly connected to FLUKA.

One recent study (Al-Affan *et al* 2015) uses FLUKA (and EGS) to model the impact of lining the walls of a bunker maze entrance with layers of lead, acting as an absorber for the low energy scattered photons from the concrete walls and thereby reducing the dose rate at the maze entrance. This study shows the power and flexibility of a Monte Carlo simulation approach as the authors were able to model only the scattered photon component, ignoring head leakage to maximize the sensitivity of their method to changes in scattered dose rate only.

Nuclear activation can be initiated in FLUKA using a card called RADDECAY. There are several ways to score the produced residual nuclei, but the important fact to underline is that the entire process involving the generation and subsequent transport of decay particles, or radiation, including time evolution and tracking, is now obtainable in one single simulation, the same simulation that generates the radio-nuclides. This has been possible using decay emission databases derived from the National Nuclear Data Center (NNDC) of the Brookhaven National Laboratory, and in some cases, when explicit data were not available, models have been used.

Some of the issues in the routine operation of particle therapy facilities using high energy protons relate to the activation of beam-line components (Infantino *et al* 2015) and the associated generation of high energy neutron fields. In proton therapy facilities delivering the beam using the passive scattering method, patient specific collimators are commonly constructed from brass because of its easy machining properties. The data in figure 6.6 show a FLUKA simulation of nuclei produced when a brass block is irradiated with 200 MeV protons (a typical energy for proton radiotherapy). It is clear that a very wide variety of nuclei are produced, with those with a high atomic number originating from the small amount of lead included in the composition of brass. These induced nuclei will decay, mostly very rapidly, and some with the emission of gamma-rays which can be a hazard for staff. These emitted gamma-ray fields can be directly calculated in FLUKA, and example calculations are shown in figure 6.7 for 50, 100 and 150 MeV protons incident on brass. Similar simulations can be performed in the case of facilities using the active scanning delivery method which still have the necessity of adapting the accelerated particle energy to the ones necessary for the therapy by placing energy modulators at the exit of the accelerator (in the case of cyclotrons) and/or range shifters close to the patient body.

It is perhaps worth noting that while the simulations above have been performed with proton radiotherapy in mind, they could just as easily have been performed for

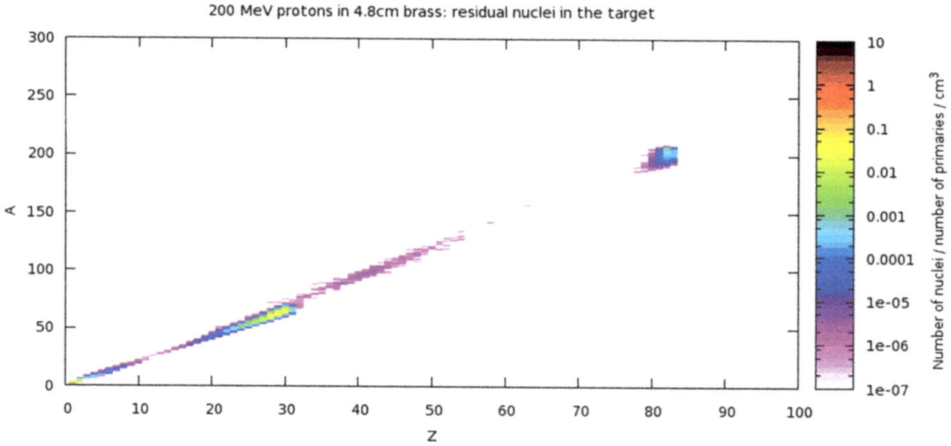

Figure 6.6. FLUKA results for the mass/charge distribution of nuclides produced during 200 MeV proton irradiation of brass.

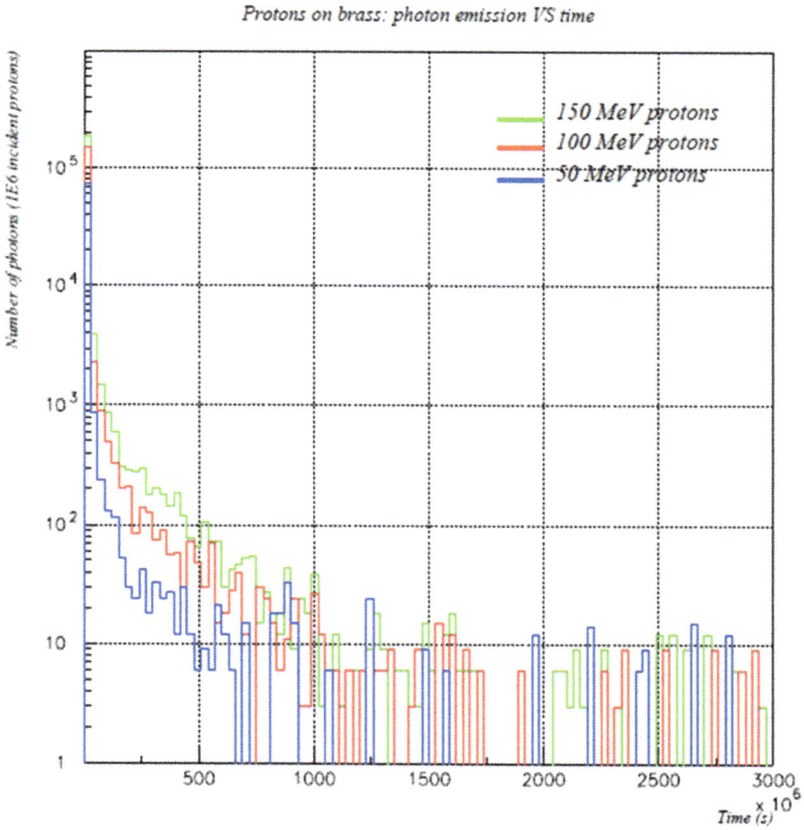

Figure 6.7. Photon emission as a function of time after an extended irradiation of brass by 200 MeV protons.

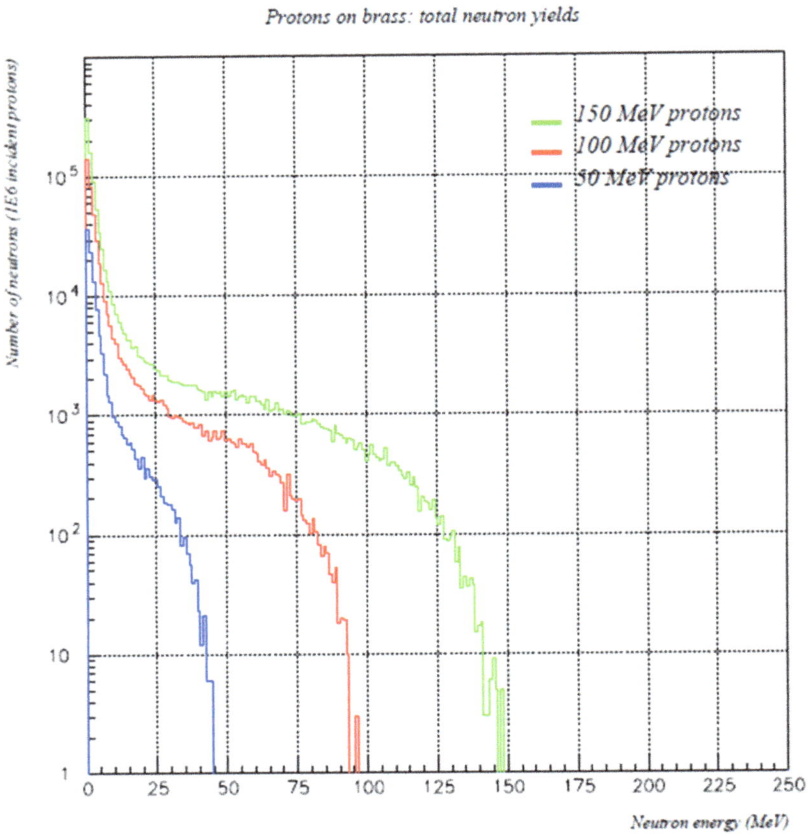

Figure 6.8. FLUKA simulations of neutron spectra produced by irradiation of brass with 50, 100 and 150 MeV protons.

the activation of components in the head of a conventional linear accelerator, for the activation of structural steel-work within the treatment room and its walls or for the activation in ion therapy facilities (Morone *et al* 2008).

It is common for high energy neutrons to be emitted as part of the nuclear reactions that result in residual active nuclei. These neutrons can produce further activations in the treatment room and represent a significant source of whole-body dose and therefore hazard to patients. The biological effectiveness of these very high energy neutrons is subject to considerable uncertainty (Brenner and Hall 2008). The accurate modelling approach that FLUKA follows means it has a better chance than many codes of reproducing these neutron spectra correctly. Figure 6.8 shows the FLUKA calculation of the neutron spectral emissions from irradiation of brass with 50, 100 and 150 MeV protons.

6.5 MCNP, induced neutrons and particle therapy

The ability to generate and model secondary neutron transport within a typical bunker is not unique to FLUKA and (as described in section 6.3) is also available in

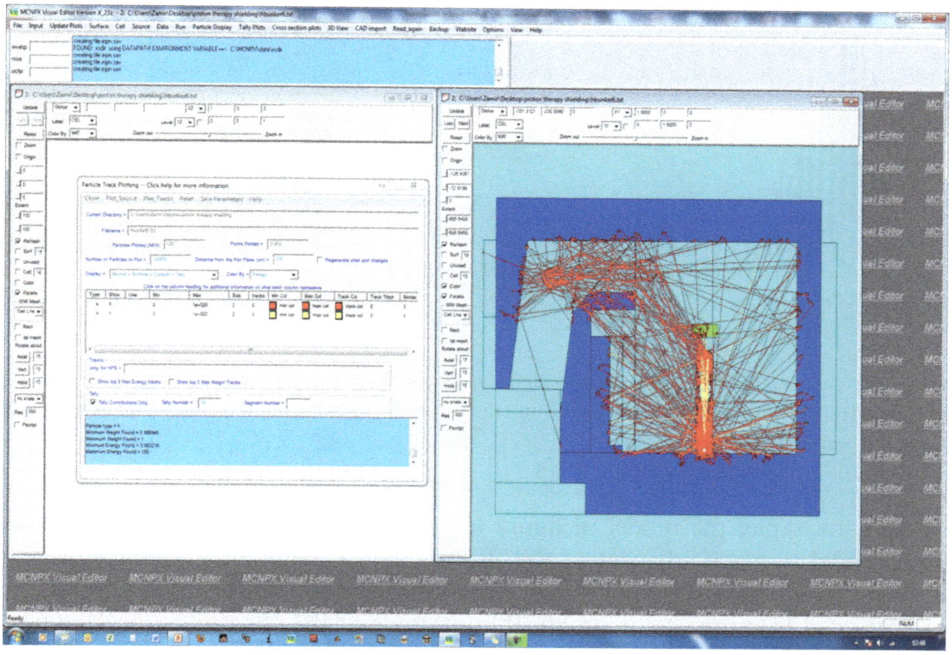

Figure 6.9. VISED representation of the neutron tracks generated by a model passive scattering proton beam nozzle within a linear accelerator bunker.

MCNP. The example in figure 6.9 shows the model of a passive scattered proton beam-line developed by Guan (2009) inserted into the linear accelerator bunker model developed many years ago in Birmingham. This is a very artificial example since the room is small (certainly by the standards of proton radiotherapy rooms) and not suitable for shielding against high energy neutrons. Nevertheless the capabilities of MCNP and VISED are demonstrated. The VISED run was designed to show only those secondary neutrons which are heading (eventually) along the maze and towards the entrance. While it is not particularly clear from figure 6.9, the results are as expected with the majority of the neutrons originating in the scattering foil and the final patient collimator.

6.6 Calculation of whole-body doses

One area where Monte Carlo codes are now especially suited is in the calculation of individual organ and whole-body radiation doses. A number of phantom models have been developed over the years, one of the most recent being that originating from the Visible Human project (Xu *et al* 2000). This has a voxel size of 0.4 mm × 0.4 mm × 1.0 mm with many segmented organs/tissues. The model is such that it can be placed anywhere within a simulation geometry and calculations can be performed in exquisite detail of the doses to different organs. While this is not usually appropriate for staff who might work in the vicinity of a linear accelerator bunker, it does provide a useful tool to investigate doses to patients during radiation therapy.

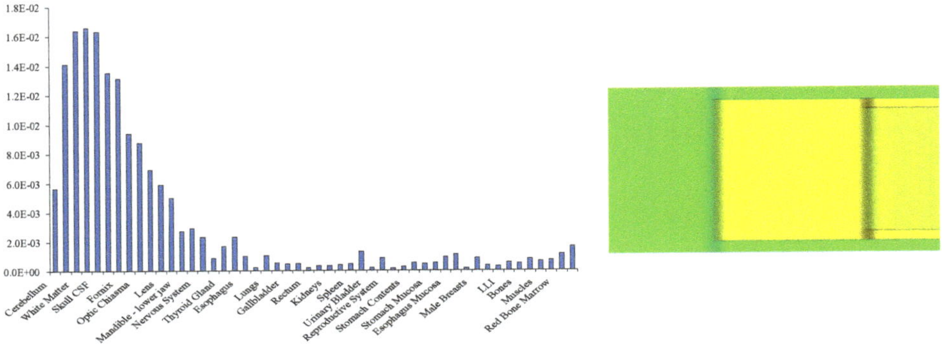

Figure 6.10. Left: a horizontal plane through the Birmingham neutron beam shaping assembly for BNCT and the Visible Human voxel model. Right: Dose rates (in Gy min^{-1}) experienced by a wide range of body organs during a typical treatment irradiation.

As an example, the model in figure 6.10 shows a section of the visible human voxel model in place adjacent to the Birmingham experimental facility for boron neutron capture therapy (BNCT; see Culbertson *et al* 2004). This particular example was designed to mimic some practical limitations of the construction of the beam-shaping assembly (BSA) which has a small gap between the two halves. This was placed in a full model of the BNCT treatment room, and the main purpose of the study was to assess the impact on organ and whole-body doses of neutron absorbent material on the walls of the room. The results on the right of figure 6.10 illustrate the very high degree of sophistication and detail which can be generated in such a model with individual organ doses (in Gy min^{-1}) during a neutron beam irradiation. Clearly the organs receiving the higher doses (mainly to the left in the figure) are in the head which is deliberately irradiated during treatment while those on the right are in the remainder of the body. The latter could be reduced if additional neutron absorbent material is placed on the walls, ceiling and floor of the treatment room.

6.7 Summary

The capabilities of Monte Carlo radiation transport codes continue to advance rapidly and to be supplemented by a growing array of sophisticated supporting programs which ease their use. Modern computing capabilities are such that it is feasible to design a radiotherapy linear accelerator bunker based only on Monte Carlo calculations.

For those considering the use of Monte Carlo codes in this application, while MCNP remains an excellent code, its licencing restrictions may continue to be problematic and the timelines for obtaining a useable version may remain long. For a department hoping to develop expertise amongst a small team of staff, the open access to codes such as FLUKA and GEANT is a substantial advantage. The available interface systems such as GATE (for GEANT) and Flair (for FLUKA) do much to reduce the learning-curve associated with these codes, and their excellent underpinning physics models should deliver accurate results when used correctly.

References

Al-Affan I A M *et al* 2015 Dose reduction of scattered photons from concrete walls lined with lead: implications for improvement in design of megavoltage radiation therapy facility mazes *Med. Phys.* **42** 606–14

Bohlen T T *et al* 2014 The FLUKA code: developments and challenges for high energy and medical applications *Nucl. Data Sheets* **120** 211–4

Brenner D J and Hall E J 2008 Secondary neutrons in clinical proton radiotherapy: a charged issue *Radiother. Oncol.* **86** 165–70

Culbertson C N *et al* 2004 In-phantom characterisation studies at the Birmingham Accelerator-Generated epithermal Neutron Source (BAGINS) BNCT Facility *Appl. Radiat. Isot.* **61** 733–8

Facure A, da Silva A X, da Rosa L A R, Cardoso S C and Rezende G F S 2008 On the production of neutrons in laminated barriers for 10 MV medical accelerator rooms *Med. Phys.* **33** 3285–92

Ferrari A, Sala P R, Fasso A and Ranft J 2005 *FLUKA: A Multi-Particle Transport Code* CERN-2005-10 (2005) INFN/TC_05/11 *SLAC-R* **773**

Guan F 2009 Design and simulation of a passive-scattering nozzle in proton beam radiotherapy *PhD thesis* Texas A&M University

Hall G 2009 Optimisation of the BNCT treatment room shielding by evaluation of neutron and photon dose in organs of VIP-Man, using MCNPX *MSc thesis* (Birmingham, UK: University of Birmingham)

Infantino A *et al* 2015 Accurate Monte Carlo modeling of cyclotrons for optimization of shielding and activation calculations in the biomedical field *Radiat. Phys. Chem.* **116** 231–6

IPEM (Institute of Physics and Engineering in Medicine) 1997 *The Design of Radiotherapy Treatment Room Facilities Report* 75 (York: IPEM)

Lei F *et al* 2002 MULASSIS: a Geant4-based multilayered shielding simulation tool *IEEE Trans. Nucl. Sci.* **49** 2788–93

Liu J C, Kase K R, Mao X S, Nelson W R, Kleck J H and Johnson S 1997 Calculations of photoneutrons from Varian Clinac accelerators and their transmission through materials SLAC-PUB-704 http://inspirehep.net/record/731803/files/slac-pub-7404.pdf (Accessed: 8 November 2016)

McGinley P H 1992a Photoneutron production in the primary barriers of medical accelerator rooms *Health Phys.* **62** 359–62

McGinley P H 1992b Photoneutron fields in medical accelerator rooms with primary barriers constructed of concrete and metals *Health Phys.* **63** 698–701

Morone M C, Calabretta L, Cuttone G and Fiorini F 2008 Monte Carlo simulation to evaluate the contamination in an energy modulated carbon ion beam for hadron therapy delivered by cyclotron *Phys. Med. Biol.* **53** 6045–53

O'Hara M E 2003 Neutron dose evaluation in the maze of a linear accelerator treatment room using MCNP4C2 *MSc thesis* (Birmingham, UK: University of Birmingham)

Perl J, Shin J, Schuemann S, Faddegon B A and Paganetti H 2012 TOPAS an innovative proton Monte Carlo platform for research and clinical applications *Med. Phys.* **39** 6818–37

Rezende G F S, da Rosa L A R and Facure A 2014 Production of neutrons in laminated barriers of radiotherapy rooms: comparison between the analytical methodology and Monte Carlo simulations *J. Appl. Clin. Med. Phys.* **15** 247–55

Theis C *et al* 2006 Interactive three dimensional visualization and creation of geometries for Monte Carlo calculations *Nucl. Instrum. Methods Phys. Res.* A **562** 827–9

Varian Medical Systems 2014 *Clinac IEC Accompanying Documents 60601-2-1 Type Test: Clinac models include Novalis Tx™, Trilogy Tx, Trilogy, Clinac iX, Clinac CX™, DMX and DHX, High Energy C-Series Clinac Silhouette edn* (Palo Alto, CA: Varian Medical Systems)

Vlachoudis V 2009 FLAIR: a powerful but user friendly graphical interface for FLUKA *Proc. Int. Conf. on Mathematics, Computational Methods & Reactor Physics* (New York: Saratoga Springs)

Wareing T A, McGhee J M, Morel J E and Paultz S D 2001 Discontinuous finite element S_N methods on three-dimensional unstructured grids *Nucl. Sci. Eng.* **138** 256–68

Xu X G, Chao T C and Bozkurt A 2000 VIP-Man: an image-based whole-body adult male model constructed from color photographs of the Visible Human Project for multi-particle Monte Carlo calculations *Health Phys.* **78** 476–86

Chapter 7

Shielding materials and construction details

D J Peet and P W Horton

7.1 Introduction

The specifications of shielding thickness and density in radiotherapy treatment rooms are made as a result of the calculations detailed in chapters 5 and 6. However, those involved in these projects should be aware of the limitations and pitfalls in the construction process. The actual construction of such a structure may have cavities, cracks, gaps or other defects. Joints between materials, e.g. between separately constructed parts of the shielding, or in block construction, or around doors, need to be designed to ensure they do not reduce the integrity of the shielding.

Furthermore the rooms have to have a number of openings in the shielding. The largest of these being for the patient, possibly on a bed or trolley, and the component parts of the equipment itself. As indicated in chapter 5, many linear accelerator bunkers incorporate a maze of some description to reduce the need for large and heavy entrance doors. Nibs and lintels can be used to reduce the level of scattered radiation reaching the bunker entrance. However, doors incorporating shielding may be used when there is insufficient room for a maze. These are described in more detail later in this chapter. Ducts through the shielding or along the maze are required for services such as air-conditioning, electrical power, water supplies and dosimetry cables. Again, their positioning and orientation needs to be considered so as not to reduce the intended radiation protection. Within the bunker the thickness of the shielding may also be reduced by the fitting of devices to the walls, floor or ceiling.

A variety of materials and construction methods have been used in the shielding around radiotherapy installations. They include:

- Concrete (poured).
- Magnetite concrete (poured).
- Concrete blocks.
- High density blocks.
- Steel/laminated barriers.

doi:10.1088/978-0-7503-1440-4ch7

- Lead.
- Forster sandwich.
- Earth.

These will each be considered in turn.

7.1.1 Poured concrete

In the UK the construction material most commonly used for linear accelerator bunkers is poured concrete. The physical density of the concrete will be specified along with the required thickness as part of the design process. In terms of radiation protection the physical density is critical and it is important that the expected value for the proposed installation is used in the shielding calculations. A typical density in the UK is 2350 kg m^{-3} but may vary with the geographical source of the constituents and can vary from supplier to supplier. The density should be checked at regular intervals during the construction of the bunker. This can be done as part of the regular taking of test cubes by the contractor and the density results made available to the radiation protection adviser (RPA).

Concrete is a mixture of aggregate, sand, cement and water. The science of concrete is complicated and the chemical constituents can be specified very precisely to change the strength, density and characteristics of the final product. The chemical composition may be of particular interest if high energy beams are used with the possibility of neutron generation if high Z atoms are present in the mix. This is more important when high density concretes with aggregates such as MagnaDense™ (see below) are used[1].

Poured concrete sets slowly over time. At the same time it shrinks although not significantly in terms of barrier thickness. The shrinkage comes from two main sources—the hydration of the cement and thermal reactions. Hydration is a chemical reaction causing some shrinkage, but this will be uniform across the poured section and any cracking from this would be due to some external restraint on the section. Because the setting reaction is exothermic, heat is generated and if the external surfaces are not insulated, the temperature will not be uniform across the section. The concrete sets at these different temperatures and as it cools to the ambient temperature internal tensions can lead to cracking. Some contractors use thermocouples to assess the temperature and use this as a guide to the timing of the next pour to avoid an excessive heat build-up. Measures to give a more uniform temperature include insulating the external surfaces of the concrete or using a concrete mix with a lower cement content that generates less heat. Thick concrete barriers are sometimes constructed with cooling pipes in the concrete. This approach is not recommended for radiotherapy facilities.

Concrete as a material is very strong in compression but weak in tension. Even small tensile stresses will cause cracking. To control cracking under tension, reinforcement is added, normally steel rods, and this allows the reinforced concrete to withstand tension. The section will still tend to crack if subjected to tension, but

[1] MagnaDense is a trademark of LKAB Minerals.

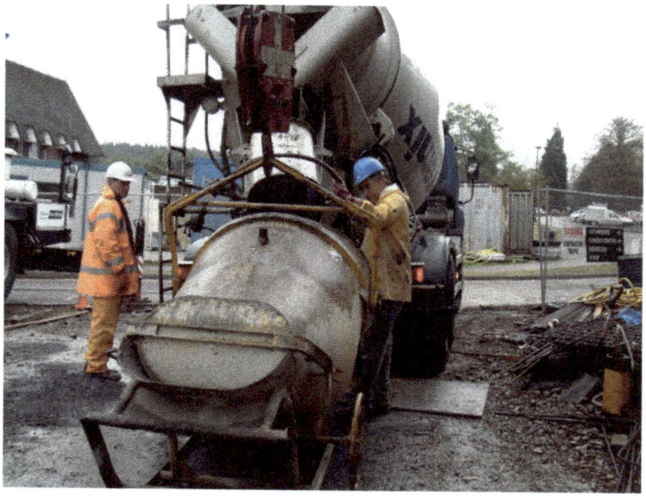

Figure 7.1. Delivery of standard concrete into a hopper to be lifted by crane over the bunker site.

this is controlled by the reinforcement and careful proportioning and siting of the reinforcement can distribute the cracking to give more small (hairline) cracks instead of fewer larger cracks. Discussions should be held with the contractor to establish exactly how the concrete will be poured. The concrete is delivered in trucks which continuously move the concrete mix, preventing it setting (see figure 7.1).

7.1.2 High density concrete

In the 1970s a number of bunkers were constructed using barytes concrete. This increased the physical density to between 3000 and 4000 kg m^{-3} (IPEM 1997). This reduces the thickness of the shielding and therefore the size of the external footprint of the bunker. However, this material is very difficult to work with and is not robust. Walls can be 'powdery'. It is unlikely to be used today but there are still bunkers in the UK and around the world which are made of this material.

A more recent development has been to use higher density natural aggregates resulting in poured concrete with a physical density of 3800 kg m^{-3}. For example, MagnaDense is a high grade aggregate manufactured by LKAB Minerals from the naturally occurring iron oxide ore, magnetite, mined and processed in the north of Sweden. This ensures a long-term reliable source of material of consistent quality. MagnaDense is used as the aggregate in the mix to produce high density concrete. This is readily produced and poured using standard concrete mixing and handling equipment. It is a little darker in appearance than standard concrete. It is more expensive than conventional concrete and less volume can be transported in standard concrete trucks due to its increased density.

This material has been used in a number of installations in the UK for all the walls and ceiling. It has also been used in the primary barriers in the walls and ceiling in some installations to reduce their thickness alongside standard density concrete wall and ceiling sections which form the secondary barriers.

7.1.3 Blocks

Precast interlocking blocks are available in a range of physical densities between 2320 kg m^{-3} and 5000 kg m^{-3} from a number of suppliers. These include NELCO (MegaShield®) and Veritas Medical Solutions (Verishield®) (figure 7.2). A number of installations in the UK have used Ledite® from Atomic International, but this company no longer operates in the UK; Ledite is said to contain fragmented steel scrap (Barish 1993). The use of blocks eliminates the additional work needed on site to ensure the quality of poured concrete by using a factory made product and speeds up the construction process. There is also the potential when the blocks are not mortared together to dismantle an installation and reuse the blocks. The blocks can be very heavy and manual handling issues are a potential concern. Most blocks have a limited range of dimensions, which may result in gaps within a wall which must be

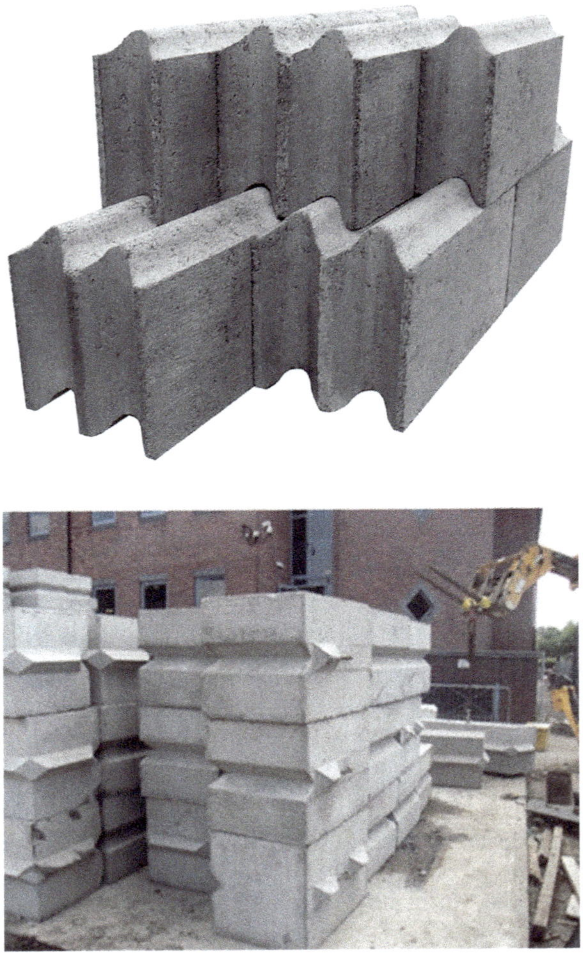

Figure 7.2. Examples of preformed interlocking blocks. Upper image courtesy of Veritas Medical Solutions; lower image courtesy of NELCO Worldwide.

filled. Some barriers are designed to be multiple layers of blocks. In this case the block positions in adjacent rows tend to be staggered, but the issue with gaps then becomes more acute.

The radiation survey of a bunker built with blocks should be done with care in case there are any zones where there have been irregularities in the blocks and any gaps between them have been filled with grout with a lower density and a higher transmission. Interlocking blocks reduce any direct lines of sight through the barrier, but standard concrete blocks can be used if for example a nib is added inside a bunker. In the UK demountable rectangular blocks have also been used. Particular care needs to be taken around the doors if a maze is not used.

7.1.4 Steel sheet

Steel sheet is often used when space is at a premium. At higher energies, neutron production is a concern so it might be considered optimal to embed the steel sheets within the concrete barrier so that any neutrons that are produced are attenuated before reaching either side of the barrier (see sections 5.11 and 6.3). Steel is expensive by comparison with concrete so steel plates of decreasing width can be used. The greatest thickness will be in the plane of the isocentre with the shortest distance between the target and the shielding and the thickness can be reduced away from the isocentre plane to take advantages of increasing obliquity and the longer attenuation path length (see figure 5.14(b)). The sheets require careful positioning during construction. The radiation survey after the installation of the treatment unit needs to be rigorously carried out with a precise knowledge of where the changes in sheet thickness occur. This type of construction is often termed a laminated barrier.

7.1.5 Lead

Lead can be used but with caution at higher linear accelerator energies for the reasons given earlier because of neutron production. It is very expensive. It is usually only used when additional shielding is required because of an equipment upgrade with higher energy or radiation output and there is no other alternative because of limited space. It can be in the form of sheet, which requires additional structural support, or interlocking blocks. It may be appropriate for shielding kilovoltage installations, where the shielding required is less and there is no neutron production.

7.1.6 Sandwich construction

The walls comprise pairs of thin precast concrete panels with an infill of dry mineral ('the sandwich'). The precast panels are made off-site. They are less prone to the cracking and the temperature variations found in large volumes of poured concrete. The required shielding is obtained by calculating the appropriate separation of the panel walls and the density of the infill material. Natural gypsum ($CaSO_4.2H_2O$), limestone ($CaCO_3$) or anorthite ($CaAlSi_2O_8$) are used as fillers suitable for accelerators working up to an end point energy of 20 MV. In the UK, calcium carbonate magnetite and blast furnace slag have been used. Roof shielding is provided by suitably thick containers of the infill material on a concrete roof to the bunker. The design and construction results in bunkers that can be demountable. The technique has been used for linear accelerators and proton therapy centres.

7.1.7 Earth

When facilities are built on a sloping site, bunkers can be set into the hillside using the Earth to reduce the thickness of the rear walls and prevent access. IPEM (1997) quotes a density of 1600 kg m^{-3} for earth fill. Caution may need to be applied if the use of the adjacent land changes and the barrier is dug away for further development.

7.2 Materials with unspecified TVLs

The TVL values for primary radiation in standard concrete, steel and lead are given in table 5.1. TVLs for secondary radiation in standard concrete are given in table 5.2. The TVLs for secondary radiation in steel and lead may be calculated from the secondary TVL for concrete by dividing by the thickness factors for equivalent radiation attenuation set out in table 7.1 (IPEM 1997).

Information on the attenuation properties of high density materials is scarce. This may be because the material is new or the data are not available for commercial reasons. In these situations it will be necessary to infer the TVL for shielding calculations using the inverse relationship between TVL and physical density. Conventional concrete is used as the reference material since its attenuation properties are well established, i.e.

$$\mathrm{TVL}_{\mathrm{material}} = \mathrm{TVL}_{\mathrm{concrete}} \times \rho_{\mathrm{concrete}}/\rho_{\mathrm{material}},$$

where ρ is the physical density.

This relationship relies on the Compton effect for the attenuation of x-ray photons and underestimates the TVL due to the additional presence of pair production as an attenuating mechanism, especially with increasing x-ray energies. Consequently it results in an overprovision of shielding thickness which helps with radiation safety.

Measurements have been carried out on MagnaDense concrete (Jones *et al* 2009) to measure the limiting TVLs for 6, 10 and 15 MV x-rays. Jones *et al* also considered the TVLs calculated using the ratio of physical densities from TVL values for standard concrete in IPEM (1997). This showed that this approach is conservative,

Table 7.1. Concrete/steel and concrete/lead thickness factors for secondary radiation (IPEM 1997, table VI.1.3).

Material	6 MV	10 MV	15 MV
Steel	3.5	3.6	3.8
Lead	6.2	6.6	7.0

Table 7.2. Measured TVLs for MagnaDense high density concrete (3800 kg m^{-3}) compared with density scaled TVLs (IPEM 1997) using standard concrete.

	6 MV		10 MV		15 MV	
	Primary	Secondary	Primary	Secondary	Primary	Secondary
Measured TVL (mm)	184	160	219	181	253	–
Calculated TVL (mm)	213	173	241	189	268	205

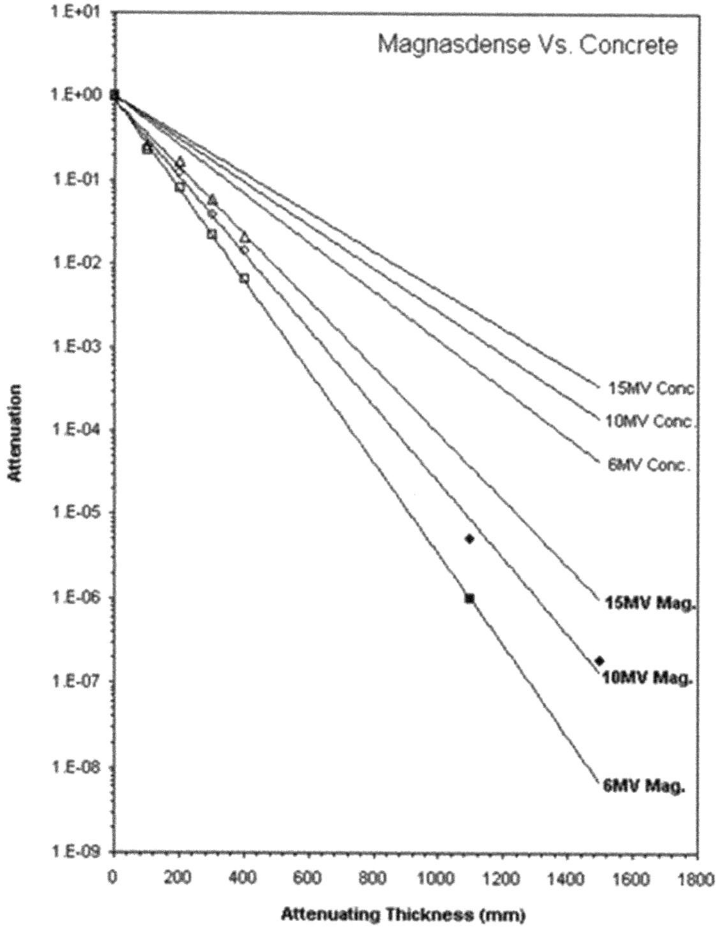

Figure 7.3. Measured TVLs for MagnaDense high density concrete (3800 kg m^{-3}).

but not excessively so, and can be used when the exact attenuation properties are unknown (table 7.2 and figure 7.3).

The scaled density approach to calculating the TVL has to be employed when checking bunker designs and only the density is available. Such an approach has

Table 7.3. Density scaled TVLs from standard concrete for some new high density materials.

Material	Density ($kg\ m^{-3}$)	Scaled TVL					
		6 MV		10 MV		15 MV	
		Primary (mm)	Secondary (mm)	Primary (mm)	Secondary (mm)	Primary (mm)	Secondary (mm)
High density concrete blocks (MegaShield)	3840	210	171	239	187	265	202
High density concrete blocks (MegaShield)	4600	175	–	199	–	221	–
Ledite blocks (no longer available)	3700–4000[a]	218	178	247	194	275	210
Verishield blocks	4000	202	164	229	179	254	194
Verishield blocks	5000	161	–	183	–	203	–

[a] The manufacturers of Ledite said they reduced the density from 4000 $kg\ m^{-3}$ to a minimum of 3700 $kg\ m^{-3}$ as they reduced the proportion of high Z material for bunkers with linear accelerators operating above 8.5 MV. It is therefore safe to assume a density of 3700 $kg\ m^{-3}$ on which the density scaled values in the table are based.

been used with a number of new materials to suggest that a proposed design will be satisfactory which has subsequently been confirmed by a satisfactory radiation survey. Values used for a number of new materials are tabulated in table 7.3.

7.3 Construction details

7.3.1 Formwork, shuttering, tie bolts and reinforcement for poured concrete

When forming the walls of the bunker, the concrete is poured into the space between strong plates called shutters (see figure 7.4). The framework of shutters outlining the wall surfaces is called formwork. The shutters are supported externally (see figure 7.5, left) but also need tie rods (see figure 7.5, right) between them to prevent bulging when full of concrete. Care should be taken in the forming of the shuttering to avoid having tie bolts in the primary shielding at isocentre height (see figure 7.4). When building a linear accelerator bunker it is essential that the tie rods are left *in situ* as they form part of the shielding. Conventional concrete structures have these rods removed after the concrete has set and the formwork has been struck (removed). Linear accelerator bunkers should have the bolts cut off the end of the tie rods and the residual holes filled with a dense mortar.

Bunker walls can be poured in layers which are gradually built up to wall height. Each layer must be joined in some way to the previous layer to avoid direct lines of sight through the wall. For horizontal joints scabbling is employed, which uses vibration to make an uneven surface on the top of the newly poured concrete as it sets. Walls can also be poured in vertical sections. The joints between sections and therefore the formwork need careful design, such as that shown in figures 7.5 (right) and 7.6. Steel reinforcement is always used for concrete structures to hold the structure together (see figure 7.7).

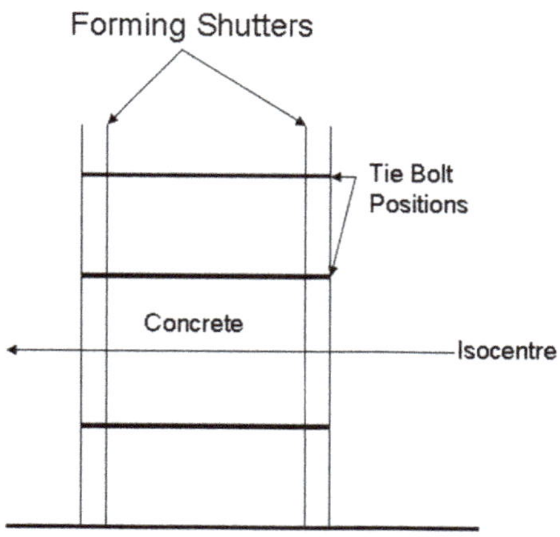

Figure 7.4. A cross-section through a bunker wall showing the shutters defining the surfaces of the wall and held together by tie bolts.

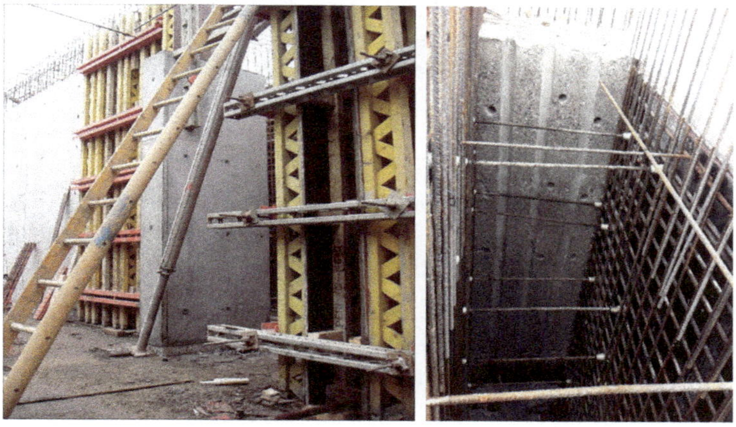

Figure 7.5. External wall shuttering (left) and internal tie rods (right). The right-hand illustration also shows the grooves in a previously poured section that will key with the next section and prevent line of sight joints.

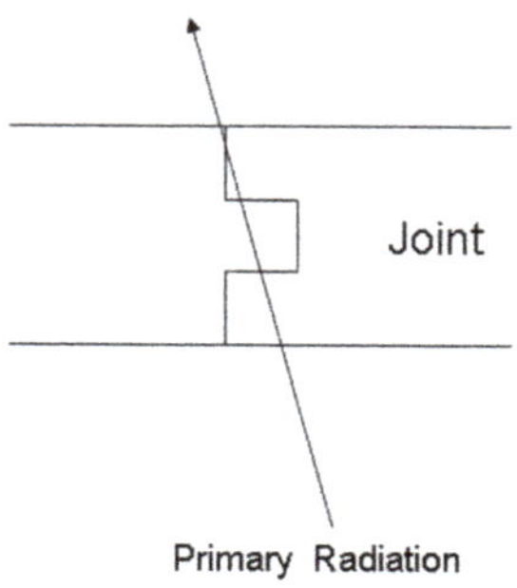

Figure 7.6. A keyed joint between vertical wall sections.

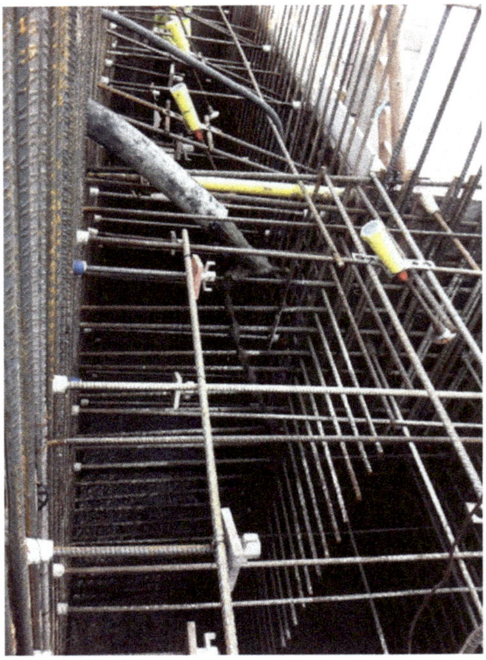

Figure 7.7. Wall space showing tie rods and reinforcement.

The issues are similar although potentially more complicated with high density concrete. For example the logistics around the deliveries and concrete pours are more complex due to the physical density of the material and greater number of deliveries.

7.3.2 Block construction

Blocks may need to be lifted into position using mechanical aids due to their size and weight. The barrier may be formed of multiple layers of blocks. Any gaps need to be infilled with material of sufficient density to maintain the intended attenuation in the barrier. If the shielding is designed to be a permanent structure, mortar can be used to join the blocks. Photographic surveys during construction can give assurance on the build quality and integrity of the construction. Figure 7.8 contains images showing the construction of a bunker using NELCO blocks.

7.3.3 Nibs in bunkers

For bunkers with mazes, nibs on the end of the inner maze wall are useful to reduce the amount of leakage and patient scattered radiation entering the maze. In figure 7.9(a), the presence of the nib reduces the area of the back wall of the bunker which can be irradiated by the radiation components originating from the isocentre. This in turn will reduce the amount of scatter entering the maze and being scattered toward the entrance, as described in chapter 5. The presence of the nib may eliminate the need for

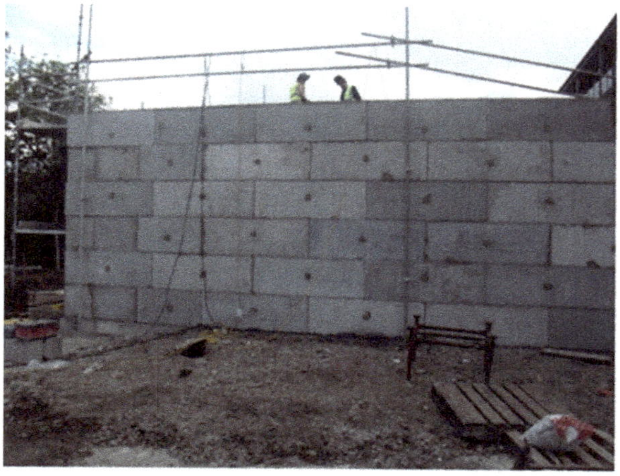

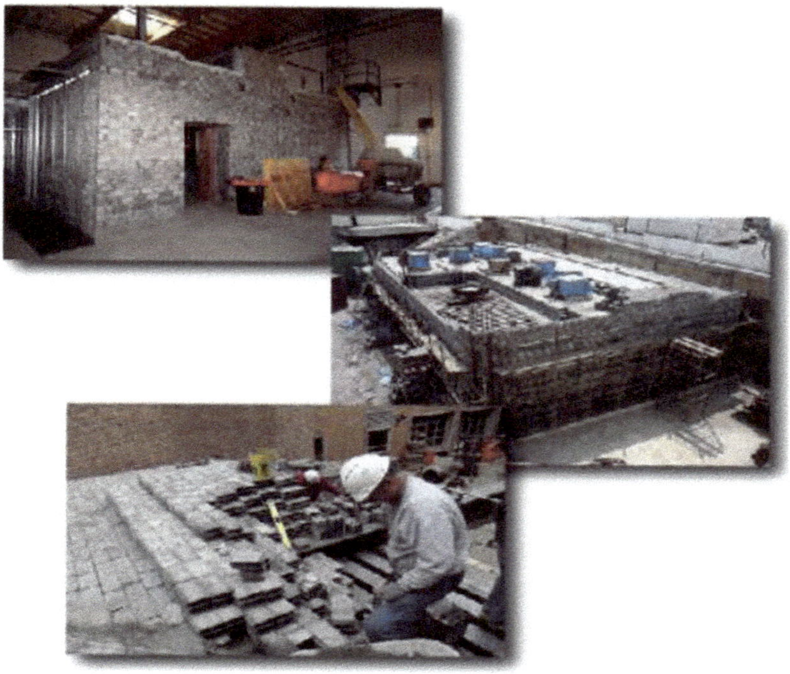

Figure 7.8. Block construction using interlocking concrete blocks. (Courtesy of John Crossman, Reading.)

a shielded door altogether, although some form of barrier is required to prevent unauthorised or accidental access during radiation exposures (see chapters 3 and 4). In designing the nib, care needs to be taken to ensure it does not interfere with the rotation of the patient couch at full extent. If space is limited and a nib is necessary to achieve acceptable doses at the maze entrance, it may be necessary to restrict the longitudinal range of the couch provided that this does not limit clinical procedures.

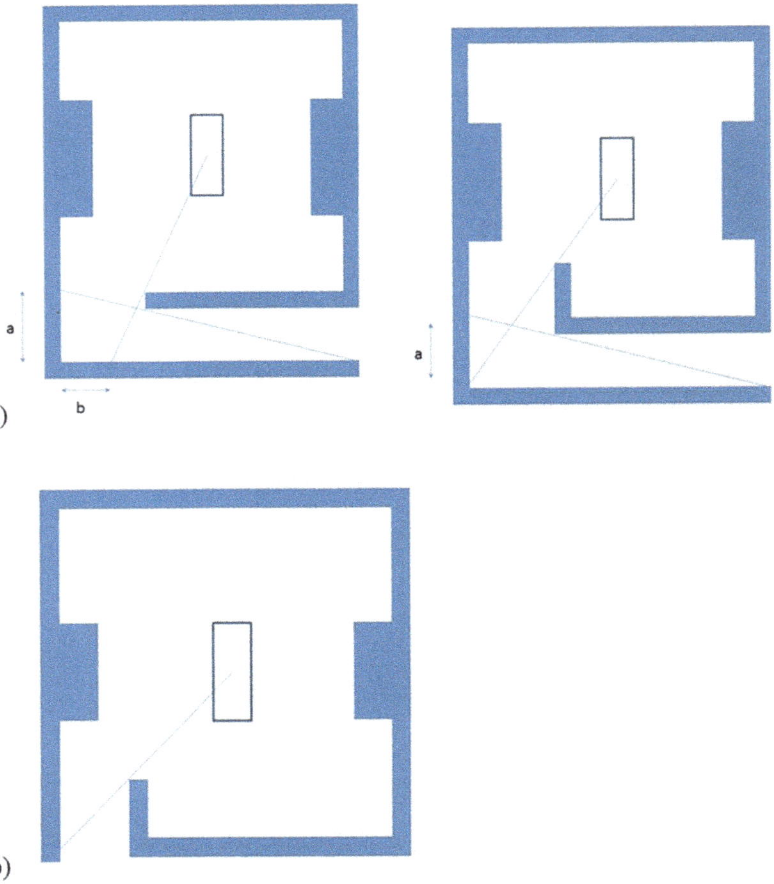

(a)

(b)

Figure 7.9. (a) Bunker with maze showing the area of scatter (with a width of a + b) reduced (to a width a) with a nib at the end of the inner maze wall. (b) Bunker with a direct door showing how a nib prevents leakage and scattered radiation directly reaching the door.

For bunkers with direct doors (figure 7.9(b)), a nib between the door and the isocentre will considerably reduce the amount of radiation reaching the door. This will reduce the shielding required in the door and its weight.

7.3.4 Lintels

Reference to the equations for calculating the dose rate at the maze entrance from scattered radiation (e.g. equation (5.12)) and from neutrons (e.g. equation (5.20)) show each is directly related to areas, in the former by the wall areas irradiated and in the latter by the cross-sectional area of the maze. To reduce the x-ray and neutron dose rates the cross-sectional area of the maze can be reduced by solid concrete lintels in the maze between the false ceiling and the concrete roof. A lintel is often placed at the inner maze entrance and a second in the first leg of the maze (see figure 7.10(a)). The lintels should be at least 500 mm thick. The height should not restrict access into the room. As noted

(a)

(b)

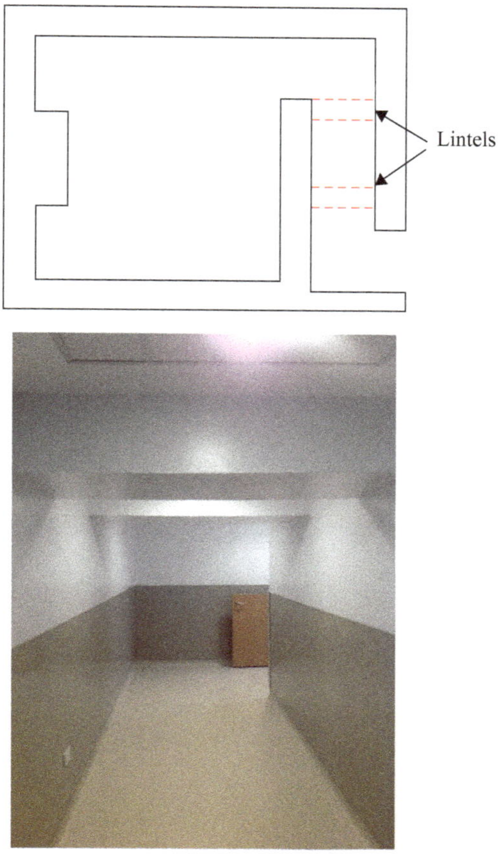

Figure 7.10. (a) Bunkers showing the position of lintels to reduce the cross-sectional area of the maze. (b) A maze with a visible lintel looking from the treatment room down the long leg of the maze towards the half door at the maze entrance.

above the area of the first wall scatter can also be reduced by a nib on the inner maze wall.

7.3.5 Ducts and cableways

The paths chosen for service ducts and cable ways should always be in secondary shielding and positioned such that they do not align with ray paths from the isocentre. Ducts through the shielding should include at least one bend if possible so that radiation cannot escape the room after only a single scatter.

Electrical power, water and possibly compressed air supplies will need to enter the treatment room and will normally be at floor level where alignment with a ray path through the isocentre is not a possibility. The generally desirable arrangement is shown in figure 7.11 (left). A cableway will be required between the treatment and control rooms for dosimetry equipment to avoid taking cables down the maze. This will normally run downhill from bench height in the control room to floor level in the treatment room and therefore not be aligned with a ray path. If necessary the

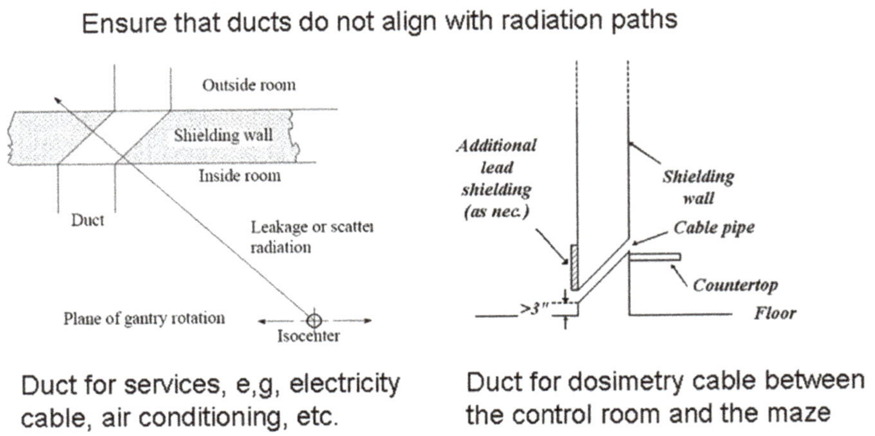

Figure 7.11. General arrangement for the alignment of service ducts (left) and a common alignment of the duct for dosimetry cables (right).

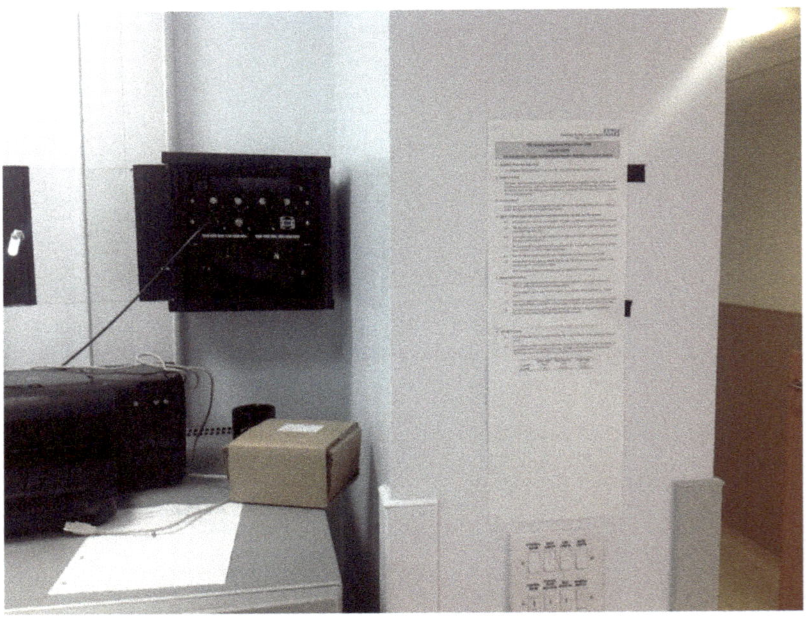

Figure 7.12. An example of a panel with the cable terminations for dosimetry equipment in the control room of a linear accelerator. (Note the Local Rules affixed to the side of the maze entrance.)

duct should be large enough to allow the passage of the large plug on the end of the multiway cable of beam data acquisition systems and incorporate a shallow bend. A suitable arrangement is shown in figure 7.11 (right). Some centres have opted for having permanent arrangements for regular dosimetry with suitable terminations at panels in the control room and treatment room. An example of such a panel is shown in figure 7.12.

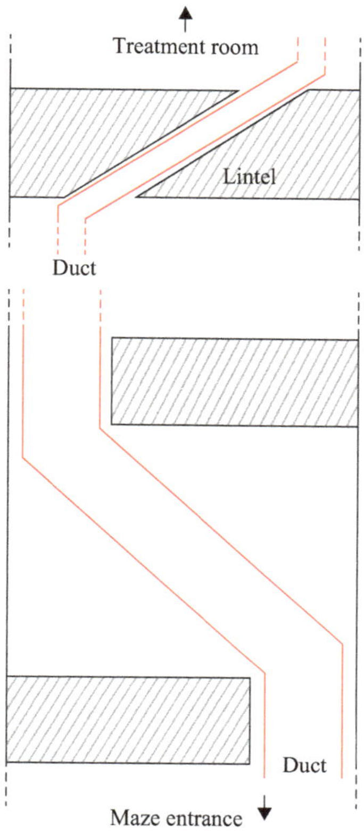

Figure 7.13. Typical arrangements to take HVAC ducts through lintels in the maze (plan view).

The passage of heating, ventilation and air conditioning (HVAC) ducts into the treatment room presents a special radiation protection problem due to their large cross-sectional area which can reduce the protection if special measures are not taken. These ducts are usually taken down the maze to avoid penetrating the primary and secondary shielding. If so they need to pass through the lintels (see above) without reducing the protection. Two common arrangements are shown in figure 7.13. In the upper diagram the duct passes through the lintel as obliquely as possible to maintain the total path length in concrete for radiation at normal incidence as much as possible along its passage. If the width of the duct and the depth of the lintel do not permit this geometry, the lintel may be split into two sections on opposite walls of the maze and the duct shaped to pass through the chicane created, as shown in the lower diagram.

The special requirements for linear accelerators equipped with magnetic resonance imaging have been discussed in section 4.1.2.1.

7.3.6 Direct doors

If doors incorporating shielding are employed at the bunker entrance, consideration needs to be given to avoiding the leakage of radiation around the edges of the

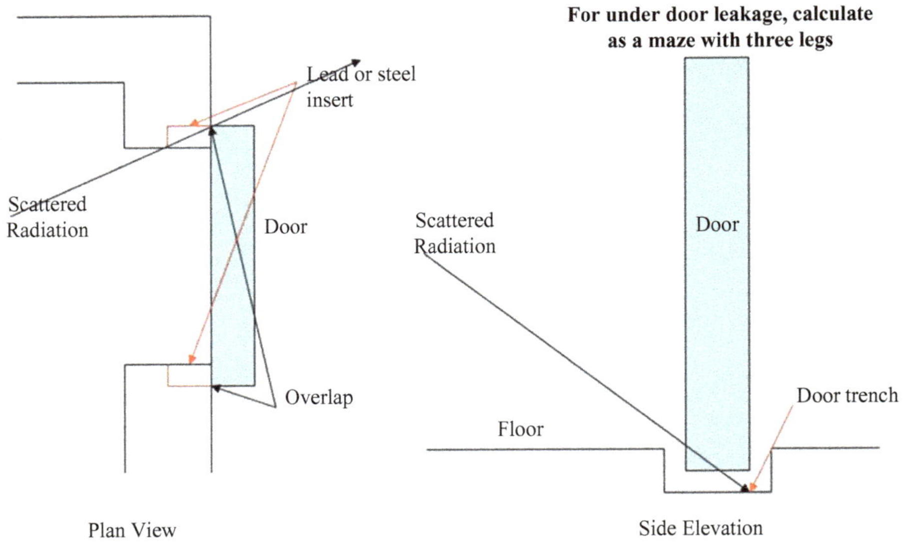

Figure 7.14. The features to be adopted with a direct door to avoid radiation leakage around the edges of the door.

door. Doors need to overlap the opening and, depending on the nature of the radiation in the direction of the door, it may be necessary to insert a high Z absorber in the edges of the door opening. To avoid radiation leaking beneath the door, it may need to run in a shallow trench; this will need an infill when the door is open to provide a flat surface. These features are illustrated in figure 7.14. These features become especially important with a CyberKnife® installation with a direct door[2].

7.3.7 Wall fixings

Items which need to be flush with the wall of the treatment room to avoid being knocked will need a recess that will reduce the barrier thickness. Protection is usually maintained with a steel plate behind the item and this should have at a minimum the same concrete equivalence as the material missing. Alignment lasers are the most common item fixed to the walls, and this is illustrated in figure 7.15.

7.3.8 Warning lights

These are ideally positioned at eye level either side of the entrance to the treatment room, but the design of many entrances means the exact positioning is sometimes above or to one side of the entrance. The wording needs to include a description of the hazard which may include x-rays, electrons and neutrons. Care is needed in

[2] CyberKnife is a registered mark of Accuray.

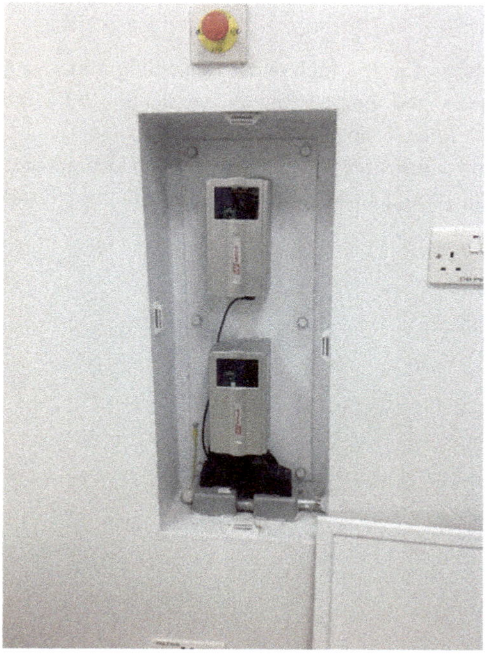

Figure 7.15. Alignment laser showing the recess in the shielding.

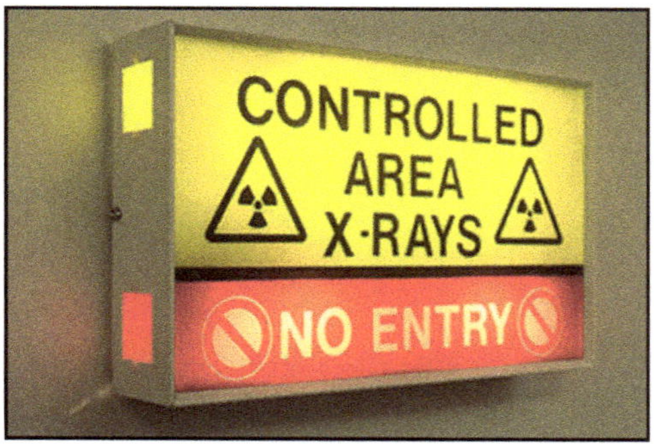

Figure 7.16. Typical radiation warning sign for an external beam radiotherapy facility.

the specification of any legend. A two stage warning light is commonly used (see figure 7.16). The upper yellow section is illuminated when the equipment is powered and can provide radiation. The red section is illuminated when radiation is being generated. Some centres use a three stage warning light with a centre section confirming to those outside the bunker when the LPO circuit has been closed. The lettering on the example shown is visible when the light is not on in the upper part and it is preferable to have the same legend on a black background.

References

Barish R J 1993 Evaluation of a new high-density shielding material *Health Phys.* **64** 412–6

IPEM (Institute of Physics and Engineering in Medicine) 1997 *The Design of Radiotherapy Treatment Room Facilities* Report 75 (York: IPEM)

Jones M R, Peet D J and Horton P W 2009 Attenuation characteristics of MagnaDense high-density concrete at 6, 10 and 15 MV for use in radiotherapy bunker design *Health Phys.* **96** 67–75

Chapter 8

Specialist applications: Gamma Knife®, TomoTherapy® and CyberKnife®

L Walton, T Soanes, T Greener, D Prior and E G Aird

8.1 The Gamma Knife®

L Walton and T Soanes

8.1.1 Introduction

The Leksell Gamma Knife[1] (Elekta AB, Stockholm, Sweden) is a dedicated unit designed for stereotactic radiosurgery of lesions within the brain. It was designed by Swedish neurosurgeon Professor Lars Leksell and physicist Borje Larson in the 1960s (Leksell 1951, Larsson *et al* 1974). A unit was first introduced into the UK in 1985 (Walton *et al* 1987) and at the time of writing there are seven units installed in the UK and around 265 units worldwide.

In the UK both Perfexion™ (Regis *et al* 2009, Lindquist and Paddick 2007) (figure 8.1) and Icon™ models of the Gamma Knife are in clinical use. Both models consist of:

- a radiation unit, which houses the radioactive cobalt-60 sources and aligned collimator systems which together produce a series of narrow beams with their intersection at a point at the centre of the radiation unit, and
- a couch assembly, which acts as the patient positioning system (PPS), to accurately position the patient such that the abnormal tissues within the brain are at the confluence of the beams during the treatment process.

The Icon model also incorporates an on-board cone beam CT (CBCT) which facilitates imaging during the course of treatment.

[1] Gamma Knife is a registered trademark of Elekta.

doi:10.1088/978-0-7503-1440-4ch8

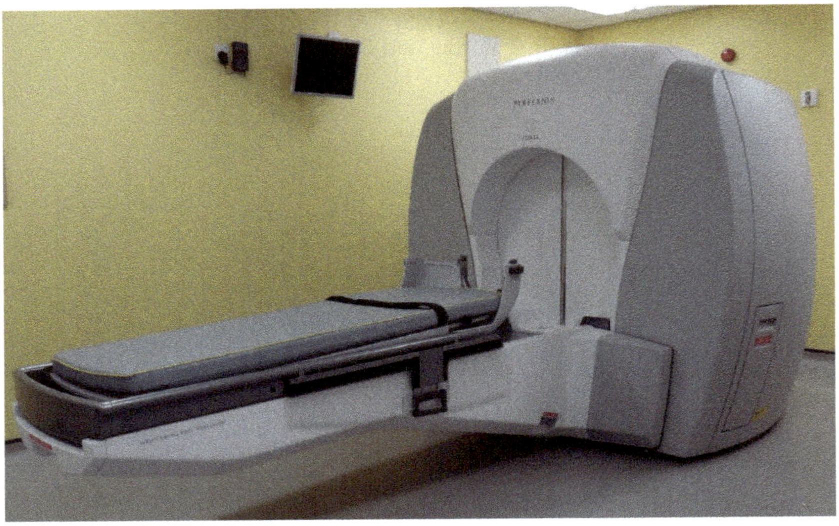

Figure 8.1. Gamma Knife Perfexion (Courtesy of The National Centre for Stereotactic Radiosurgery, Sheffield).

Gamma Knife bunker design needs to ensure that radiation protection measures cater for the routine patient use of the unit, including the use of the CBCT and also for the initial on-site loading of its cobalt-60 sources and future periodic source exchange processes.

8.1.2 Sources and source loading

The Perfexion and Icon models of the Gamma Knife have 192 individual cobalt-60 sources, each of which has an activity of ~1.16 TBq resulting in a total activity of around 233 TBq. The sources figure 8.2(a) are each triple encapsulated in stainless steel, housed in an aluminium source bushing and delivered to site separately from the treatment unit within an approved type B(U) container, shown in figure 8.2(b) (Croft Associates Limited 2015), in order to simplify the requirements of the transport regulations.

Once on site the external cover of the transport container is removed and an inner flask containing the sources is moved into the treatment room, the sources are then loaded into the radiation unit via a specially designed loader which is attached to the radiation unit. Figure 8.3 shows the source loader and radiation unit.

Once the source loading process is complete, the unit can be installed and prepared for clinical use. Following installation the equipment should satisfy the requirements of the *Ionising Radiation Regulations* 1999 (IRR 1999), the *Environmental Permitting Regulations* 2016 (EPR 2016), the *Radioactive Substances Act* 1993 (RSA 1993) and *Medical Electrical Equipment: Particular Requirements for the Basic Safety and Essential Performance of Gamma Beam Therapy Equipment: Particular Requirements for the Basic Safety and Essential Performance of Gamma Beam Therapy Equipment* (IEC 2013), which define the safety and security features that should be operative and the tolerable levels of leakage radiation in the surrounding treatment room.

During the installation period the manufacturer will perform wipe tests of essential components including the source delivery cask at the beginning and end

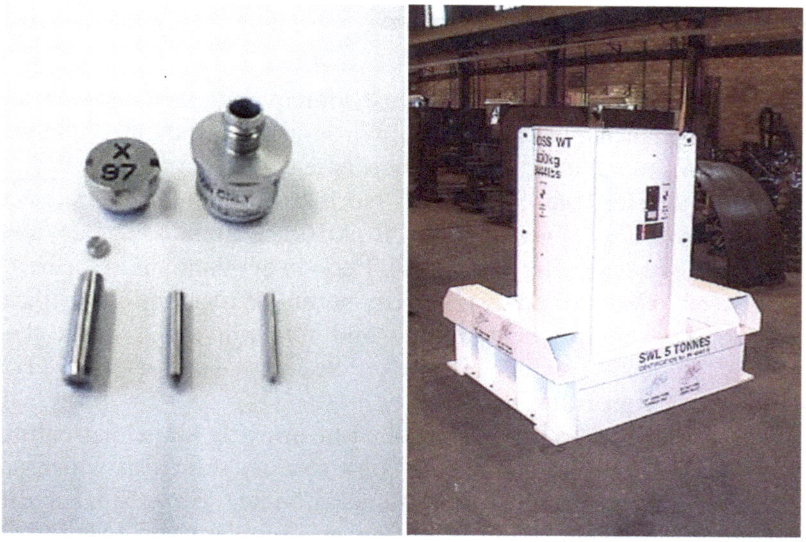

(a) (b)

Figure 8.2. A dummy source (a) showing the three stainless steel tubes which encapsulate the cobalt-60 and the aluminium bushing which houses the source. (Courtesy of Elekta Instruments AB). All sources and bushings are assembled prior to delivery to site in an approved transport container (b).

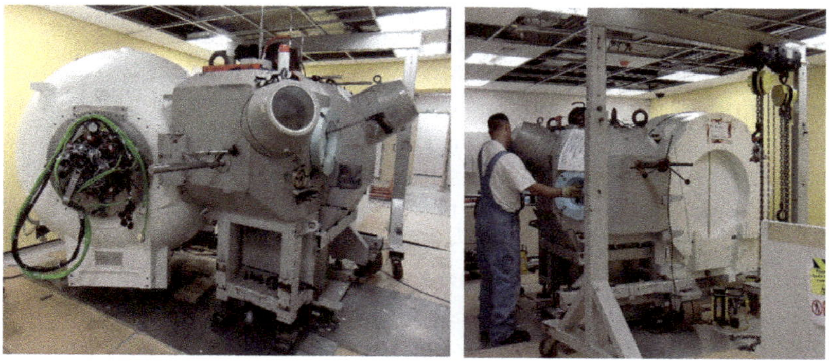

Figure 8.3. The source loader attached to the radiation unit in preparation for the on-site loading of the 192 cobalt-60 sources.

of the source loading period to ensure that there is no leakage from the cobalt sources. Further tests are performed during installation and include wipe tests of the collimator cap within the central body of the radiation unit and also of the sector drive shafts at the rear of the unit. Further periodic wipe tests should be performed by hospital staff at intervals not exceeding two years to satisfy Regulation 27(3) of the *Ionising Radiation Regulations* (IRR 1999) and to meet the International Standard: *Radiation Protection—Sealed Radioactive Sources—Leakage Test Methods* (ISO 1992). The surfaces chosen are selected to be the closest accessible surfaces to the sources.

8.1.3 Treatment room design considerations

8.1.3.1 Security requirements

The sources are classified as high activity sources and their storage and use is regulated by the environment agencies (Environment Agency in England, Natural Resources in Wales, the Scottish Environment Protection Agency, and the Environment and Heritage Service in Northern Ireland) and subject to the *Environment Permitting Regulations* (EPR 2016) in England and Wales and to the *Radioactive Substances Act* 1993 (RSA 1993) in Scotland and Northern Ireland. The sources need to be covered by a security permit or registration certificate issued by the appropriate environment agency and this will require that the suite is inspected by the local Counter Terrorism Security Advisor (CTSA) who will approve the security measures in place.

It is advised that the CTSA be consulted at an early stage of treatment room design and their advice obtained on the latest security standards which need to be applied. These are outlined in the National Counter Terrorism Security Office document *Security Requirements for Radioactive Sources* (NaCTSO 2011) and the Gamma Knife currently falls in the category requiring the highest levels of security. The sources need to be protected from unauthorised access by two physical security measures with a timely detection of unauthorised access by a remotely monitored intruder alarm with a police response to a verified alarm. The document specifies the standards which define the applicable security ratings of the suite doors, locks and walls. CCTV monitoring of the suite and its approaches is advisable.

Figure 8.4 shows two of the many possible suite configurations. The bold lines indicate the boundary of the secure area which needs to meet the defined security standards. In (a) the secure area encloses the control area and its walls and ceiling will therefore need security protection. The doors to the control area will need to be reinforced. In (b) the control area is more open without added security and the concrete walls and roof of the treatment room itself define the boundary of the secure area. The walls provide ample security but the doors to the room will need to be reinforced steel doors to satisfy the security requirements.

8.1.3.2 Routes of access and floor loadings

Routes of access for delivery of the treatment unit also require careful consideration at the design stage and may determine the siting of a treatment suite. The radiation unit which houses the sources is approximately spherical with a 1.8 m diameter and a weight of 18 tonnes; the source flask is 4.3 tonnes and the loader is 12 tonnes. Routes of access will also need to be able to withstand the floor loading associated with these individual components and be sufficiently wide to allow the equipment to be manoeuvred. Minimising the distance to the point of delivery is clearly advantageous.

The floor of the suite itself will need to support the combined weight of the radiation unit, source flask and the source loader during the source loading procedure. The process of source loading will need to be repeated every 6–8 years so careful thought at the design stage will minimise disruption. Some suites are designed adjacent to roadways with a removable roof hatch which allows the heavy

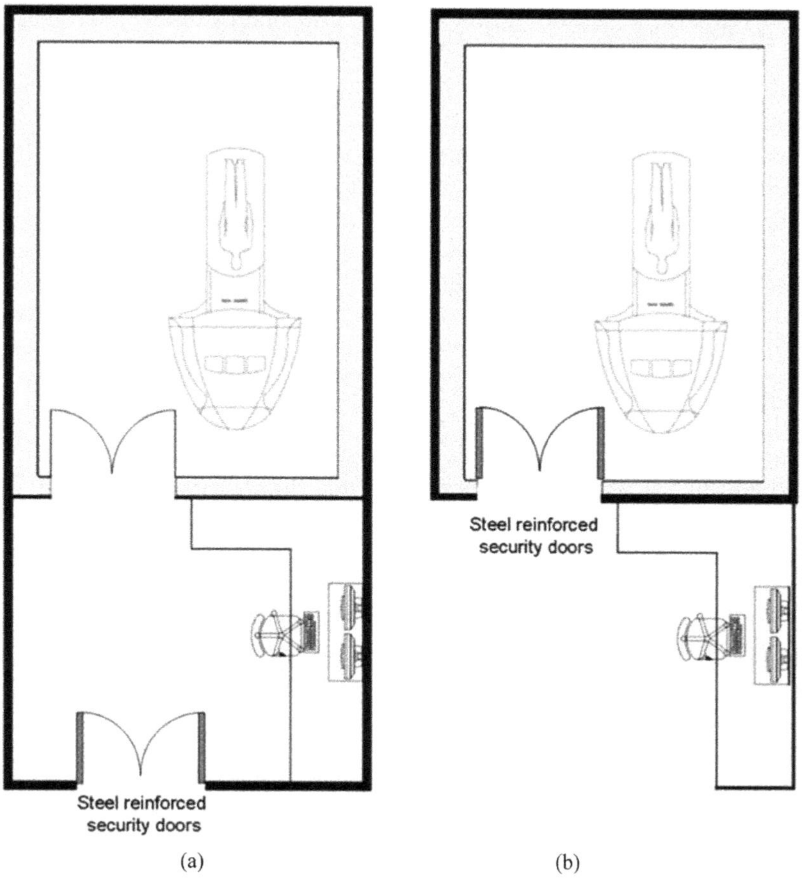

Figure 8.4. Schematic diagram showing two possible layouts for Gamma Knife treatment rooms. The bold line illustrates the limits of the secure area and the possible positions of the reinforced security doors are shown.

items to be craned directly into the suite. The manufacturer publishes site planning guides for Perfexion and Icon models (Elekta Instruments AB 2011, 2015) and will provide support in the design process.

8.1.3.3 Treatment, control and planning areas

The treatment room should be large enough to accommodate the Gamma Knife with sufficient space to manoeuvre a hospital bed alongside the treatment couch for patient transfer.

Because about 5% of cases require treatment under general anaesthetic, the treatment room will need to be equipped with piped medical gases and have space to accommodate an anaesthetic machine. Facilities for remote monitoring of the life support systems will also need to be incorporated into the control area.

The control area will be occupied by radiographic and physics staff, but should also be sufficiently large to accommodate other staff including support workers, visitors, the anaesthetist, operating department practitioners, etc, who may be involved in the procedure.

A treatment planning station will be provided with the unit and connects via the hospital network to the Gamma Knife. It is advisable that this is accommodated in a room which is separate from the control area. It may be close to the treatment suite but it is worth noting that input and advice from other staff such as neuro-radiologists (who will demarcate the tissues for treatment), oncologists and neuro-surgeons will be required at various stages in the treatment planning process and an alternative site may assist in establishing an efficient workflow.

8.1.3.4 Treatment room access

The layout of the treatment suite will largely determine the requirements for the treatment room doors including any security and shielding requirements.

Figure 8.4(a) shows a situation in which the treatment room entrance is wholly contained within the confines of the control area, thus forming a self-contained suite with steel reinforced security doors at the control room entrance. Between the control area and the treatment room, a short maze may be incorporated or doors may be used. Careful positioning of the treatment room entrance towards the rear or adjacent to the side of the radiation unit will reduce or eliminate the need for additional shielding (see section 8.1.4.3). With an entrance in the position shown the radiation levels (beam on) are less than 2 $\mu Sv\ h^{-1}$ (see figure 8.5). This permits some flexibility in the design of the treatment room doors and an open approach with half height doors or a light barrier can be considered. The manufacturer suggests that a viewing window can be incorporated into the room design but its position needs to be carefully considered as some locations may not provide a useful view.

Figure 8.4(b) illustrates an alternative layout with the steel reinforced doors at the entrance to the treatment room satisfying the security requirements whilst also providing radiation protection at the entrance.

8.1.4 Shielding considerations

8.1.4.1 Source loading

In preparation for loading the sources, the flask containing the sources is positioned at the centre of the source loader. The sources are then individually removed from the flask, manipulated using special tooling and engaged in position in one of the sectors within the radiation unit. The process of loading all the sources takes around 6 h and should be carried out under the supervision of a hospital radiation protection adviser.

When source exchange is taking place, the spent sources are first extracted from the radiation unit, removed from their aluminium bushings and temporarily stored in the loader. The new sources can then be loaded into the radiation unit the following day and the spent sources are moved into the flask ready for return to their manufacturer for disposal.

Radiation exposure rates at the walls of a treatment room with dimensions 4.5 m × 6.5 m would be expected to be less than 10 $\mu Sv\ h^{-1}$, with exposure rates at the

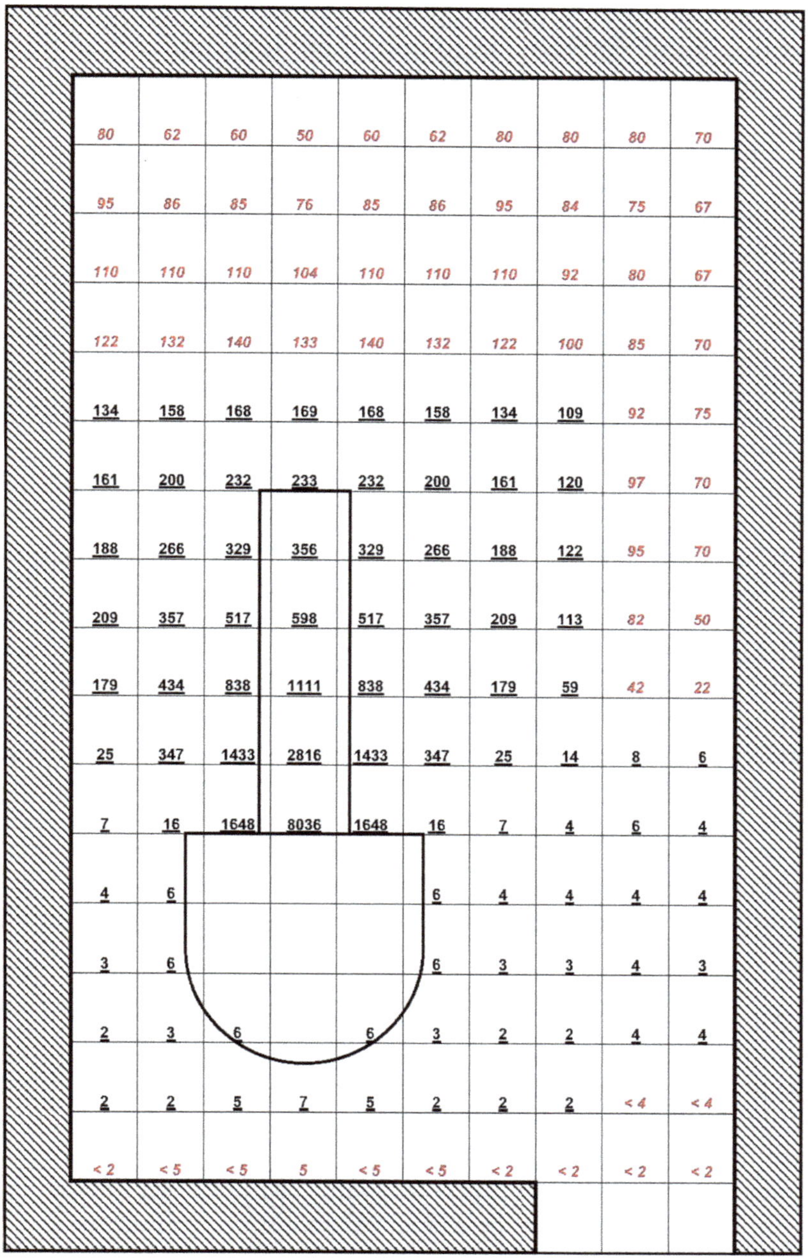

Figure 8.5. Radiation field in a Perfexion treatment room with a total source activity of 233 TBq, with the beam on, shutter doors open and the 16 mm collimator field size selected (Elekta 2011). Values are shown on a grid with 0.5 m spacing, are in $\mu Sv\ h^{-1}$ and are at 1 m above floor level. Measured values are underlined, others are extrapolated values. *Note: These figures are for illustration purposes only—for reference data consult the manufacturer's documentation.* (Courtesy of Elekta Instruments AB.)

surface of the source flask of 250 μSv h^{-1} (Elekta Instruments AB 1999). The exposure rates within the room reduce as the sources are moved from the flask into the radiation unit with its superior shielding. These levels are significantly lower, by at least a factor of 10, than those experienced during normal operation of the Gamma Knife.

8.1.4.2 Routine use

The installed Gamma Knife unit consists of the radiation unit with integral shutter doors and attached couch assembly for patient support. All sources and collimator systems are housed within the radiation unit and the sources move to align with a chosen collimator during treatment delivery.

In the 'beam off' state the sources are retracted to a home position and are well shielded, the patient couch is withdrawn, the shutter doors are closed and the CBCT is turned off. Despite the shielding, there will be some leakage through the walls of the radiation unit and the treatment room should therefore be designated as a permanently controlled area.

In the 'beam-on' state the shutter doors are open, the patient couch has moved into position and the sources are aligned with the selected collimators. A beam-on state is also indicated when the CBCT is operating. Radiation levels in the treatment room are highest when the largest 16 mm field size is selected. Figure 8.5 (Elekta Instrument AB 2011) shows a matrix of exposure rate values measured around the treatment unit with the 16 mm collimator field size[2]. The values are in μSv h^{-1} and are measured 1 m above floor level; the underlined values are measured values and the other values are extrapolated. Further matrices showing the radiation levels during a CBCT scan, in different planes and with the 'beam off' are also available within the site planning guide to assist in shielding barrier design. Shielding barriers will be required for all walls, floor and the roof of the treatment room. Consideration should also be given to ensure that the x-ray beams from the CBCT are adequately shielded.

8.1.4.3 Entrance

The entrance to the treatment room from the control area can be positioned in the wall behind or to the side of the radiation unit where the radiation levels are low. Depending on the positioning of the entrance, the size of the room and the occupancy of the area immediately outside the entrance, it may not be necessary to add radiation protection to the room doors. The use of half-height doors or a short maze at the entrance may be considered and will reduce the sense of isolation felt by a patient who may spend several hours in the treatment room.

8.1.4.4 Calculation of barrier thickness

Calculations of barrier thickness are based on the principles outlined elsewhere in this report. The orientation of the individual beams of cobalt gamma rays within the

[2] The values shown are for illustration purposes only and should not be used as reference data. Readers are directed to the latest version of the Elekta Site Planning Guide for reference values.

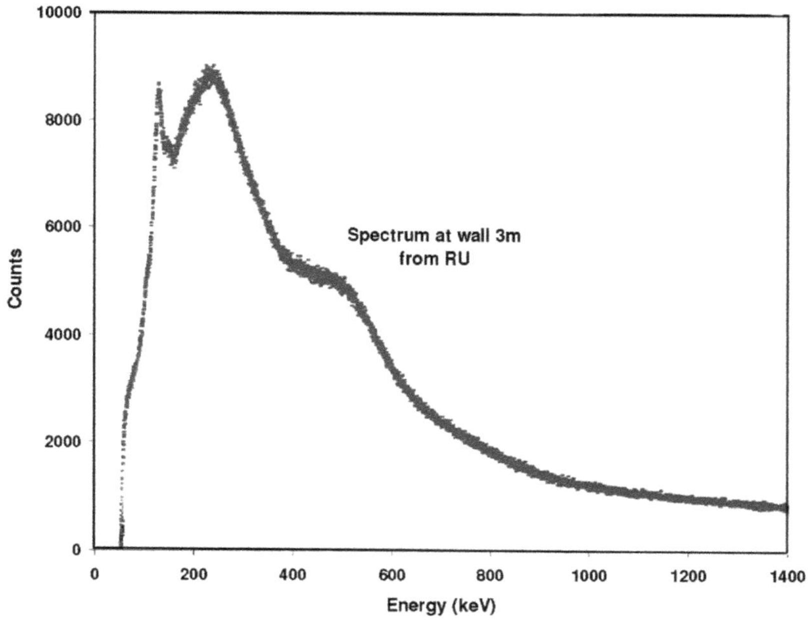

Figure 8.6. Gamma ray spectrum showing the distribution of detected energies in the Perfexion treatment room at Marseille. (Courtesy of Elekta Instruments AB.)

radiation unit is such that none of the primary beams exit through the shielding doors. Radiation escaping into the treatment room through the open shutter doors on a Perfexion is therefore predominantly scatter. Although the dose rate data provided by Elekta (2011) is for scattered radiation rather than the primary beam, some conservatism can be built into the barrier calculation by assuming that the energy of the radiation reaching the barriers is at the same energy as the primary beam. Dryzmala *et al* (2001) have interrogated the gamma-ray spectrum within a treatment room equipped with an earlier B model of the Gamma Knife and found a mix of scatter and primary beam with an angular dependence related to the mean energy of the emitted spectrum. Elekta have performed similar spectral measurements around the Perfexion model installed in Marseille and figure 8.6 shows the spectrum obtained with barely discernible characteristic peaks at 1.17 and 1.33 MeV energies. Elekta have plans to obtain further data and with the aid of movable shielding barriers aim to derive 'effective tenth value layer' (TVL) values for use in future shielding calculations. This may help to reduce the barrier thickness in future installations.

McDermott (2007) describes his approach to bunker design for a Gamma Knife. He warns that care should be taken in extrapolating the data provided and advises that where this is needed the extrapolation should be along ray lines from the unit centre.

Radiation workload

The length of a Gamma Knife treatment varies considerably depending on the shape and size of the target tissues and to some extent on the planning preferences of the hospital, but typically ranges from 20 min to 5 h per patient. There is increasing use of the unit for the treatment of multiple metastases and these treatments can be particularly lengthy. A treatment with new sources would average around 75 min. A busy treatment centre would treat 4–5 patients per day, giving an average beam-on time of around 6.25 h/day depending on case mix. The use of this figure includes two safety margins: first, the treatments may extend beyond a normal 8 h day, and second, a large proportion of the beam-on time will be delivered with the 4 mm and 8 mm collimators, resulting in lower exposure rates at the barrier than those shown for the 16 mm collimator in figure 8.5. As the sources decay the beam-on times will become proportionately longer, but this will be accompanied by a reduction in exposure rates within the room. Calculations of barrier thickness can therefore safely be done on the basis of a new unit with new sources.

Barrier thickness calculation

The following steps should be followed:

- Determine the maximum permissible dose or dose rate beyond each of the barriers taking into account regulatory requirements and levels of occupancy of the adjacent areas. Where adjacent areas will be occupied by members of the public or staff who are not routinely exposed to radiation:
  - the barrier thickness should be specified such that a design constraint of 0.3 mSv/year can be achieved and
  - instantaneous (IDR) or time averaged dose rates (TADRs) should be such that designation of adjacent areas as either controlled or supervised radiation areas is avoided.

  These criteria may be relaxed where the exposed persons beyond the barrier are staff who are routinely exposed to radiation and are individually monitored. The *Medical and Dental Guidance Notes* (IPEM 2002) contain flowcharts in appendix 11 which will help determine whether designation as a radiation area is required.
- Determine the maximum workload of the unit taking into account any future changes in workload. Potential workloads for a busy centre are given above. Using the tables provided in the site planning guide determine cumulative doses over an appropriate time period (e.g. per working day or per year) for each barrier. The dose rates used in the calculation should be based on the largest sized collimator available. This will be the unshielded dose or dose rate over a given time period.
- Calculate the ratio of these to determine the required attenuation factors for each barrier. The thickness of the barrier, in terms of half-value layer (HVL), can then be determined using natural logarithms as outlined below:

$$\text{Barrier thickness in terms of HVL} = \frac{-\ln\left(\dfrac{\text{max permissible dose rate}}{\text{unshielded dose rate}}\right)}{\ln(2)}.$$

  This value can then be multiplied by the HVL of the appropriate construction material to determine the thickness of the barrier.

Table 8.1. HVL and TVL values from Elekta (2011, 2015), based upon ICRP (1991). (Note: the TVL values are slightly different from those in table 5.1 taken from NCRP (2005).)

Material	Density (kg m^{-3})	HVL (mm)	TVL (mm)
Concrete	2350	61	203
Steel	7900	20	67
Lead	11 340	10	34

The site planning guidance (Elekta 2011, 2015) quotes HVL values for concrete, steel and lead. These are given in table 8.1. In practice, deriving the barrier thicknesses as outlined above will be conservative as the following assumptions lead to overestimates:

- the energy of the radiation field is based on primary radiation from Co-60 (however, the energy spectrum does not show any significant emissions at Co-60 energies),
- the direction of the radiation field is assumed perpendicular to the walls and
- use of the largest sized collimator (the majority of treatments will use the smaller size collimators).

Where space or cost is at a premium, it may be appropriate to take into account the energy spectrum and determine the required attenuation assuming a lower energy than cobolt-60.

Following installation or source loading, a dose rate survey using a dosimeter calibrated in terms of ambient dose equivalent should be undertaken to verify the adequacy of the barriers.

8.2 TomoTherapy®

T Greener and D Prior

8.2.1 Introduction

A TomoTherapy[3] treatment unit (figures 8.7 and 8.8) comprises a 6 MV standing waveguide accelerator mounted in line with the x-ray target. From a radiation protection point of view the key differences to a conventional C-arm type linear accelerator, operating at the same energy, arise as a result of

- longer treatment delivery times and
- a primary beam stopper.

Treatment delivery times for TomoTherapy can be as much as ten times longer when compared with simple static conformal field delivery on conventional linear accelerators. This differential will be less when comparing to more advanced

[3] TomoTherapy is a registered trademark of Accuray.

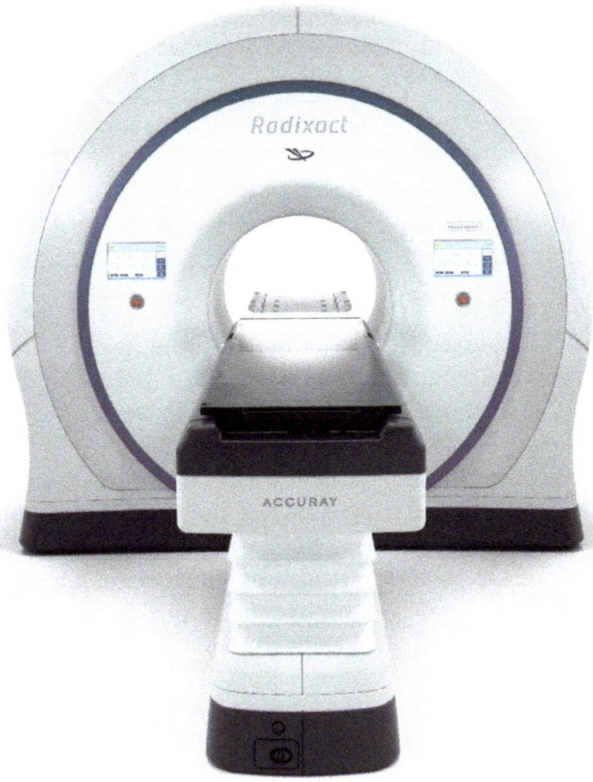

Figure 8.7. TomoTherapy Radixact System (Courtesy of Accuray Inc.)

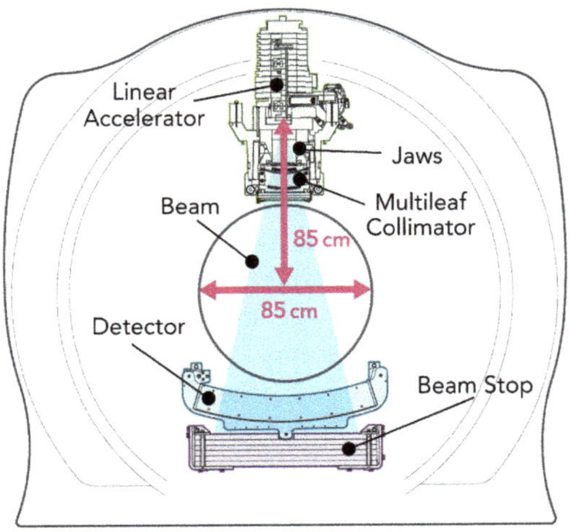

Figure 8.8. Schematic of the standard TomoTherapy Hi-Art Unit.

delivery methods such as intensity modulated radiotherapy (IMRT) and volumetric intensity modulated arc therapy (VMAT). A primary beam stopper mounted on the opposite side of the source reduces the shielding requirements for primary radiation. As a result leakage radiation becomes the major shielding consideration in TomoTherapy room design. The reasons for and consequences of these differences will be explained along with examples and a case study involving the installation of a TomoTherapy unit in an old cobalt-60 unit bunker.

8.2.2 Basic operation

The TomoTherapy treatment system (Mackie *et al* 1993, Beavis 2004) uses helical TomoHelical™ and topographic mode TomoDirect™ to deliver IMRT[4]. Helical tomotherapy generates a 6 MV slit beam of flattening filter free radiation perpendicular to the length of the patient that continuously rotates on a slip ring gantry while the patient slowly moves through the beam on the treatment couch.

The maximum radiation beam size is 40 cm in the transverse direction. A primary set of moveable tungsten jaws defines discrete slice widths (1, 2.5 or 5 cm) for treatment and 1 mm for megavoltage CT imaging in the superior–inferior direction of the patient (the IEC 1217 (IEC 2011) Y direction). TomoEDGE™ dynamic jaw technology is also available on more recent TomoTherapy systems[5]. This technology moves the appropriate primary jaw during the beginning or end of delivery to reduce the penumbra in the superior–inferior treatment direction. For some treatment sites this enables a larger field width to be chosen, e.g. 5 cm instead of 2.5 cm, without compromising beam modulation, which can significantly reduce treatment times.

The primary beam is further collimated by 64 interleaved adjustable binary leaves, i.e. either fully closed or open, each projecting a transverse width of 6.25 mm at the isocentre. This pneumatically driven multi-leaf collimator (MLC) in conjunction with the synchronous rotational delivery is able to produce the beam modulation required for IMRT. TomoDirect is a topographic mode of operation that generates a 6 MV slit beam of radiation at discrete static gantry angles, while the patient moves through the beam. Relevant shielding design characteristics are summarised in table 8.2.

TomoTherapy machines have evolved through various platforms from the Hi-Art model through to the H-Series and more recently the Radixact™ treatment delivery system[6].

8.2.3 Machine calibration

During factory set up and on site commissioning TomoTherapy units are matched to the 'standard' data set in the treatment planning system. Beam energy, output and profile distributions from one unit to the next will therefore be very similar. Referencing monitor units (MU) to treatment dose is achieved by 'calibrating' the

[4] TomoHelical and TomoDirect are trademarks of Accuray.
[5] TomoEDGE is a trademark of Accuray.
[6] Radixact is a trademark of Accuray.

Table 8.2. Relevant TomoTherapy shielding design characteristics. Data taken from TomoTherapy (2011) unless separately referenced.

Parameter description	Value
Treatment energy	6 MV
Megavoltage CT energy	3.5 MV (Shah *et al* 2008)
Field delivery	Helical: gantry continuously rotates Direct: static gantry
Focal spot to isocentre distance	85 cm
Nominal reference dose rate (1.5 cm depth at isocentre, 40 cm × 5 cm field)	8.80 Gy min^{-1}
Maximum field size	40 cm × 5 cm at isocentre
Primary beam stop	130 mm lead (Balog *et al* 2005)
Primary transmission through beam stop	0.4% of isocentric output
Primary TVL	340 mm of concrete (density 2.3 g cm^{-3})
Leakage TVL	290 mm concrete (density 2.3 g cm^{-3})

unit against a set of standard plans produced on the TomoTherapy planning system. The machine parameters are adjusted so that the measured doses agree with those expected averaged across these standard plans. In essence the machine is calibrated to the planning system output.

8.2.4 Shielding considerations

Shielding considerations for helical tomotherapy were first discussed by Balog *et al* (2005). These were based on measurements performed around the Hi-ART II TomoTherapy machine with results reported in the TomoTherapy *Site Planning Guide* (TomoTherapy 2004). In this work primary, leakage and scatter radiation contributions were quantified. Comparable results were obtained by Ramsey *et al* (2006) using similar methods. Wu *et al* (2006), using data in the *Site Planning Guide* (TomoTherapy 2004), presented shielding calculations for a TomoTherapy unit sited in an existing linear accelerator bunker. Baechler *et al* (2007) presented shielding calculation formulae, largely based on the measurements of Balog *et al* (2005) and using methodology drawn from NCRP Report 49 (NCRP 1976). This included a model to estimate leakage radiation as a function of the angle relative to the rotation axis and distance from the isocentre.

8.2.5 Workload

100 MU approximates to 1 Gy at the isocentre under static beam reference measurement conditions. However, equating delivered MU to treatment dose in helical TomoTherapy is not as straightforward as for single direct beams with a stationary patient, and explains why treatment times are longer. Due to the

Table 8.3. Typical parameters for a range of helical TomoTherapy treatments.

Treatment site	Dose per fraction (Gy)	Beam-on time (min)	Field width (cm)	Leaf open time (%) (100/MF)
Prostate[a]	2.0	4	2.5	41
Prostate[b]	2.0	2–3	2.5	70
Whole brain[b]	3.0	3.5	2.5	60
Nasopharynx[b]	2.1	6.3	2.5	54
Whole central nervous system[b]	1.5	8.0–13.5	5.0	55
Breast[b]	2.67	10–13	5.0	40–55
Lower gastro-intestinal[b]	1.8	3–6	2.5	55
Head and neck[c]	2.0	8.3	2.5	30.4

[a]TomoTherapy (2011).
[b]GSTT.
[c]TomoTherapy (2014).

continuous translation of the patient on the treatment couch and the slit beam arrangement a point within the treatment target is only in a position to be irradiated for a proportion of the overall treatment. In addition to this the binary MLC leaves continuously open and close to modulate the field and so a point of interest will be shielded for some of the time from certain beam projection angles, even though it lies within the radiation field. This effect is called the modulation factor (MF), defined as the ratio of the maximum leaf opening time divided by the mean leaf opening time for those leaves that open during a treatment. With TomoTherapy the MF is a user-defined value, chosen at the time of planning, typically between 1.2 and 3.5 to improve beam conformance. However as the MF increases the beam-on time has to increase because on average the leaves are closed for a longer proportion of the treatment. A typical average MF for TomoTherapy patients would be around 2.0. Table 8.3 shows some typical parameters for a range of helical treatments. As for conventional linear accelerators estimation of the yearly workload will depend on the projected case mix and working hours. TomoTherapy beam-on times are longer than conventional linear accelerators with a typical range of around 3–4 min for prostate treatments to 10–15 min or more for treatments that may consist of one or more combinations of high MF, smaller field width (1 cm) and extended treatment length. For some cases, such as total body treatments, treatment times can exceed 30 min.

Workload examples

For a 40 h week and beam-on time of 16 min h^{-1} (e.g. four prostate treatments):

$$\begin{aligned}\text{radiation workload} &= 16\text{ min} \times 40\text{ h} \times 8.80\text{ Gy min}^{-1}\\ &= 5.63\text{ kGy/week} \times 50\text{ weeks}\\ &= 282\text{ kGy/year.}\end{aligned}$$

For a 40 h week and beam-on time of 30 min h^{-1} (e.g. three complex cases), annual workload would equate to 528 kGy.

Balog *et al* (2005) proposed a weekly workload of 700 min beam-on time. Baechler *et al* (2007) reviewed several sites and adopted a weekly workload of 1000 min. This gave a workload of 10 kGy/week or 500 kGy/year based on an approximate dose rate of 10 Gy min^{-1} at the isocentre. This is typically 5–10 times that of a conventional linear accelerator. TomoDirect treatment times also need to be considered if these are likely to increase the beam-on time.

8.2.6 Leakage

Because of the helical operation and primary beam stopper, leakage radiation from the treatment head is the major shielding consideration (see section 8.2.8 for the detailed reasoning for this conclusion). Careful head design seeks to minimise leakage radiation with the linear accelerator unit surrounded by interlocking lead shielding disks and the x-ray target encompassed within a tungsten fitting. The TomoTherapy site planning guides present leakage data measured both for continuous helical rotation and static gantry angle cases. Helical leakage measurements were performed with the jaws and all MLC leaves closed with a gantry rotation period of 20 s. Data are presented as a function of angle and radial distance measured, in a horizontal (IEC 1217 (IEC 2011) XZ) plane, from the isocentre with zero degrees as the direction from the isocentre to the treatment couch (figure 8.9). The static leakage data were collected in a similar manner but with the gantry at 0 degrees. Table 8.4 gives example data measured during helical operation. Similar data are available in the TomoTherapy planning guides for static operation.

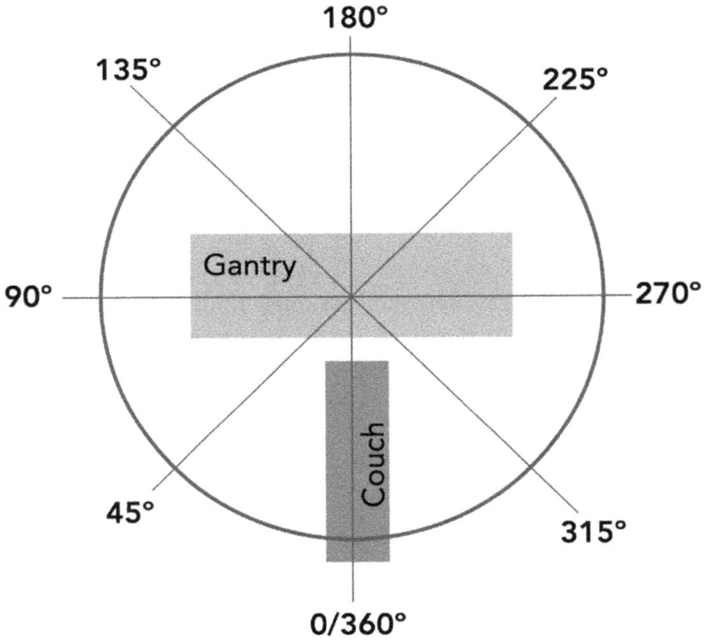

Figure 8.9. Top view of the room angles defined for the room leakage measurements. (Courtesy of Accuray Incorporated.)

Table 8.4. Fraction of the leakage radiation (at 1, 2 and 3.5 m) and leakage plus scattered radiation (at 2 m) relative to isocentre output versus radial distance from the isocentre for various room angles with *continuous* helical rotation of the gantry. Data reproduced from TomoTherapy (2011) table 3.1. Refer to the most recent planning guide specific to the machine model for the latest data.

Degrees from IEC-1217 Y direction	Distance from isocentre (m)			
	1	2	3.5	2
	Leakage Jaws and leaves closed			Leakage + scattered Jaws and leaves open
0	3.59×10^{-5}	1.09×10^{-5}	5.08×10^{-6}	7.81×10^{-5}
15	3.35×10^{-5}	1.36×10^{-5}	6.62×10^{-6}	8.21×10^{-5}
30	6.72×10^{-5}	2.27×10^{-5}	9.32×10^{-6}	1.01×10^{-4}
45	5.93×10^{-5}	2.33×10^{-5}	1.10×10^{-5}	1.14×10^{-4}
60	1.35×10^{-4}	3.42×10^{-5}	1.16×10^{-5}	1.22×10^{-4}
75	1.94×10^{-4}	4.25×10^{-5}	1.24×10^{-5}	1.31×10^{-4}
90	3.47×10^{-4}	5.74×10^{-5}	1.49×10^{-5}	8.44×10^{-5}
150	1.60×10^{-5}	7.80×10^{-6}	4.38×10^{-6}	5.73×10^{-5}
180	–	2.30×10^{-6}	–	5.79×10^{-5}

In the TomoTherapy *Site Planning Guide* (TomoTherapy 2011) measurements were performed using a large volume ion chamber with portable cylindrical lead collimator to prevent the chamber from measuring low energy scatter radiation from the walls. It is not clear whether a build-up cap was used to perform these measurements. It is noted that these leakage values are typically two to five times less than corresponding values presented in earlier guides (TomoTherapy 2003, 2004) and reported by Balog *et al* (2005) and Ramsey *et al* (2006). The *Site Planning Guide* for the TomoTherapy H-Series units (TomoTherapy 2014) presents new leakage and scatter data based on the latest machine design with reported leakage values lower than those in table 8.4. The maximum leakage at 1 m from table 8.4 is 0.035%, compared to a corresponding value of 0.014% in the TomoTherapy H-Series *Site Planning Guide* (TomoTherapy 2014). A typical value of 0.1% is used for conventional linear accelerators and for some TomoTherapy installations (e.g. Brighton and Sussex University Hospitals NHS Trust) this more conservative value has been adopted.

Does the inverse square law apply to leakage radiation?

The helical leakage radiation emanates from a ring source of radius 0.85 m so calculation of the leakage reduction at extended distances is less straightforward than assuming an inverse square fall off. Baechler *et al* (2007) performed a ring source integration as a function of distance from the isocentre (a_p) and angle (θ), to

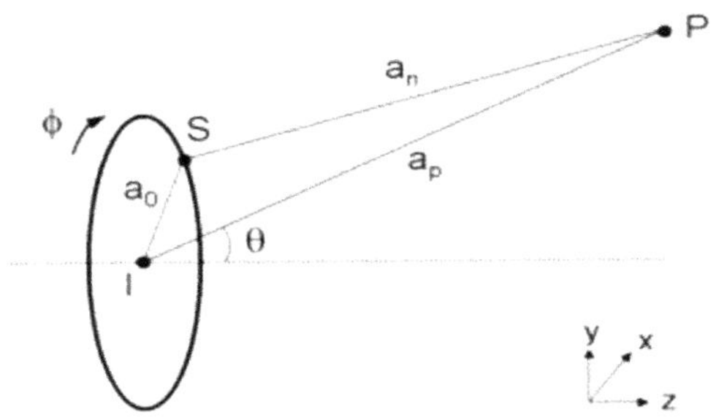

Figure 8.10. Schematic view of the TomoTherapy unit for calculation of the mean distance of a_n as the source S rotates around the isocentre I and generates leakage (and scatter radiation) at point P. (Reproduced from Baechler *et al* (2007) *Phys Med Biol* **52** 5057 © Institute of Physics and Engineering in Medicine. Reproduced by permission of IOP Publishing. All rights reserved.)

calculate a mean distance for which the dose decreases with the square of the distance (figure 8.10):

$$\bar{a}_n(a_p, \theta) = \left(\left(a_0^2 + a_p^2\right)^2 - \left(2a_p \times a_0 \times \sin\theta\right)^2\right)^{0.25}.$$

In practice, this treatment does not change the amount of shielding required significantly compared to the simple use of the inverse square law with the isocentre as the 'source', as assumed for conventional linear accelerators. Readers should refer to Baechler *et al* (2007) if they wish to pursue this line of calculation.

8.2.7 Scatter

Under normal clinical conditions scatter from the patient to the walls of the room is small compared to the leakage radiation. The planning guide presents data for leakage plus scatter radiation (see table 8.4). At first glance, the scatter component appears greater than leakage but clinically relevant situations will exhibit smaller scatter increases. Using an example from the *Site Planning Guide* (TomoTherapy 2011) as an illustration, table 8.4 shows that the increase in measured radiation due to scatter from the patient is 47% (100 × ([8.44/5.74] − 1)) at 90° and a radial distance of 2 m from the isocentre. Assuming that clinical cases use an average field width of 2.5 cm rather than the maximum of 5 cm, an average of 16 rather than 64 open leaves per projection and 50% leaf open time (MF = 2.0), the additional scatter would be reduced by a factor of 16 bringing the scatter increase down to only 2.9% (47%/16) above the leakage value.

8.2.7.1 Scatter down the maze

The method for calculating the scattered radiation down a maze is the same as for conventional linear accelerators. Baechler *et al* (2007) calculated scatter fractions for TomoTherapy based on the original data measured by Balog *et al* (2005). Derived scatter fractions, defined as the percentage of radiation scatter at 1 m from the patient per m^2 at the isocentre, were reported to be in the range 0%–2%.

Example. Calculation of the scatter fraction at 75° using data from table 8.4.

Irradiated area = 40 cm × 5 cm = 0.02 m^2
Scatter at a distance of 2 m and angle 75° = (1.31 − 0.425) × 10^{-4} = 0.885 × 10^{-4}
Scatter at distance of 1 m and angle 75° = 3.5 × 10^{-4} (assume inverse square law)
Scatter fraction = 3.5 × 10^{-4}/0.02 = 1.8%.

Baechler *et al* (2007) adopted the conservative value of 2% for any room angle and also adopted this as the reflection coefficient for both second scatter and scattered leakage radiation. For the wall scattered leakage radiation Baechler *et al* (2007) also used the maximum helical leakage dose rate incident on the wall irrespective of direction. If a maze door is required some estimation of the likely beam spectra for leakage and scatter has to be made. Radiation following a second scatter will have a lower energy spectrum than the wall scattered leakage radiation. This is discussed further in the detailed case study.

8.2.8 Primary beam

It is important to demonstrate that the shielding required for primary and leakage radiation is similar in extent for helical operation. If TomoDirect (i.e. static) beams are planned, then the primary shielding may need to be greater than in helical use only.

The primary beam stopper consists of 130 mm of lead which is opposite the source and reduces the transmitted beam to 0.4% of the dose at the isocentre (table 8.2). There are several other factors that contribute to a further reduction in primary beam intensity. These are:

- low use (or orientation) factor for helical delivery (since the source is continuously rotating) and
- the beam MFs.

8.2.8.1 Use or orientation factor

The use factor for helical delivery has been evaluated by several authors. The maximum primary beam size at the isocentre distance of 85 cm is 40 cm × 5 cm, corresponding to an opening angle of 27° in the transverse direction. Adding a 5° margin to each side to allow for high energy scattered radiation at small angles, the use factor becomes 0.10 (Baechler *et al* 2007). Wu *et al* (2006) proposed an analytical expression dependent on the distance between the calculation point and the isocentre to produce use factors in the range 0.08–0.1. Robinson *et al* (2000) derived a use factor of 0.09. For TomoDirect the effect of fixed gantry angles will need to be considered by increasing the use factor appropriately in certain directions.

Example. Comparing the helical leakage and primary radiation intensities relative to the isocentre at a distance of 3.5 m from the isocentre with the gantry at 90°:

Leakage fraction at 3.5 m = 1.49 × 10^{-5} (table 8.4)

Primary fraction at 3.5m = 0.04 × $(0.85/(0.85 + 3.5))^2$ × 0.10 = 1.53 × 10^{-5}, where

0.04 = the transmission of the primary beam stopper
$(0.85/(0.85 + 3.5))^2$ = the inverse square law correction from the isocentre to the calculation point
0.10 = the use factor for a rotational source.

For an annual workload of 500 kGy and a dose constraint of 0.3 mSv per annum the concrete thickness required to satisfy the dose constraint from leakage radiation only would be:

$$\text{Concrete thickness} = -\ 290 \times \log(0.3 \times 10^{-3}/5 \times 10^{5} \times 1.49 \times 10^{-5}) = 1275 \text{ mm},$$

where the TVL in concrete for leakage radiation is 290 mm.

The primary dose for this thickness of concrete using a TVL for primary radiation of 340 mm will be

$$\text{Dose/year} = 1.53 \times 10^{-5} \times 10^{-1275/340} \times 5 \times 10^{5} = 1.36 \text{ mSv}.$$

Using these values means the primary beam dose would predominate due to its larger TVL, requiring more shielding than in this simple leakage calculation. However, further corrections may be applied to the primary dose calculation to account for beam modulation.

8.2.8.2 Beam modulation

A reduction factor of 1/16 was recommended in the TomoTherapy *Site Planning Guide* (TomoTherapy 2011) to account for beam modulation of the primary beam. This incorporated:

- A mean leaf MF of 2 on the assumption that on average leaves are open for 50% of the time (reduction factor = 0.5).
- For typical clinical cases only 16 of the 64 leaves would be open per projection (reduction factor = 0.25).
- The average field width is 2.5 cm rather than the maximum of 5.0 cm (reduction factor = 0.5).

Unlike the scatter example presented above it is suggested that this value should be 1/8 rather than 1/16, since reducing the primary beam width from 5 cm to 2.5 cm has no effect on barrier thickness calculation along the beam central axis. Balog *et al* (2005) also recommend a reduction factor of 1/8 to the effective contribution of the primary beam.

Combining these additional factors reduces the primary dose contribution:

$$\text{Primary dose per annum} = 1.36 \times 0.50 \times 0.25 = 0.17 \text{ mSv},$$

where

MF = 0.5
beam size reduction = 0.25.

In this example the primary contribution is less than that due to leakage (0.3 mSv) but not negligible with the combined total of 0.47 mSv exceeding the design constraint and requiring additional shielding. It is interesting to note that the larger magnitude leakage data presented in earlier planning guides would have produced a thicker barrier based on leakage only but would have made the primary component less in a similar example.

8.2.9 Summary of practical considerations for shielding

For any installation the design calculations follow similar methodology to a conventional linear accelerator but using the more detailed information described above, outlined as follows:

- Determine dose constraints.
- Calculate the annual workload.
- Draw a line from isocentre to the point of interest and calculate leakage contribution at this point as a function of distance and angle using the data in the site planning guide.
- Determine required wall and ceiling thicknesses to meet the design constraint at each point, making appropriate allowance for obliquities.
- Check the primary barrier is adequate and increase leakage barrier thickness if necessary.
- Calculate maze doses using a similar methodology to conventional linear accelerators and choosing appropriate reflection coefficients and leakage data (see example below).

Wu *et al* (2006), using data from the *Site Planning Guide* (TomoTherapy 2004) presented shielding calculations for a TomoTherapy unit installed in an existing treatment room that had contained a Varian 600 C linear accelerator, which operates with an end point energy of 6 MV. It was found that existing shielding was adequate apart from one region in the control area requiring an additional 180 mm of concrete equivalent.

Because of the significantly higher leakage from TomoTherapy units it can never be assumed that the secondary barriers of an existing bunker are adequate.

8.2.10 Case study: installation into an existing cobalt-60 bunker

8.2.10.1 Overview

A TomoTherapy Hi-Art unit, helical delivery only, was installed into an existing cobalt-60 bunker at Guy's and St Thomas' NHS Hospital Foundation Trust (GSTT), London, in 2010. This case study describes the methods employed locally at the time to design the new facility. Large sections of the existing bunker wall shielding were inadequate and due to severe space constraints had to be increased using interlocking lead blocks fixed to the inside of the room. The ceiling shielding, particularly above the isocentre, was also inadequate. Rolled steel joints (RSJ) were installed below the existing ceiling to provide a false ceiling. Steel plates were placed on these RSJs and additional lead then placed on top of the steel plates. To accommodate the false ceiling and provide the minimum clearance for the machine, the floor level of the existing bunker was lowered with the maze floor sloping down into the room. The existing maze nib was reduced by 0.5 m in length in order to allow access for the machine. The increased leakage and scattered radiation from the TomoTherapy unit necessitated additional shielding along the existing maze and the introduction of an 18 mm lead door at the end of the maze.

In the maze lead lined panels were introduced above head height, where service ducts entered the room, to reduce scattered and leakage radiation. These consisted of two lead sheets mounted on plyboard and hung vertically in the roof space and separated by 2 m. The lead sheets were cut around the service ducts and the spacing between the two sheets helped to remove a large proportion of the remaining scattered radiation. Specialised lead shapes were designed and made to accurately shield points of weakness in the construction of the false ceiling, particularly where the RSJs were supported by steel angles running along the walls on the sides of the room and maze. A schematic room plan is shown in figure 8.11.

8.2.10.2 Data

Annual dose constraints:

- 1 mSv at 100% occupancy for control desk area.
- 2 mSv at 50% occupancy for brachytherapy suite next door (itself a controlled area).
- 1.5 mSv at 20% occupancy for the door area.
- 1.5 mSv at 20% occupancy for waiting and corridor areas.
- 0.3 mSv at 100% occupancy for Medical Records and floor above.

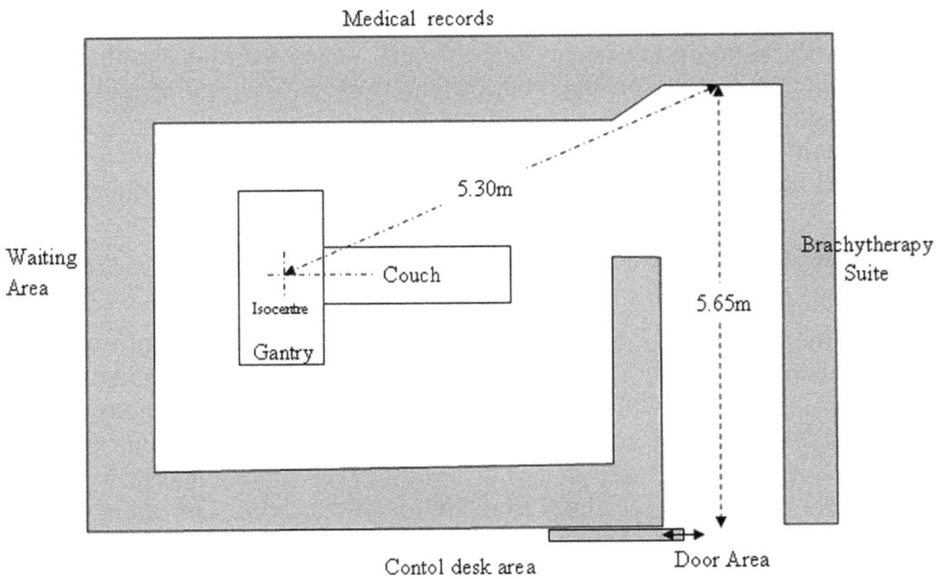

Figure 8.11. Schematic room plan of the TomoTherapy unit (not to scale).

Workload = 500 kGy per year.

Transmission as per table 8.2 (*Site Planning Guide*, TomoTherapy 2009).

Leakage data. The leakage data from the TomoTherapy *Site Planning Guide* (TomoTherapy 2003) and Balog *et al* (2005) was used. It was recognised that this might overestimate the dose by a factor of 2 to 5 times leading to more shielding than perhaps necessary based on the more recent planning guide values in table 8.4.

Scatter and primary radiation. These were confirmed as negligible and effectively ignored as outlined above.

8.2.10.3 Method

- Draw a line from the isocentre to the point of interest. Distance = a_p (m).
- Determine the length of line passing through the existing concrete wall L (mm) and calculate the transmission through the concrete. TVL is the tenth value layer for leakage radiation.

  $$\text{transmission factor} = 10^{-L/\text{TVL}}.$$

- Estimate the transmitted leakage dose per annum, D_t (mSv) at the point of interest:

  $$D_t = \text{workload} \times (D_L/D_R)_{3,\theta} \times (3/a_p)^2 \times \text{transmission factor},$$

  where

  $(D_L/D_R)_{3,\theta}$ = ratio of leakage dose rate (D_L) at a distance of 3 m to the reference dose rate at the isocentre (D_R) as a function of the room angle θ in the IEC 1217 (IEC 2011) XY plane (figure 8.9). These values were derived from data presented in table 8.4.

  $(3/a_p)^2$ = inverse square correction to account for the fall off in leakage radiation intensity from 3 m to extended distance a_p. Using the ring integration method of Baechler *et al* (2007), this would more correctly be calculated as $(a_n(3,\theta)/a_n(a_p,\theta))^2$.

- Estimate the additional oblique thickness of concrete required T (mm) to meet the required dose constraint:

  $$T = -\text{TVL} \times \log(\text{dose constraint}/D_t).$$

- Calculate the required perpendicular thickness of extra concrete correcting for oblique incidence using the method described in NCRP 151 (NCRP 2005) by adding an additional perpendicular thickness to remove side scatter within the barrier for larger angles of incidence, i.e. add 1, 2 and 3 HVLs for angles of incidence of 50, 60 and 70 degrees, respectively. To make spreadsheet implementation easier this was approximated using the formula $((1.8/\cos\Phi) - 1.8)$ where Φ is the angle of incidence.
- Convert the additional concrete thicknesses to steel and lead by dividing by 3.5 and 6.2, respectively (IAEA 2006).

8.2.10.4 Maze calculation

Scattered radiation down the maze was calculated in a similar manner to Baechler *et al* (2007) except that the leakage radiation reflection coefficient was taken as 0.01, as for conventional linear accelerators, and also the leakage radiation in the direction of the scattering wall (30°) was taken rather than the maximum value at any angle:

Workload per year (W) = 5×10^8 mSv
Distance from isocentre to back wall = 5.30 m
Distance from back wall to maze entrance (D_w) = 5.65 m
Area of back wall, ceiling and floor irradiated (A_w) = 24.6 m^2
Leakage reflection coefficient = 0.01 m^{-2}
Scatter reflection coefficient = 0.02 m^{-2}.

Leakage fraction hitting the first wall:

For angle (θ) = 30°, the leakage fraction[7] at 1 m = 3.41×10^{-4}
Mean distance from the rotating source[8] = 5.33 m
Calculated leakage fraction at wall = $3.41 \times 10^{-4}/5.33^2 = 1.2 \times 10^{-5}$.

Scatter fraction hitting the first wall:

Largest area of beam at scatterer = 40 cm × 5 cm = 0.02 m^2
Worst case scatter fraction = 0.02 m^{-2}
Scatter fraction at 1 m = 4×10^{-4}
Scatter fraction at wall = $4 \times 10^{-4}/5.30^2 = 1.42 \times 10^{-5}$.

At the maze entrance:

$$\text{Leakage} = (W \times \text{leakage fraction} \times A_w \times \text{reflection coefficient})/D_w^2$$
$$= (5 \times 10^8 \times 1.2 \times 10^{-5} \times 24.6 \times 0.01)/5.65^2 = 46.2 \text{ mSv},$$
$$\text{Scatter} = (5 \times 10^8 \times 1.42 \times 10^{-5} \times 24.6 \times 0.02)/5.65^2 = 109 \text{ mSv}.$$

Door shielding thickness

It was assumed that the energy of the scattered leakage radiation is equivalent to a 500 kVp broad beam and the energy of the second scatter radiation is equivalent to a 400 kVp broad beam. The *Handbook of Radiological Protection* (RSAC 1971) was used to derive shielding values of $TVL_{500\ kVp}$ = 1 cm lead and $TVL_{400\ kVp}$ = 0.5 cm

[7] This value was taken from an earlier planning guide. The corresponding value in table 8.4 from a more recent site planning guide (TomoTherapy 2011) is 6.72×10^{-5}.

[8] The ring integration correction by Baechler *et al* (2007) was used to calculate the mean distance taking into account the rotating source. It can be seen that in reality this makes negligible difference to the inverse square fall off (1.1% in this case) than using the distance from the isocentre.

lead. Using these TVL values a door shielding thickness of 17 mm lead produces a total transmitted dose of about 1 mSv as shown below:

Transmitted leakage radiation = $46.2 \times 10^{-17/10} = 0.92$ mSv

Transmitted scatter radiation = $109 \times 10^{-17/5} = 0.04$ mSv

Total = 0.96 mSv

Allowing for a possible further 0.5 mSv at the door entrance from wall transmission, this meets the dose constraint of 1.5 mSv for the door area.

A final door thickness of 18 mm lead was chosen. The spectrum of the leakage radiation down the maze is a major uncertainty. Assuming a 400 kVp broad beam for both leakage and scatter components would have reduced the required door thickness to 12 mm of lead.

8.2.10.5 Survey

Optically stimulated luminescence dosimetry badges were positioned at a range of locations outside the bunker and left for three months with the unit in full clinical operation. All results were well within the design constraints.

A TomoTherapy unit with a workload of 500 kGy per year equates to around 1000 h beam-on time per annum. The IDR in a 0.3 mSv per year area is therefore around 0.3 μSv h^{-1}, lower than for a conventional linear accelerator. If the dose is integrated over 3 min, corresponding to nine rotations for a 20 second gantry rotation period, an instrument capable of measuring to 15 nSv with an acceptable degree of accuracy (typically ±20%) is required.

Acknowledgements

The authors would like to thank P J Rudd and D Gallacher for the original calculations presented in the case study.

8.3 CyberKnife®

E G Aird

8.3.1 Introduction

The CyberKnife[9] is a 6 MV linear accelerator mounted on a robotic arm that delivers stereotactic precision using multiple small fields. The gantry holding the accelerator can point in almost any direction; but currently cannot point upwards more than 18–22 degrees above the horizontal. The gantry does not have an isocentre. The centre of treatment is defined by the centre of the imaging system (termed 'the room imaging centre'). The imaging system consists of two x-ray tubes mounted on the ceiling of the room together with two digital imaging plates located in the floor. The position of the patient is monitored by image matching and the

[9] CyberKnife is a registered trademark of Accuray Incorporated.

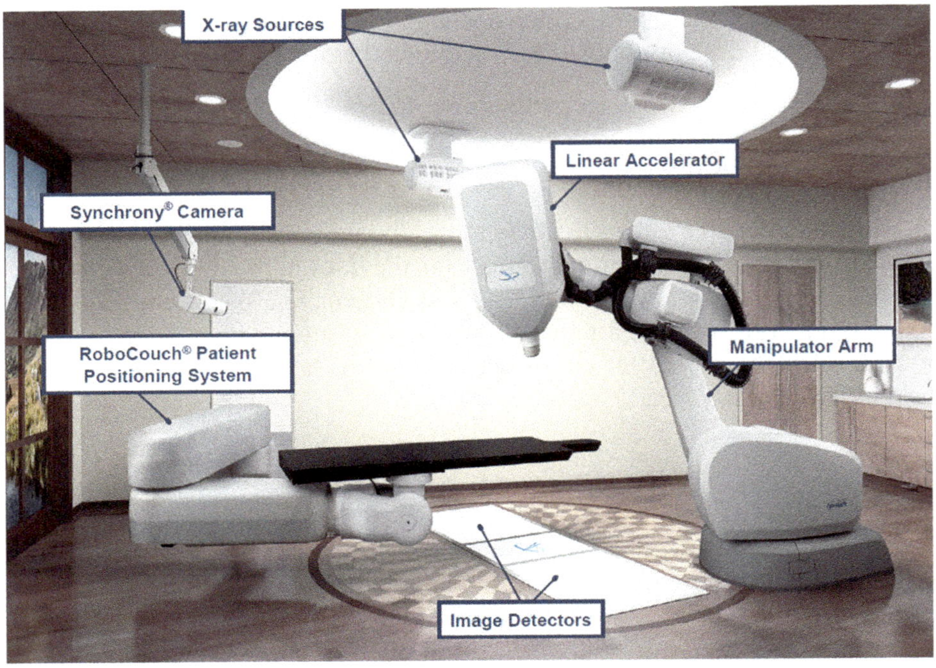

Figure 8.12. A typical CyberKnife installation. (Courtesy of Accuray Inc.)

position corrected by movement of the treatment couch with either three or six degrees of freedom and by the robot arm itself. A typical installation is illustrated in figure 8.12.

Most treatments are given using only 1–5 fractions with 5–30 Gy per fraction. This means that the number of monitor units is very high for each fraction, but the number of patient treatments per day is much less than a conventional linear accelerator.

8.3.2 CyberKnife specification

The *source to axis distance* (SAD) is variable (65–100 cm), but it is recommended to use 85 cm when calculating shielding requirements.

The *dose rate* (at 80 cm) is typically 800 MU min^{-1} (calibrated to give 1 cGy MU^{-1} at 1.5 cm depth using the 60 mm collimator), but can be increased to 1000 MU min^{-1}.

The *maximum field size* at 80 cm is 60 mm (using the fixed collimator assembly).

The 'iris' variable size collimator is designed to closely replicate the 12 fixed collimator aperture sizes. Recently an MLC has been developed, the 'InCise MLC', with a variable aperture and a maximum field size of 9.75 cm × 11.0 cm at 80 cm SAD.

Beam directions

This is a complex issue. The direction of beams is determined by the nodes (see figure 8.13) that have been selected at commissioning. A typical treatment has

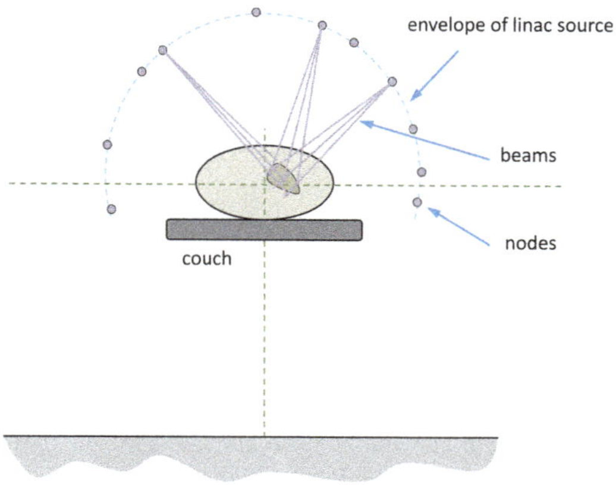

Figure 8.13. Transverse plane showing the positions of the beam nodes. (Courtesy of M Folkard.)

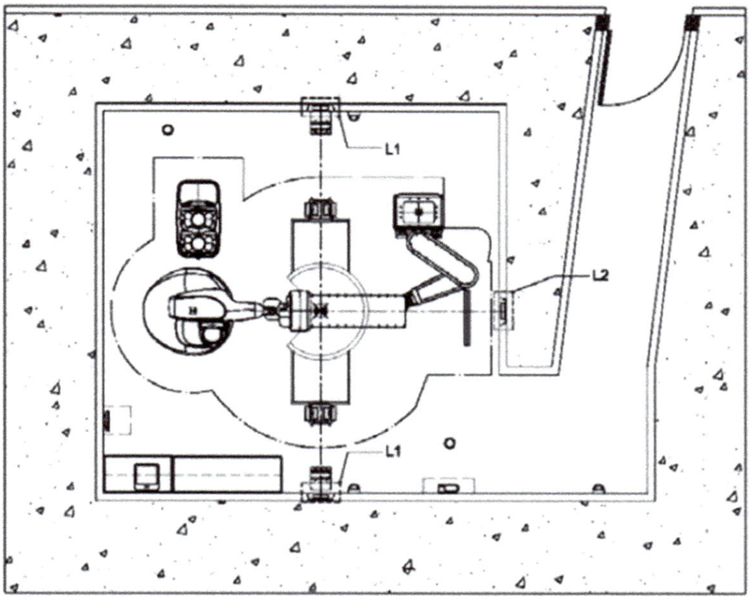

Figure 8.14. CyberKnife bunker with a maze and primary barrier walls.

120–180 beams and around 102–180 nodes (Accuray Inc. 2016). A bunker can either be designed to allow all nodes in which case all the walls of the bunker must be designated as primary barriers (see figures 8.14 and 8.15). Alternatively a bunker similar to that required for a conventional linear accelerator ('gantry linac bunker') can be designed which only allows nodes to be used that are in conventional gantry directions towards a primary barrier (see figure 8.16). As stated above, upward directed beams are not currently enabled and all beams pass within 10 cm of the room imaging centre.

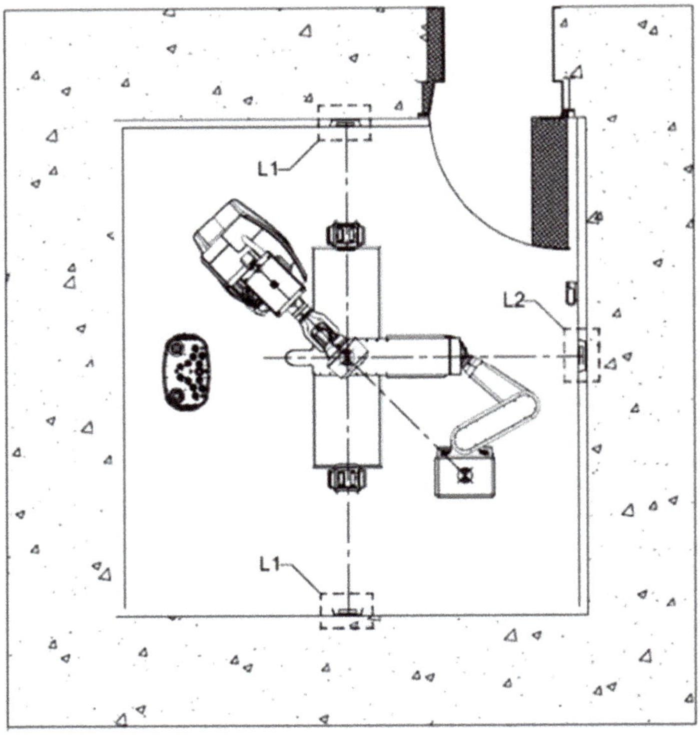

Figure 8.15. Typical CyberKnife bunker floor plan with a directly shielded door (Courtesy of Accuray Inc.)

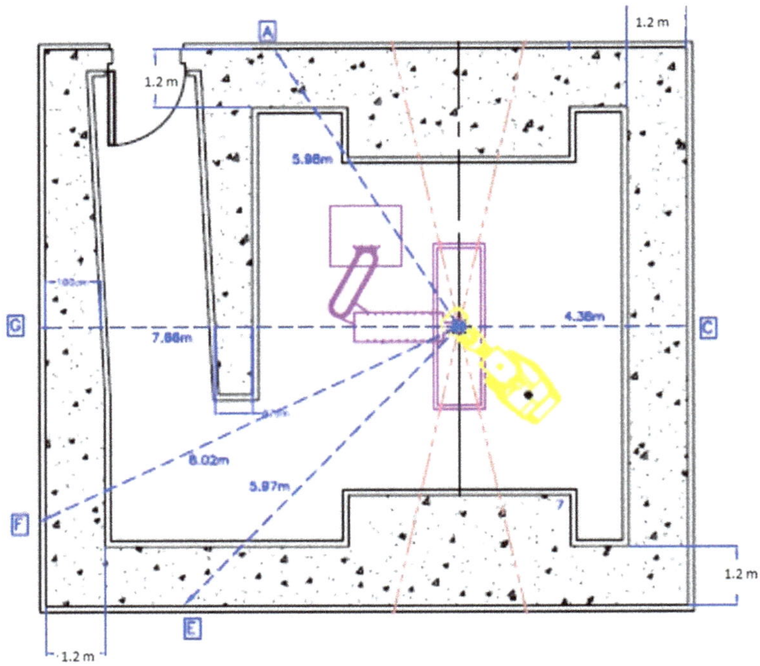

Figure 8.16. CyberKnife in a conventional linear accelerator bunker with limited primary barrier walls.

Table 8.5. CyberKnife IMRT factors.

Site	Total dose (Gy)	No. of fractions	MU/ fraction	MU cGy^{-1}
Intracranial	24.6	3.3	10 072	**12.4**
Spine	26.7	4.3	14 522	23.2
Lung	46.3	3.4	12 424	9.0
Prostate	35.6	4.3	16 431	18.5
Others	–	–	–	14.0
Extra cranial average				**16.1**
				12.3 (weighted by frequency)

IMRT factor

This is the parameter that determines the MU from the dose for a typical set of patient treatments and is used to determine the thickness of the barrier to shield against leakage radiation. A conservative figure of 15 MU cGy^{-1} has been suggested for fixed and iris collimators and 7 MU cGy^{-1} for the MLC (Accuray Inc. 2016) although the data in a previous publication (Accuracy Inc. 2009) (see table 8.5) suggests a value weighted by the frequency of treatments of 12.3. A more recent publication found an even lower value of 7.4 in clinical practice (Yang and Feng 2014).

Use factor

This is an estimate of the typical dose delivered in any given direction and leads to differences between calculations based on IDR and average dose rate (see below). The average value of the use factor is typically taken as 0.05 (Rodgers 2005). The CyberKnife *Site Planning Guide* M6 (Accuray Inc. 2016) quotes a value of 0.05 for fixed and iris collimators and 0.075 for the InCise MLC. Experience at Mount Vernon Cancer Centre, London, has shown that unusual fractionations such as treating single brain metastases can give values as high as 0.12. Yang and Feng (2014) used the primary workload on each section of the walls to calculate individual thicknesses. This is not recommended because this leads to room shielding for a particular machine and its current clinical use and does not provide for possible future changes in clinical use.

Workload

Various estimates of the typical or worst case workload have been made. For example, the CyberKnife *Site Planning Guide* M6 (Accuray Inc. 2016) estimates giving six head and six body treatments per day to give 445 Gy/week @ 100 cm. This is based on the information in table 8.6. However, the average time per fraction given for the fixed collimator system is about 50 min, so it would require a 10 h day to achieve this throughput. For iris and MLC fitted systems the time per fraction is shorter but only the latter permits an 8 h working day with this workload.

Table 8.6. Radiation workload (Accuray Inc. 2016).

Site	Average dose per fraction	Total dose over 5 day week @ 100 cm	Average time per fraction (fixed collimator/iris)
Head	8 Gy @ 80 cm	154 Gy	51/34 min
Spine/body	9.7 Gy @ 100 cm	291 Gy	53/35 min

Other estimates of radiation workload/week @ 100 cm are:

- NCRP (2005): 320 Gy
- Queen Elizabeth Hospital, Birmingham (2016): 400 Gy
- Yang and Feng (2014): 160 Gy
- Mount Vernon Cancer Centre, London: 150 Gy.

It should be noted that the workload dose in grays is the prescribed dose and not the dose at the centre of the treated volume which will be higher. However, this is the easiest way of calculating total dose per working week; otherwise factors such as attenuation in the body need to be considered for primary beam calculations though not for leakage.

8.3.3 Typical CyberKnife bunker features

Primary barriers

The TVLs quoted by Accuray Inc. (2009) are lower than for the standard end point energies on the assumption that the nominal energy is slightly lower than for conventional linear accelerators. For standard concrete of 2350 kg m^{-3} the equilibrium TVL is given as 324 mm, and for lead 55 mm. To meet regulatory dose rates for the USA (typically 20 μSv/week for an uncontrolled area) Accuray Inc. (2009) recommends 1.52 m concrete for all primary barriers and 1.07 m for all secondary barriers. In the UK, barriers have been based on a maximum IDR of 7.5 μSv h^{-1} in most installations. For 7.5 μSv h^{-1}, a typical primary barrier will need to be 1.9–2.1 m (see section 8.3.4). When occupancy and use factors are taken into account, the values will be lower. For example, to achieve a TADR of 7.5 μSv h^{-1} in figure 8.14 would require a primary barrier of 1.6 m.

Secondary barriers

The large IMRT implies that the leakage radiation will be large. The manufacturer recommended value of 0.1% of the primary x-ray beam at 0.8 m may be used but this will generally overestimate the amount of leakage radiation. A value of 0.05% has also been suggested (Accuray Inc. 2009, Yang and Feng 2014). The TVL for leakage radiation is lower than for the primary beam because of the reduced energy; Accuray Inc. (2009) quotes 292 mm for standard concrete or 53 mm for lead. A typical secondary barrier will be at least 1.2 m thick (see figure 8.16).

Scattered radiation
The intensity of scattered radiation from the patient is negligible compared with leakage radiation due to the small field sizes.

Use of lead
Lead can be used to replace concrete where necessary. The relevant TVLs for primary and secondary barriers of lead are given above. Lead is much more expensive but where it has to be used to save space it is possible to make use of the extra path length provided by obliquity with oblique ray paths to reduce the overall thickness required. Measures may need to be taken against groundshine (see section 5.5).

Room layout
A classical maze entrance can be used. But the orientation of the maze needs careful consideration if only one leg is included; unlike a conventional linear accelerator the CyberKnife is not confined to coplanar gantry angles. It is possible to reduce both leakage and primary radiation striking the far wall of the maze by appropriate use of the inner maze wall (see figure 8.14). If this is not possible, it may be necessary to use 5–30 mm thick lead in the door depending on distances and the angle of first order scatter impinging on the door. A direct access door will need to contain enough steel or lead to be equivalent to a secondary barrier (assuming it is positioned so that the primary beam cannot be directed towards it), i.e. 180–220 mm lead depending on the dose rate at the door.

Room size
The following dimensions are specified in Accuray Inc. (2016):

- Recommended area: 7.32 m × 6.40 m (or 7.14 m × 6.58 m, if machine sited diagonally).
- Minimum area: 6.40 m × 4.83 m (or 6.20 m × 5.67 m, if machine sited diagonally).
- Height: recommended 3.35 m to rough ceiling; 3.0 m to finished ceiling within the treatment manipulation operating area.

Imaging
When setting up the patient, the two imaging systems can be used without a door interlock, if strict systems of work are followed. The dose rate at the door when imaging only is very low.

8.3.4 Worked example: primary barriers

The simplest bunker for a CyberKnife (figure 8.14) is to ensure all the walls and possibly the roof are primary barriers. This provides future-proofing for upward directed beams and changes in beam patterns. The ceiling can be a secondary barrier provided there is no occupancy above. With the maze shown, the door should contain at least 5 mm lead (assuming no scattered photons greater than 0.5 MeV).

The thickness of the primary barrier will depend on whether the TADR is taken into account or not. For the layout in figure 8.16, the following can be deduced, assuming:

$$\text{Output} = 6.4\ \text{Gy min}^{-1}\ @\ 100\ \text{cm}\ (1000\ \text{MU min}^{-1}\ @\ 80\ \text{cm})\ \text{and}$$

$$\text{TVL(concrete)} = 324\ \text{mm}.$$

For the primary beam, wall thicknesses of 2.0 m will be equivalent to 6.17 TVLs. If the dose rate at 1 m is 6.4 Gy min^{-1}, the IDR at 5 m on the far side of the wall will be about 10 μSv h^{-1}. A wall thickness of 2045 mm will result in an IDR of 7.5 μSv h^{-1}, given by

$$(6.4 \times (1/10^{-(2045/324)}) \times 60 \times 10^{6})/5^{2} = 7.5\ \mu\text{Sv h}^{-1}.$$

However, at any given position the beam is only incident for 2–3 min every hour (even in the busiest centre) which would greatly reduce this dose rate to about 10–15 μSv/week given by

$$(2 - 3 \times 7.5 \times 40)/60.$$

Alternatively, using the worst case workload (445 Gy/week) and use factor (0.05) listed above the average dose rate in the same position gives an even lower value:

$$\text{Dose rate} = (445 \times 0.05 \times (1/10^{-(2045/324)} \times 10^{6})/5^{2}) = 0.4\ \mu\text{Sv/week}.$$

Both these calculations demonstrate that using the TADR could theoretically reduce the thickness of primary barriers, but this does not allow for any future changes in working practice. For example, to achieve a TADR of 7.5 μSv h^{-1} over 8 h day would require a primary barrier of only 1.623 m thickness, given by

$$(6.4 \times 0.05 \times (1/10^{-(1623/324)}) \times 60 \times 10^{6})/5^{2} = 7.5\ \mu\text{Sv h}^{-1}.$$

Figure 8.15 shows how the CyberKnife can be used in a room with a direct access door, which can be considered a secondary barrier provided the beam cannot be directed at it.

8.3.5 Worked example: secondary barriers

These only exist in rooms that are converted from conventional linear accelerator bunkers (see figure 8.16). It is possible to use this form of room as long as (a) the original secondary barriers are sufficiently thick (see calculation below) and (b) the 'treatment nodes' are selected so that there is no possibility of the primary beam striking a secondary barrier during treatment. The secondary barriers may have thinner walls than the primary barriers but thicker than those present in conventional bunkers, (where the secondary barrier is typically half of the primary barrier thickness). This is because of the much greater number of MUs used with CyberKnife due to the high IMRT factor of 15.

Suppose a TVL in standard concrete of 292 mm and a head leakage of 0.1% of the primary beam at 0.8 m are assumed. The unattenuated dose/week for the worse case workload (445 Gy/week) at 5 m is given by

$$(445 \times 10^{-3} \times 15)/5^2 = 267 \text{ mSv/week}.$$

If the dose per week is limited to 20 μSv (for staff to have a limit of 1 mSv/year or for members of the public in an area with an occupancy of 0.3 or less to have a limit of 0.3 mSv/year) then the secondary barrier attenuation is given by

$$20/(267 \times 10^{-3}) = 7.49 \times 10^{-5} = 4.1 \text{ TVLs} = 1.2 \text{ m concrete}.$$

The IDR will be given by

$$(10 \times 10^{-3} \times 10^{-(1170/292)} \times 60 \times 10^6)/5^2 = 2.4\ \mu\text{Sv h}^{-1}.$$

References

Accuray Inc. 2009 *Tenth-value layer measurements of leakage radiation and secondary barrier shielding calculations for the CyberKnife robotic surgery system* (Sunnyvale, CA: Accuray Inc.)

Accuray Inc. 2016 *CyberKnife M6 Series Site Planning Guide 11.0 EN 501035* Revision A (Sunnyvale, CA: Accuray Inc.)

Baechler S, Bochud F, Verellen D and Moeckli R 2007 Shielding requirements in helical tomotherapy *Phys. Med. Biol.* **52** 5057–67

Balog J, Lucas D, DeSouza C and Crilly R 2005 Helical TomoTherapy radiation leakage and shielding considerations *Med. Phys.* **32** 710–9

Beavis A W 2004 Is Tomotherapy the future of IMRT? *Brit. J. Radiol.* **77** 285–95

Croft Associates Limited 2015 *Safshield Package Design* No 2773A (Abingdon: Croft Associates Limited) http://www.croftltd.com/products/type-b-package-designs.php Accessed: 18 January 2017

Dryzmala R, Sohn J, Guo C, Sobotka L and Purdy J 2001 Angular measurement of the Cobalt-60 emitted radiation spectrum from a radiosurgery irradiator *Med. Phys.* **28** 620–8

Elekta Instruments AB 1999 *Loading Machine LM3: Loading and Unloading Cobalt Sources in Leksell Gamma Knife* Document Art No 008114, Rev 00 (Stockholm: Elekta Instruments).

Elekta Instruments AB 2011 *Leksell Gamma Knife Perfexion: Site Planning Guide* Document No 1019394, Rev 02 (Stockholm: Elekta Instruments).

Elekta Instruments AB 2015 *Leksell Gamma Knife Icon Site Planning Guide* Document No 1516109 Rev 01 (Stockholm: Elekta Instruments)

EPR 2016 *The Environmental Permitting (England and Wales) Regulations* SI 2016/1154 (London: The Stationery Office)

IAEA (International Atomic Energy Agency) 2006 *Radiation Protection in the Design of Radiotherapy Facilities* Safety Reports Series no. 47 (Vienna: IAEA)

ICRP (International Commission on Radiological Protection) 1991 *1990 Recommendations of the International Commission on Radiological Protection* Report 60, Ann ICRP 21(1-3)

IEC (International Electrotechnical Commission) 2011 *Radiation Equipment—Coordinates, Movements and Scales* 61217 (Geneva: IEC)

IEC (International Electrotechnical Commission) 2013 *Medical Electrical Equipment—Part 2-11: Particular Requirements for the Basic Safety and Essential Performance of Gamma Beam Therapy Equipment* 60601-2-11 (Geneva: IEC)

IPEM (Institute of Physics and Engineering in Medicine) 2002 *Medical and Dental Guidance Notes: a Good Practice Guide to Implementing Ionising Radiation Protection Legislation in the Clinical Environment* (York: IPEM)

IRR 1999 *The Ionising Radiation Regulations* SI 1999/3232 (London: The Stationery Office)

ISO (International Organisation for Standardisation) 1992 *Radiation Protection—Sealed Radioactive Sources—Leakage Test Methods* ISO 9978:1992 (Geneva: ISO)

Larsson B, Liden K and Sarby B 1974 Irradiation of small structures through the intact skull *Acta Radiol.* **13** 511–33

Leksell L 1951 The stereotaxic method and radiosurgery of the brain *Acta Chir. Scand.* **102** 316–9

Lindquist C and Paddick I 2007 The Leksell Gamma Knife Perfexion and comparisons with its predecessors *Neurosurgery* **61** 130–40

Mackie T R, Holmes T, Swerdloff S, Reckwerdt P, Deasy J O, Yang J, Paliwal B and Kinsella T 1993 Tomotherapy: a new concept for the delivery of dynamic conformal radiotherapy *Med. Phys.* **20** 1709–19

McDermott P N 2007 Radiation shielding for gamma stereotactic radiosurgery units *J. Appl. Clin. Med. Phys.* **8** 147–57

NaCTSO (National Counter Terrorism Security Office) 2011 *Security Requirements for Radioactive Sources* (London: NaCTSO)

NCRP (National Council on Radiation Protection and Measurements) 1976 *Structural Shielding Design and Evaluation for Medical Use of X-Rays and Gamma Rays of Energies up to 10 MeV* Report 49 (Bethesda, MD: NCRP)

NCRP (National Council on Radiation Protection and Measurements) 2005 *Structural Shielding Design and Evaluation for Megavoltage X- and Gamma-ray Radiotherapy Facilities* NCRP 151 (Bethesda, MD: NCRP)

Ramsey C, Siebert R, Mahan S, Desai D and Chase D 2006 Out-of-field dosimetry measurements for a helical tomotherapy system *J. Appl. Clin. Med. Phys.* **7** 1–11

Regis J, Tamura M, Guillot C, Yomo S, Muraciolle X, Nagaje M, Arka Y and Porcheron D 2009 Radiosurgery with the world's first fully robotized Leksell Gamma Knife Perfexion in clinical use: a 200-patient prospective randomized, controlled comparison with the Gamma Knife 4C *Neurosurgery* **64** 346–56

Robinson D M, Scrimger J W, Field G C and Fallone B G 2000 Shielding considerations for tomotherapy *Med. Phys.* **27** 2380–4

Rodgers J E 2005 CyberKnife treatment room design and radiation protection *Robotic Radiosurg* **1** 41–50

RSA 1993 *Radioactive Substances Act* (London: The Stationery Office) SI 1993/0012

RSAC (Radioactive Substances Advisory Committee) 1971 *Handbook of Radiological Protection* (London: The Stationery Office)

Shah A P, Langen K M, Ruchala K J, Cox A, Kupelian P A and Meeks S L 2008 Patient dose from megavoltage computed tomography imaging *Int. J. Radiat. Oncol. Biol. Phys.* **70** 1579–87

TomoTherapy Inc. 2003 *Helical Tomotherapy Radiation Leakage and Shielding Considerations* T-INT-HB0010A-0304 (Madison, WI: TomoTherapy Inc.)

TomoTherapy Inc. 2004 *TomoTherapy Hi-Art System Site Planning Guide* 1204 T-SPG-HB5001 (Madison, WI: TomoTherapy Inc.)

TomoTherapy Inc. 2009 *TomoTherapy Hi-Art System Site Planning Guide* T-SPG-HB6000-K (Madison, WI: TomoTherapy Inc.)

TomoTherapy Inc. 2011 *TomoTherapy HD System Site Planning Guide* T-SPG-0000B (Madison, WI: TomoTherapy Inc.)

TomoTherapy Inc. 2014 *TomoTherapy H Series Site Planning Guide* T-SPG-00725 (Sunnyvale, CA: Accuray Inc)

Walton L, Bomford C K and Ramsden D 1987 The Sheffield Stereotactic Radiosurgery Unit, physical characteristics and principles of operation *Bri. J. Radiol.* **60** 897–906

Wu C, Guo F and Purdy J 2006 Helical tomotherapy shielding calculation for an existing LINAC treatment room: sample calculation and cautions *Phys. Med. Biol.* **51** N389–92

Yang J and Feng J 2014 Radiation shielding evaluation based on five years of data from a busy CyberKnife center *J. Appl. Clin. Med. Phys.* **15** 313–22

Chapter 9

Kilovoltage therapy and electronic brachytherapy

C J Martin and D J Eaton

9.1 Superficial and orthovoltage therapy

C J Martin

9.1.1 Introduction

Superficial and orthovoltage therapies employ conventional x-ray tubes for treating shallow lesions. They are used to treat various forms of skin cancer, including melanoma, basal cell carcinoma and squamous cell carcinoma, as well as other skin lesions such as keloids. The treatment fields are delineated using applicators attached to the tube housing, with lead inserts customized to the treatment area on the patient's skin. Particular filters to harden the x-ray beam will be used for specific treatments and interlocks prevent incorrect combinations of kVp, mA and filtration being employed. Therapy units will often be used for both superficial and orthovoltage treatments up to about 300 kV. However, since superficial therapy units (operating up to 150 kVp) are available and their use is closely linked to specialist applications, dedicated designs may sometimes be required. A separate note on shielding for superficial units is therefore included here.

9.1.2 Superficial therapy

Superficial therapy units operate between 50 and 150 kVp with beam qualities equivalent to half value layers (HVLs) of 0.5–8 mm of aluminium. Units are used with cone applicators for treating skin lesions up to about 7 cm across. The energy range coupled with the low workload mean that extensive shielding is not usually required and methodologies similar to those used for diagnostic x-rays can be applied. Comprehensive coverage of shielding for diagnostic facilities is given in

doi:10.1088/978-0-7503-1440-4ch9

Sutton *et al* (2012). The x-ray beam can in principle be pointed in any direction, so the walls, ceiling and the floor all need to provide shielding against the primary beam, unless restrictions are placed on beam orientation. Scatter calculations for tube potentials between 50 and 150 kV can be derived from the product of the primary air kerma incident on the skin surface and the area treated, using scatter factors (S_{kV}) dependent on tube potential from the equation

$$K_S = \sum_{kV}\left[S_{kV} \times \sum_{i}(K_{Pi} \times A_{Pi})_{kV}\right] \tag{9.1}$$

where K_S is the total scatter air kerma at 1 m from the patient; K_{Pi} is the primary beam air kerma for each treatment of skin area A_{Pi} and the products are summed for each tube potential (kV).

Scatter factors derived by Sutton *et al* (2012) are in close agreement with those reported by Trout and Kelley (1972) for tube potentials between 50 and 150 kV and applied to orthovoltage shielding calculations in NCRP (1976). Scatter factors are usually specified in therapy texts as the ratio of scatter air kerma at 1 m from the patient divided by the incident primary air kerma for a beam of a specific area. Therefore factors in both forms representing the direction with the highest scatter level are given in table 9.1.

Brick, concrete or lead sheet are all suitable for protecting superficial therapy rooms and methods of calculating thicknesses required where the workload is high are described in Sutton *et al* (2012). Because the scatter rates are comparatively low, the control area does not necessarily have to be outside the treatment room for superficial therapy, although this is the better option. The shielding for the control area will depend on the range of tube potentials used and the workload, and a substantial protective screen will always be required with either a window or closed circuit television (CCTV) for viewing the patient.

The x-ray beam energies used in superficial therapy are such that lower energy photons are attenuated to a greater extent through photoelectric interactions, so that

Table 9.1. Ratios between scatter air kerma at 1 m from the patient and the incident primary air kerma.

Tube potential (kVp)	Scatter factor S_K (μGy Gy^{-1} cm^{-2})	Ratio of (scatter at 1 m)/(primary) for a beam of area 100 cm^2 (μGy Gy^{-1})
50	4.0[a]	400
70	4.7[a]	470
100	5.6[a]	560[b]
125	6.4[a]	640[b]
150	7[a]	700
200	7	700[b]
300	7	700[b]

[a] Sutton *et al* (2012).
[b] Trout and Kelley (1972).

Table 9.2. Coefficients with which transmission curves can be generated using equations (9.1) and (9.2).

Material	Tube potential (kVp)	$\alpha(\text{mm}^{-1})$	$\beta(\text{mm}^{-1})$	γ
Lead	50	8.801	27.28	0.296
	70	5.369	23.49	0.588
	100	2.500	15.28	0.756
	125	2.219	7.923	0.539
Concrete (2350 kg m^{-3})	100	0.0395	0.0844	0.519
	125	0.0350	0.0711	0.697

the assumption of a fixed HVL may not be appropriate. Equations have been developed by Archer *et al* (1983) to describe the transmission curves for different materials and beam energies based on sets of three coefficients (α, β and γ). The equation for the transmission of material thickness (x) has the form

$$B = [(1 + \beta/\alpha) \times \exp(\alpha\gamma x) - \beta/\alpha]^{-1/\gamma}. \quad (9.2)$$

The inverse of this equation can be used to calculate the thickness of material to give a required transmission

$$x = \frac{1}{\alpha\gamma} \ln\left[\frac{B^{-\gamma} + (\beta/\alpha)}{1 + (\beta/\alpha)}\right]. \quad (9.3)$$

A selection of coefficients are given in table 9.2 and a more complete set is included in Sutton *et al* (2012).

9.1.3 Orthovoltage therapy

Orthovoltage therapy is defined as the range 150–500 kVp with beam qualities equivalent to HVLs of 0.2–5 mm of copper, but the majority of units only operate up to 300 kVp. Orthovoltage therapy can be used for treating deeper skin lesions and bone metastases using either applicators or a diaphragm. A ceiling suspended x-ray tube is usually employed, and the generator sited within the treatment room. However, the control area will need to be outside the treatment room and the patient viewed via CCTV. The x-ray beam can in principle be pointed in any direction, so the walls, ceiling and the floor all need to provide shielding against the primary beam, unless restrictions are placed on beam orientation.

Scatter levels can be calculated as for superficial therapy using the scatter factors given in table 9.1. The allowable leakage is 10 mGy h^{-1} at 1 m from the target (IEC 2009). Although measured values tend to be much lower, this is the value that should be used in calculations. The time is based on the number and length of treatments. As with other therapy modalities, the primary beam will only be directed towards any single wall for a limited portion of the time, so use factors relating to the clinical workload can be employed.

Concrete is likely to be the lowest cost option for walls, ceiling and floor. Values for the HVL and tenth value layer (TVL) for concrete and lead are given in table 9.3. Calculation methods are similar to those described in chapter 5 for other external

Table 9.3. Approximate values for the limiting HVL and TVL thicknesses for broad beam x-ray transmission for concrete (density = 2350 kg m^{-3}) and lead.

Tube potential (kVp)	Concrete HVL (mm)	Concrete TVL (mm)	Lead HVL (mm)	Lead TVL (mm)
50[a]	7.7	25.4	0.08	0.3
70[a]	14	46	0.13	0.43
100[a]	18	59	0.28	0.9
125[b]	20	66	0.29	0.95
150[b]	22.4	74	0.31	1.0
200[c]	25	84	0.52	1.7
250[c]	28	94	0.88	2.9
300[c]	31	104	1.47	4.8

[a] Sutton *et al* (2012).
[b] British Standards (1971), taken from graphs.
[c] Trout and Kelley (1972).

beam treatment units. Primary barriers are likely to be 400–500 mm thick and secondary ones 200–350 mm. Brick or stud walls may be lined with lead ply, but thicknesses of 15–20 mm may be required for 300 kV x-rays. Another alternative is barytes plaster, but the thicknesses required are likely to limit the usefulness as thicker layers are difficult to apply. If a therapy room is being installed in an existing building and the shielding in the walls, floor or ceiling needs to be upgraded, lead may be the preferred option particularly if space is limited.

The door of the treatment room will require to be shielded by lead. It is advantageous to restrict the orientation of the x-ray tube to avoid directing the primary beam towards the door in order to reduce shielding requirements. This can be done using either mechanical or electrical interlocks with little impact on clinical usage. The operation of a door containing several millimetres of lead is difficult and it may sometimes need to be power-operated because of the weight. A sliding door is an option that is often adopted, particularly with power driven doors. Particular care is needed in ensuring that gaps in the lead protection around the edges and underneath the door are kept to a minimum, with overlaps where possible, as they can be a source of significant radiation leakage. For example, a layer of low attenuation material on the surface of the floor will create a gap through which the scatter dose rate could be significant, and a strip of lead may need to be inset into the floor to avoid any problem. These areas should be reviewed during installation if possible and tested for leakage during the critical examination.

9.1.4 Example of superficial/orthovoltage room protection

An example plan for an orthovoltage/superficial therapy treatment room is given in figure 9.1. The control area is adjacent to the room entrance to provide good visibility for controlling room access and the protection is designed to allow staff to be present in the control area throughout all treatments. The patient is viewed through CCTV cameras, so no viewing window is required.

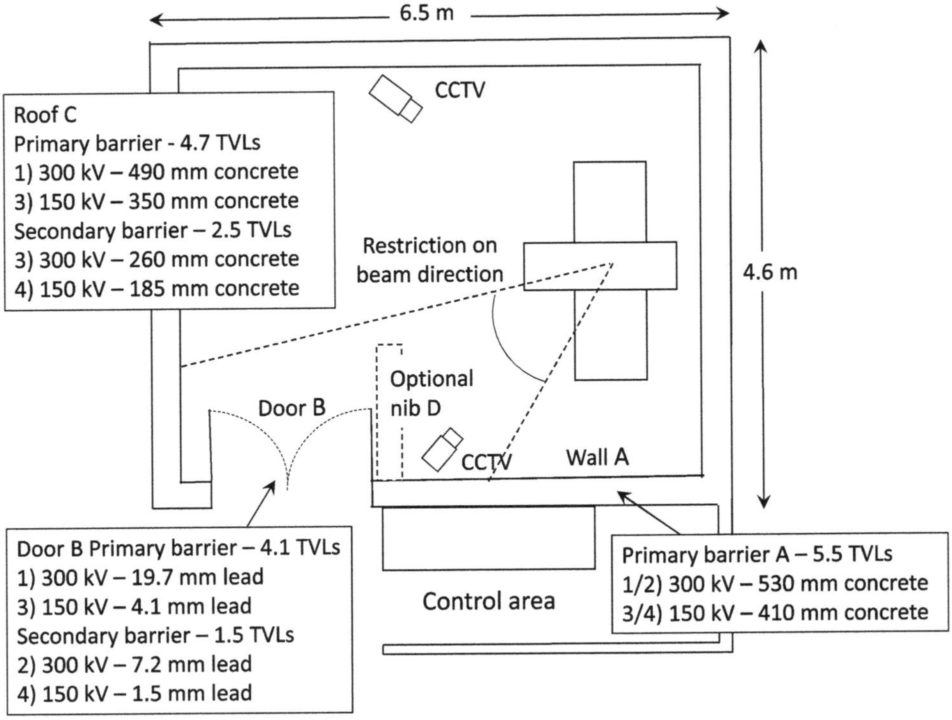

Figure 9.1. Example orthovoltage/superficial voltage treatment room with examples of protection that might be required with the four different use options.

Calculations and shielding requirements are given for four different treatment options:

1. 300 kV orthovoltage treatment unit with no restriction on beam direction.
2. 300 kV orthovoltage treatment unit with restrictions on the beam pointing toward the door and ceiling.
3. 150 kV superficial treatment unit with no restriction on beam direction.
4. 150 kV superficial treatment unit with restrictions on the direction of the beam pointing toward door and ceiling.

The unit is on solid ground and consequently the floor requires no shielding. The area above the unit has 100% occupancy and consequently the ceiling requires full protection, but this can be reduced if restrictions are placed on directing the beam upwards. The corridor outside the room entrance has 10% occupancy.

If the annual treatment workload is 2000 Gy and the average field size is 100 cm^2, then the annual scatter air kerma at 1 m would be (2000 × 700 μGy) = 1.4 Gy for both energy options (table 9.1). When there is no restriction on primary beam direction, it is assumed to be directed towards each wall for 1/4 of the treatments and towards the roof for 1/8 of the time in determining the shielding requirements. No account has been taken of occupancy of adjacent areas in the calculation and this would normally be used to reduce shielding requirements. The requirements for protective barriers for the different options are included in figure 9.1, based on the following calculations.

Wall A (distance 2.34 m)

Primary air kerma incident on wall $= \dfrac{2000}{4 \times 2.34^2} = 90.9$ Gy.

Barrier transmission to reduce annual air kerma to 300 μGy = 3.3×10^{-6} (i.e. 5.5 TVLs).

Door B (distance 3.74 m, occupancy factor 0.1)

Primary air kerma incident on door $= \dfrac{2000}{4 \times 3.74^2} = 36$ Gy.

Door transmission to reduce annual air kerma to 3 mGy = 8.3×10^{-5} (i.e. 4.1 TVLs).

If the primary beam was not directed towards the door, then the shielding in the door would just be required to protect against scatter air kerma.

Scatter air kerma at door $= \dfrac{1.4}{3.74^2} = 0.1$ Gy.

Door transmission to reduce annual air kerma to 3 mGy = 0.03 (i.e. 1.5 TVLs). 4 mm of lead would be required in the door and frame to protect against the primary 150 kV beam, but this can be reduced to 1.5 mm by restricting the gantry angulation so that the beam was not directed at the door. A 4 mm lead door may require to be power driven. The installation of a 300 kV unit would require a power driven door. Another option that might be used to avoid both the primary beam and secondary scatter being incident directly on the door would be to include a nib at D, if space allowed (see figure 9.1).

Roof C (distance 4 m)

Primary air kerma incident at the floor above $= \dfrac{2000}{8 \times 4^2} = 15.6$ Gy.

Ceiling slab transmission to reduce annual air kerma to 300 μGy = 1.9×10^{-5} (i.e. 4.7 TVLs).

If the direction of the primary beam was constrained so that it could not be directed at the ceiling, the calculation for scatter air kerma would be:

Scatter air kerma at floor above $= \dfrac{1.4}{4^2} = 0.087$ Gy.

Ceiling slab transmission to reduce annual air kerma to 300 μGy = 3.4×10^{-3} (i.e. 2.5 TVLs).

Protection measures for the four scenarios are shown in figure 9.1.

9.2 Electronic brachytherapy and intra operative radiotherapy

D J Eaton

9.2.1 Intraoperative (x-ray) radiotherapy

Currently, two devices have been used for photon intraoperative radiotherapy (IORT) across a range of anatomical treatment sites: INTRABEAM[1] (Carl Zeiss)

[1] INTRABEAM is a registered trademark of Carl Zeiss Meditec Inc.

and Xoft Axxent[2] (iCAD) (Debenham *et al* 2013). The mean energy for both these devices is approximately 30 keV for the clinical situation where the source and applicator are positioned inside the patient. Therefore much of the radiation is absorbed within the patient and shielding requirements are similar to iodine-125 seeds (see section 10.6). However, the dose rate from the un-attenuated source may be much higher, if there are gaps between the patient tissues or the applicator is partially exposed. Therefore shielding sheets to cover the surface of the patient around the source entry point may be used to reduce external dose rates.

No permanent modification of the operating theatre should be necessary to maintain time averaged dose rates within limits. Typical beam-on times and workloads are given in table 9.4. If staff remain to operate the console, or monitor the patient, then lead screens or aprons are usually used to reduce staff doses. Because of the low energy and isotropic emission of the radiation, scatter around a barrier will far exceed transmission for intervening lead equivalent shielding with a thickness of greater than 0.3 mm. For the INTRABEAM system, radiation protection was comprehensively investigated by Eaton *et al* (2011), including the monitoring of dose rates for 40 breast patients. They found instantaneous dose rates (IDRs) behind a standard 2 mm lead screen to be less than 5 μSv h^{-1} and staff doses to be negligible in this position. Without the screen, the IDR at 1 m from the source was approximately 600 μSv h^{-1}, and behind a single standard door IDR values ranged from 0 to 30 μSv h^{-1} depending on the room arrangement. Behind concrete walls, floor and ceiling values the dose rates were negligible. It is recommended that a prospective survey is performed with the specific equipment to be used as part of the prior risk assessment. Detailed calculations of expected dose rates behind existing barriers (walls, ceiling, etc) may not be required in this case, although these authors also found that attenuation for INTRABEAM could be accurately modelled by standard data for 50 kVp diagnostic units (Sutton *et al* 2012).

Another possibility would be to use an operating theatre which is already used for radiation procedures such as fluoroscopy. Specific risk assessments are still required for IORT, but the shielding is likely to be sufficient. In this case, operators may stand outside the main room, and observe through a window. Further details of these examples can be found in Eaton *et al* (2011) and Eaton and Schneider (2014).

9.2.2 Superficial x-ray brachytherapy

Electronic brachytherapy devices are also being used to treat skin lesions and a range of compact mobile units have recently come to market, e.g. the Elekta Esteya™ unit[3]. They may be employed in settings where staff and/or management are unfamiliar with the hazards of therapy level sources, such as dermatology clinics

The Oraya IRay™ system[4] is designed specifically for the treatment of age related wet macular degeneration using x-ray equipment operating at a fixed potential of

[2] Xoft and Axxent are registered trademarks of iCAD Inc.
[3] Esteya is a registered trademark of Elekta Instrument AB.
[4] IRay was a registered trademark of Oraya Therapeutics Inc.

Table 9.4. Summary of electronic brachytherapy practice.

Treatment	Source used	Source energy	Typical dose rate	Typical treatment time/dose	Facilities required	Typical maximum workloads
Electronic brachytherapy	x-ray	~50 kV	Up to 1 Gy min^{-1}	10–40 min	Screen or aprons if staff remaining in operating theatre. No permanent modification. No workload restriction.	2–4 patients per day per theatre 50–250 patients per year.
Mobile electron linear accelerators	Electrons	4–12 MeV	10–30 Gy min^{-1}	10–25 Gy/patient	Beam stopper integral to unit. May be able to use standard facility with workload restriction, or with mobile shielding panels.	5–6 patients per week.

100 kV. The beam is highly collimated with each treatment comprising three small overlapping radiation fields that target the affected part of the retina and can be delivered in under 5 min. It has been designed to be given as a single treatment as an out-patient procedure. The unit has been designed so that the primary beam cannot be directed at anything other than the patient (or the beam blocker during calibration) and the positioning of the tube with respect to the patient is fixed. Only secondary radiation barriers are necessary. Staff normally sit at the control panel behind a protective lead screen, a few millimetres thick. The main hazard arises from scatter from the patient and leakage from the unit housing.

Further information on the physics and clinical practice of electronic brachytherapy devices can found in Eaton (2015). Radiation protection advisers (RPAs) should approach these situations with an understanding of the application and the characteristics of the equipment. If possible, they should become involved at an early stage of development, and be able to advise or provide appropriate radiation protection training.

9.2.3 Small animal irradiators

Kilovoltage units may also be used to irradiate small animals for research purposes. For example, the SARRP system (XStrahl Ltd)[5] uses accelerating potentials up to 225 kV, with collimated beam sizes from 1 mm × 1 mm to 40 mm × 80 mm. High positioning accuracy is achieved through diffuse optical tomography and cone beam CT scanning within the unit, and advanced techniques such as gating and intensity-modulation can be delivered. Most of these units are completely self-shielding with lead casing and interlocks to prevent unintended irradiation. Therefore radiation protection requirements are minimal.

9.2.4 Intraoperative (electron) radiotherapy (IOERT)

Various commercial systems are available to deliver IORT using mobile electron-only linear accelerators with nominal energies in the range 4–12 MeV and high dose per pulse. These devices are all fitted with beam stoppers, so the main consideration is scatter and leakage radiation. Scattered electrons have limited penetration into typical wall materials. The practice recommended by the American Association of Physicists in Medicine is to perform a survey of dose rates with the specific unit and operating theatre(s) and then limit the workload to achieve acceptable exposure levels (Beddar *et al* 2006). Workload calculations should include warm-up and daily quality assurance (QA) checks as well as the number of expected patient treatments. Commissioning and annual checks are better performed elsewhere in a shielded environment, e.g. a linear accelerator bunker.

Detailed investigations have been described for the Mobetron (IntraOp Medical)[6] (Krechetov *et al* 2010) and Liac (Sordina) systems[7] (Soriani *et al* 2010). They suggest

[5] SARRP is a trademark of XStrahl Ltd.
[6] Mobetron is a registered trademark of IntraOp Medical Inc.
[7] Liac is a registered trademark of Sordina IORT Technologies SpA.

that typical workloads of a few patients per week can be safely accommodated in buildings of standard construction or that mobile shielding panels can be used instead of permanent shielding. Neutron exposure levels were found to be very low, even for energies above 10 MeV. They also provide isodose plots which can be used to plan other centres.

A summary of electronic brachytherapy practice is given in table 9.4.

References

Archer B R, Thornby J I and Bushong S C 1983 Diagnostic x-ray shielding design based on an empirical model of photon attenuation *Health Phys.* **44** 507–17

Beddar A S *et al* 2006 Intraoperative radiation therapy using mobile electron linear accelerators. Report of AAPM Radiation Therapy Committee Task Group No 72 *Med. Phys.* **33** 1476–89

BSI (British Standards Institution) 1971 *Recommendation for Data on Shielding from Ionizing Radiation. Shielding from X-radiation* BS 4094-2 (London: BSI)

Debenham B J, Hu K S and Harrison L B 2013 Present status and future directions of intraoperative radiotherapy *Lancet Oncol.* **14** e457–64

Eaton D J 2015 Electronic brachytherapy—current status and future directions *Br. J. Radiol.* **88** 20150002

Eaton D J and Schneider F 2014 Radiation protection *Targeted Intraoperative Radiotherapy in Oncology* ed M Keshtgar, K Pigott and F Wenz (Berlin: Springer)

Eaton D J, Gonzalez R, Duck S and Keshtgar M 2011 Radiation protection for an intraoperative x-ray device *Br. J. Radiol.* **84** 1034–9

IEC (International Electrotechnical Commission) 2009 *Medical Electrical Equipment—Part 2-1: Particular Requirements for the Safety of Electron Accelerators in the Range 1 MeV to 50 MeV* 60601-2-1 2nd edn (Geneva: IEC)

Krechetov A S, Goer D, Dikeman K, Daves J L and Mills M D 2010 Shielding assessment of a mobile electron accelerator for intra-operative radiotherapy *J. Appl. Clin. Med. Phys.* **4** 263–73

NCRP (National Council on Radiation Protection and Measurements) 1976 *Structural Shielding Design and Evaluation for Medical Use of x-rays and Gamma Rays of Energies up to 10 MeV* Report 49 (Bethesda, MD: NCRP)

Soriani A *et al* 2010 Radiation protection measurements around a 12 MeV mobile dedicated IORT accelerator *Med. Phys.* **37** 995–1003

Sutton D G, Martin C J, Williams J R and Peet D J 2012 *Radiation Shielding for Diagnostic x-rays* 2nd edn (London: British Institute of Radiology)

Trout E D and Kelley J P 1972 Scattered radiation from a tissue-equivalent phantom for x-rays from 50 to 300 kVp *Radiology* **104** 161–9

Chapter 10

Brachytherapy

D J Peet, M Costelloe and T Soanes

10.1 Treatment modes

Brachytherapy is the treatment of cancer by positioning sealed radiation sources within or on the patient's body for a predetermined time or by permanent implantation close to or within the cancer, i.e. treatment at close range. The term is derived from the Greek word, *brachys*, meaning short distance.

In the UK, the most common form of brachytherapy is high dose-rate (HDR) afterloading. This uses a high activity sealed source of 350–450 GBq of iridium-192 or 70–80 GBq of cobalt-60 which is cable driven into an applicator or a number of applicators in turn under computer control. The applicator(s) are positioned in the patient prior to irradiation and this enables them to be placed accurately either in or close to the tumour site without radiation present. This reduces the potential radiation dose to staff. The position of the source is accurately known and by varying the dwell time at each stopping point a dose distribution that matches the treatment plan can be built up. Treatment times are generally short, but dependant on source activity can vary from 5 to 30 min for a gynaecological implant and up to 90 min for a complex head and neck or prostate treatments. Treatments can be delivered in a number of daily fractions—typically between 1 and 5. The dose rates within the treatment room are high, so staff are outside the shielded room at the control unit during the treatment, giving rise to the term remote afterloading. As the source decays the treatment time will increase. Iridium-192 sources are usually replaced every three months to avoid long treatment times; cobalt-60 sources are replaced at longer intervals.

Other forms of remote afterloading are available. In low dose-rate (LDR) afterloading, multiple low activity sources of caesium-137 or cobalt-60 are used and this results in treatment times measured in days. The sources are loaded at the start of treatment into a number of applicators together with inactive spacers

doi:10.1088/978-0-7503-1440-4ch10

(the whole assembly being termed a 'source train') to give the required dose distribution; three applicators are often used to treat gynaecological cancers. The source trains are withdrawn at the end of treatment or temporarily during nursing care. The radiobiological effect of HDR treatments is different from LDR treatments and adjustment has to be made to the total dose given in HDR treatments. LDR afterloading has now largely been phased out in favour of HDR afterloading and to a lesser extent by pulsed dose rate (PDR) afterloading.

PDR afterloading comprises one or two treatment sessions each consisting of hourly 'pulses' of radiation over a total period of 1–2 days, whilst HDR treatments are usually one fraction every day for up to five days. This technique combines the benefits of reliable single source delivery with a lower overall dose rate for the treatment, comparable with LDR dose rates. The same total dose is given to the patient in the same total period of time as the equivalent LDR treatment. This is done by irradiating the patient for a pre-determined time every hour, e.g. for 3–20 min. The source activity is higher than that of the caesium-137 or cobolt-60 sources used in LDR treatments and is typically 37 GBq of iridium-192, but can range from 19 GBq to 74 GBq. This technique is generally used for gynaecological treatments, where the overall treatment time is up to two days. For other treatment areas the treatment time will depend on the dose to be delivered. This technique also employs a computer controlled afterloader to control the dwell times of the source in the applicators. The time between the pulses will shorten as the source decays, so the source is usually replaced every three months to ensure that there are adequate intervals between successive pulses. Nursing care takes place in the intervals between the pulses but the treatment can be interrupted from the control unit and the source withdrawn for a medical emergency.

Manual afterloading using iridium wire is no longer carried out as the wire is no longer available.

Brachytherapy may also involve direct insertion of sources into the patient. This may be permanent or temporary. Permanent implantation of iodine-125 seeds into the prostate is an example of this procedure. The radiation hazard is low due to the low photon energy (35 keV) of iodine-125.

Some brachytherapy sources are incorporated into surface applicators to treat skin or eye conditions. These temporary implants are removed at the end of treatment. This technique is now largely confined to eye plaques using strontium-90 or ruthenium-106. Since both these radionuclides are β-emitters, the radiation hazards are low.

X-ray sources can also be used to deliver dose from within the body, either following surgical resection (termed intra-operative radiotherapy (IORT)) (Debenham *et al* 2013) or for rectal treatments, and to the skin. These devices have been called electronic brachytherapy because of the similar surface placement and insertion of sources inside a body cavity, lumen or tissue (Eaton 2015). IORT may also be delivered using mobile electron-only linear accelerators (Beddar *et al* 2006). These practices and the radiation protection measures required are considered in greater detail in section 9.2.

A summary of basic protection considerations is given in table 10.1 and the physical characteristic of radionuclides commonly used in brachytherapy in table 10.2.

Table 10.1. Summary of basic protection considerations for common brachytherapy modalities.

Treatment	Source used	Source energy	Typical treatment time	Facilities required	Typical maximum workloads
HDR afterloader	Iridium-192	612 keV	Up to 20 min dependent on source activity.	Shielded treatment room for delivery of treatment. Operator's console area.	Total dwell time of 15 min per treatment for source of 370 GBq.
	(Cobalt-60)	(1.33 MeV)		Secure storage for afterloader and exchange sources with two physical methods of securing source.	50–200 patients per year.
				Procedures may require the treatment room to have theatre facilities, e.g. piped medical gases.	Three fractions per patient
				Standard theatre for applicator insertion; facilities may depend upon the treatment area, e.g. prostate, bronchus.	Five treatments per day of 3–7 Gy.
PDR afterloader	Iridium-192	612 keV	Pulses of several minutes per hour over several days.	Shielded patient treatment room suitable for a stay of a few days with operator's console outside the room.	50–200 patients per year.
	(Cobalt-60)	(1.33 MeV)		Secure storage for afterloader and exchange sources with two physical methods of securing source.	60 Gy delivered over 3–4 days or
				Standard theatre for applicator insertion.	20 Gy in up to two treatment sessions of 10–15 pulses each over 1–2 days.

(Continued)

Interstitial brachytherapy	Iodine-125 seeds	35 keV	Permanent implant.	Secure storage. Clean environment for seed preparation. Standard theatre for seed insertion with appropriate radiation protection measures.	Three patients per session. Typical seed activity 15 MBq. Up to 120 seeds per implant.
External brachytherapy	Ruthenium-106	3.54 MeV	Temporary eye plaques.	Secure storage. Shielded facility for surface sterilisation. Facility for patients to remain in hospital overnight.	Occasionally requiring an inpatient stay of several days.
	Strontium-90	546 keV		Secure storage.	Occasional day case with treatment time of minutes.
	(Yttrium-90)	(2.27 MeV)		Shielded facility for surface sterilisation.	

Table 10.2. Physical characteristics of some radionuclide commonly used in brachytherapy.

Source	Maximum activity	Half life	Maximum photon energy (MeV)	Maximum electron energy (MeV)	Air kerma rate (μGy h^{-1}) at 1 m GBq^{-1}	TVL in concrete (mm)	TVL in lead (mm)
^{125}I	40 MBq per seed	60 days	0.035	–	33[a]	10.2	0.1[a]
^{137}Cs	450 GBq	30 years	0.662	1.17	78[a]	157[a]	21[a]
^{192}Ir	555 GBq	74 days	0.612	0.67	113[a]	147[b]	15[a]
^{60}Co (to ^{60}Ni)	75 GBq	5.27 years	1.332	1.48	309[a]	206[a]	40[a]
^{90}Sr–$^{90}Y(\beta)$	few GBq	29 years	–	2.27	–	–	–
^{106}Ru	~10 MBq	374 days	–	3.54	–	–	–

[a] IPEM (1997).
[b] NCRP (1976).

Brachytherapy is a rapidly changing field with potential applications outside the traditional boundaries of the radiotherapy department. Multidisciplinary teams are required to ensure best and safe use is made of the techniques. Regulatory requirements and training need to be addressed before clinical work starts.

10.2 Regulatory considerations

10.2.1 Use of radioactive material

Permits are likely to be required to hold radioactive material under the relevant regulatory regime—*Environmental Permitting Regulations* 2016 (EPR 2016) in England and Wales and the *Radioactive Substances Act* (RSA 1993) in Scotland and Northern Ireland. These impose a number of conditions covering for example security, storage, records, disposal and emergency arrangements. Most of these conditions are also included in the *Ionising Radiation Regulations* 1999 (IRR 1999).

10.2.2 Work with ionising radiation

Notification, registration and/or licensing may be required in addition to the requirements of the *Environmental Permitting Regulations* under the new *Ionising Radiation Regulations* when the new *Basic Safety Standard Directive* (EC 2013) is implemented in 2018. Prior risk assessments, room design, engineering controls, signs and warning lights and handling of sources all require consideration. Contingency plans not only have to be in place for foreseeable emergencies, e.g. fire, theft, death of a patient, equipment failure or medical emergency, but have to be regularly rehearsed as well. Leak tests are required for all sealed sources, although in practice those that remain on site for only a few months may not need additional testing whilst in the radiotherapy centre.

10.2.3 Patient protection

The current *Medicines (Administration of Radioactive Substances) Regulations* (MARS 1978) and the *Ionising Radiations (Medical Exposure) Regulations* (IRMER 2000) are to be revised in the new *Ionising Radiation Regulations.* Currently IRMER (2000) covers all medical exposures and the administration or application of radioactive sources has to be done by an ARSAC certificate holder—usually a radiation oncologist for brachytherapy. IRMER procedures need to be reviewed and possibly amended for new brachytherapy procedures.

10.3 Room design

10.3.1 General considerations

The workload needs to be clearly understood to enable a safe design to be developed. A knowledge of the types of treatment and doses to be given with each is essential. The duration of exposure for a known source activity will inform the total length of time the source is exposed. This will enable a project team including the Radiation Protection Adviser (RPA) to evaluate the measures required for patient, staff and public safety and be compliant with the relevant regulations. The workload should be conservative but not unrealistic.

The layout of the facility should primarily be for the effective and safe treatment of patients. The room size must be adequate for the treatment unit, patient couch or bed, emergency source container, other equipment including anaesthetic machines, imaging equipment and the number of staff including trainees, who will be involved in delivering the treatment. Ancillary functions, such as patient preparation and recovery rooms, utility rooms and scrub areas, might also need to be incorporated.

A simple maze might be recommended to prevent direct radiation falling upon the door. If space does not permit this then as for external beam treatment units, a shielded door is possible but may be heavy to operate for the operators entering and leaving the room. On occasions a motorised door may be required.

Specific radiation protection requirements for each treatment type are described in sections 10.4–10.7 below.

10.3.2 Engineering controls

Warning lights, radiation monitors and interlocks may form part of the engineering controls associated with the treatment room. Any cable ducts for monitoring or dosimetry equipment should be designed so that radiation levels are kept to the design constraint outside the room.

10.3.3 Security

Security measures are likely to be required under the *High Activity Sealed Source Regulations* (HASS) requirements of EPR (2016) to deter, delay and respond to any unauthorised access. Some of these may affect the space required within the treatment room or adjacent areas. The delivery and regular change-over of sources may also need to be considered. It is advised that the local Counter Terrorism Security Advisor (CTSA) be consulted at an early stage of treatment room design and their advice obtained on the latest security standards which need to be applied. These are outlined in the National Counter Terrorism Security Office document *Security Requirements for Radioactive Sources* (NaCTSO 2011)

10.4 High dose-rate afterloading

10.4.1 Workload

HDR afterloading units are used to treat a variety of body sites with interstitial (using cannulae), intraluminal, intracavitary or external treatment (using surface plaques). Within the UK the number of brachytherapy patients treated per annum was typically between 50 and 400 per centre, based on a survey by the Royal College of Radiologists (RCR 2012). The College recommended that to maintain staff skills the minimum number of patients treated with HDR in a brachytherapy centre is 50 per annum, a minimum of 25 interstitial prostate iodine-125 seed implants and ten patients requiring treatment with intrauterine applicators. A hospital with an HDR unit will use it to treat a substantial part of the brachytherapy workload.

The brachytherapy workload within a hospital must always be assessed on the basis of local demands and future plans, but should accommodate a minimum of 50 patients.

An estimation of the treatment time per fraction, maximum number of treatment fractions per day and per annum should be made with an allowance for quality assurance and maintenance exposures. An allowance for future workload growth should be made. In the absence of any other figures a 3% growth in workload over ten years will result in an increase of 35%, and a 5% increase will result in a 60% increase over ten years.

An example of the expected workload for an HDR unit is given in table 10.1.

10.4.2 Room layout

A common layout of an HDR room is shown in figure 10.1. Particular features that need to be considered are:

- It should not be possible to position the source near the inner maze entrance, even when the treatment unit is placed with the cables linking it to the control panel stretched at their fullest extent, and the source transfer tubes further extended towards the entrance. If necessary, the movement of the treatment unit must be restricted. This may be necessary as part of the security measures.
- The room should be arranged such that if the operator has to manually retract the source in an emergency they can access the unit as quickly as possible.
- An emergency source container needs to be located in the room and should be sited close to the treatment unit with its lid open whilst treatment is in

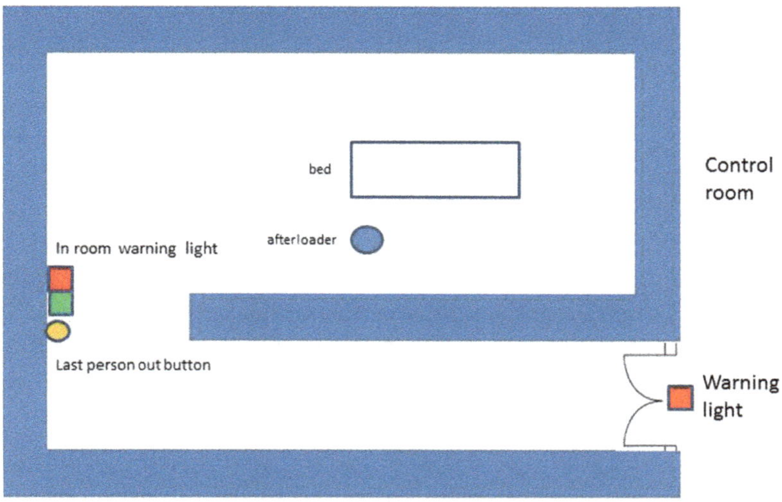

Figure 10.1. A HDR brachytherapy room.

progress so that in the event of the source sticking and unable to be retracted manually, it can be withdrawn from the patient and placed into the container quickly.

- The room is normally designed to meet infection control standards for a treatment room or ward side room. However it is possible to design the room to have an operating theatre environment if this is required.

10.4.3 Calculation of shielding thickness

Once the internal layout and space requirements have been agreed, the requisite shielding around the facility can be calculated to meet the specified design constraint in the surrounding areas. Occupancy can be applied but caution may be needed for rooms which may later change their use. These calculations can be part of an iterative process as projects usually specify the external limits of the area available. This may dictate the material used for walls, floors and ceilings. It is not usual to allow any windows in brachytherapy treatment rooms but to use closed circuit television (CCTV).

When designing a room a dose constraint is set, typically 0.3 mSv or 1 mSv per annum.

The length of time the source is exposed each year can be calculated from the number of patients treated and the treatment times for a known source activity. Care needs to be taken for units that operate on only a few days per week so that shielding is not underspecified should the workload increase.

The dose to a critical point outside the room can be derived from the activity of the source and knowledge of the reference air kerma rate (RAKR) for the radionuclide concerned. During source decay treatment times will become longer to correct for the decay in activity.

The distance between the source and the calculation points can be difficult to determine as the source can be in different positions in the room. A pragmatic choice might be the centre of the patient couch, especially if the position is fixed. It may be appropriate to select a number of worst case positions and calculate the required thicknesses under each of those conditions.

The dose per annum at the calculation points without any shielding in place is calculated from the product of the RAKR (μGy h^{-1} m^{-1} GBq^{-1}), activity A (GBq), the number of patients/week and the treatment time per patient in hours, corrected using the inverse square law for distance. For a worst case scenario, two hours exposure per week from a 370 GBq source can be used; this would be an overestimate in most facilities. The total exposure time per week, T, is the product of the number of patients/week and the treatment time per patient in hours, and may need to encompass a number of different clinical procedures each with different exposure periods. In this case T is given by

$$T = \sum n_i t_i, \tag{10.1}$$

where n_i is the number of patients/week undergoing the ith procedure and t_i is the source exposure time of the ith procedure.

Table 10.3. Calculation of annual treatment time for a HDR brachytherapy unit.

Body site	Max number of treatments per day	Max treatment time for 370 GBq source (min)	Max treatments per year = (no. of patients × no. of fractions)	Treatment time per annum (hours)
Example	4	15	100 × 3 = 300	75
Breast				
Bronchus				
Cardiac				
Gynaecological	3	10	70 × 3 = 210	35
Head and neck				
Skin				
Rectum/anal canal				
Prostate	2	10	50 × 3 = 150	25
Intravascular				
Other/quality assurance	1	30	50	25
Total				**85**
Allowance for 50% workload growth				**130**

An example of calculating the total exposure time per annum for a number of clinical techniques is given in table 10.3.

The unattenuated annual dose D_p at a point at a distance d_p (m) from the source 0.3 m beyond the barrier concerned is given by

$$D_p = \mathrm{RAKR} \times A \times T \times 50/d_p^2. \tag{10.2}$$

The required barrier transmission factor B is then given by the annual dose constraint D_{acc} divided by the unattenuated annual dose D_p, i.e.

$$B = D_{acc}/D_p. \tag{10.3}$$

Occupancy factors can be taken into account at this point as described in chapters 3 and 5 which may reduce the thickness of shielding required.

The thickness of shielding (d_s) required to reduce the transmission to this factor is derived from the number of tenth value layers (TVLs) (n) required, given by

$$n = \log_{10}(1/B) \tag{10.4}$$

and

$$d_s = n \times \mathrm{TVL} \tag{10.5}$$

This ignores any absorption in the patient and this can be justified for HDR sources as the source will be exposed in air for quality assurance or other purposes on a regular basis.

For lower energy emissions from these radionuclides the assumption of a constant half value layer (HVL) may not be justified due the increasing presence of photo-electric absorption. Archer *et al* (1983) developed equations to describe the transmission curves for different materials and beam energies based on three coefficients (α, β and γ). The expression for the transmission (B) through material of thickness, x, is given by

$$B = [1 + \beta/\alpha)\exp(\alpha\gamma x) - \beta/\alpha] - 1/\gamma. \quad (10.6)$$

Papagiannis *et al* (2008) have used Monte Carlo techniques to examine the effect of beam hardening by preferential absorption of low energy photons where a radionuclide has a spectrum of energies, e.g. iridium-192, and beam softening by the production of scatter as the radiation is transmitted through a thick absorber. α, β and γ were calculated by fitting a curve to the Monte Carlo calculated transmission data. A subset of the coefficient data is listed in table 10.4. Reference to the original work with transmission graphs and a comprehensive description of the methodology is advised before using this method of calculation.

10.4.4 Maze/door calculations

A typical situation showing the scatter path to the maze entrance is illustrated in figure 10.2. The dose rate at the calculation point at the door DR_d can be calculated and converted to annual dose from the treatment time and occupancy factors using scatter coefficients. DR_d is given by

$$DR_d = (A \times RAKR \times \acute{\alpha} \times AR)/(d_1^2 \times d_2^2), \quad (10.7)$$

where $\acute{\alpha}$ is the reflection coefficient for the radionuclide and angle of incidence and AR is the irradiated area on the end wall visible from the maze entrance.

Table 10.4. Attenuation coefficients for equation (10.5) and first and equilibrium TVLs calculated by Papagiannis *et al* (2008).

Radionuclide	Material	α	β	γ	TVL_1 (mm)	TVL_e (mm)
Ir-192	Concrete (2300 kg m^{-3})	1.666×10^{-2}	-9.368×10^{-3}	1.159×10^{0}	180	139
	Steel	3.542×10^{-2}	-1.654×10^{-3}	9.608×10^{-1}	48	41
	Lead	1.194×10^{-2}	1.552×10^{-1}	4.943×10^{-1}	11	19
Cs-137	Concrete	1.433×10^{-2}	-7.381×10^{-3}	8.375×10^{-1}	214	161
	Steel	4.826×10^{-2}	-2.337×10^{-3}	8.206×10^{-1}	63	48
	Lead	1.126×10^{-1}	-2.455×10^{-2}	6.767×10^{-1}	23	20
Co-60	Concrete	1.095×10^{-2}	-5.377×10^{-3}	8.25×10^{-1}	276	210
	Steel	3.542×10^{-2}	-1.654×10^{-3}	9.608×10^{-1}	84	65
	Lead	5.81×10^{-2}	-1.814×10^{-3}	9.608×10^{-1}	46	40

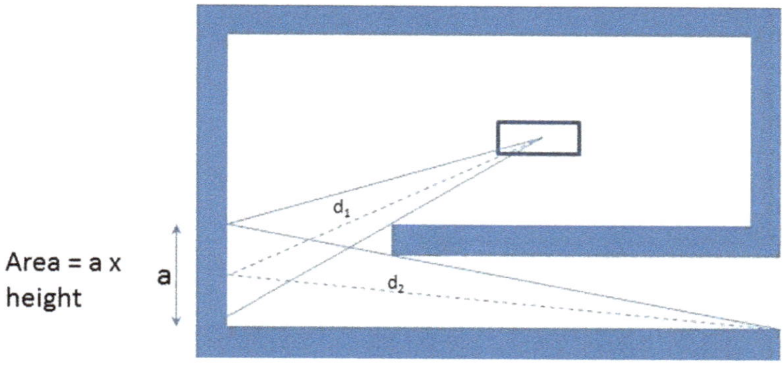

Figure 10.2. Scatter areas and distances for the calculation of the annual dose and IDR at the maze entrance.

Reflection coefficients are plotted in figure 10.3. The annual dose should be compared with the annual dose constraint. This calculation should be repeated for a number of source positions to determine the closest the source can approach the maze entrance without exceeding the dose constraint. If the source is exposed for only a few days a week, the instantaneous dose rate should be reviewed and considered whether it might be significant in relation to the treatment times as discussed in chapter 3.

10.4.5 Engineering controls

The following controls are required:

- Emergency off buttons sited at suitable locations.
- Room warning lights should be linked to the control unit of the afterloader, showing:
  - 'Controlled Area—Radiation' illuminated when the control system has power applied and is ready to operate.
  - 'Do Not Enter' illuminated when all interlocks are set and the source can be exposed from the control unit.

  For details of sign operation, please refer to the signage section in section 3.8.

  When the afterloader is being used with more than one applicator, the 'Do Not Enter' illumination should come on as the source enters the first applicator and go out as the source returns to the safe from the last applicator. It should not go out as the source returns briefly to the safe between applicators.
- Interlocks on the doors to prevent inadvertent access during source exposure. Treatment should not restart by closing the door but by resetting the last person out button and at the control desk.
- A radiation detector with an audible alarm, independent of the treatment unit, in the treatment room as an independent means of knowing that the source has returned safely to the safe when treatment is interrupted or is complete. It must be set to detect the source when it is out of its shielded position, wherever it is in the room. The detector must be linked to a display

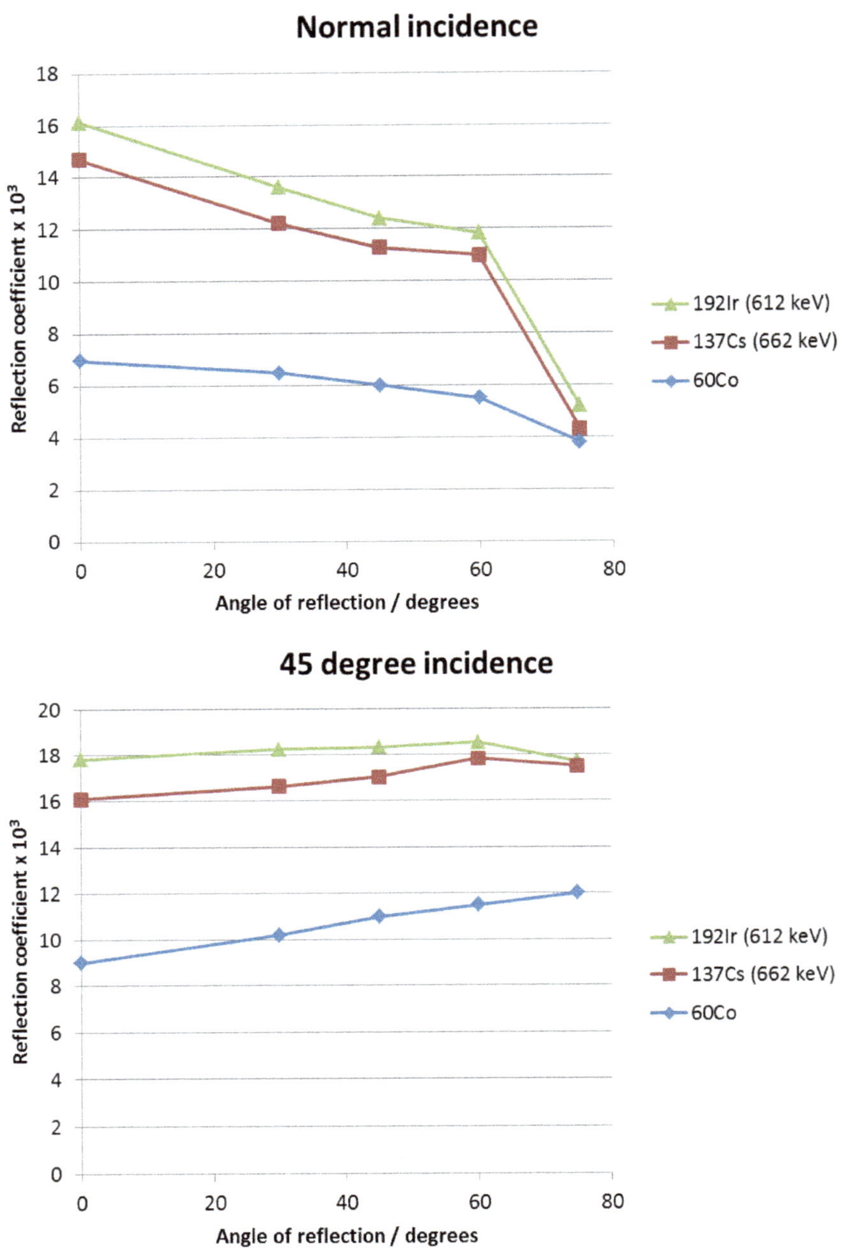

Figure 10.3. Wall reflection coefficients for Ir-192, Cs-137 and Co-60 (interpolated from graphical data in Shultis and Faw (2000)).

at the control panel; a traffic light system with green for safe and red for danger is easy to observe.

- CCTV to monitor the patient during treatment. This should be colour TV to enable the anaesthetist to properly monitor the patient's condition if treatment takes place under a general anaesthetic.

The afterloader should also be fitted with the following safety devices by the manufacturer:

- a battery back up to return the source to the safe and safely terminate the treatment in the event of failure in the electricity supply and
- a manual means of returning the source to the safe if the source sticks in an applicator in an exposed position.

10.5 Pulsed dose-rate afterloading

10.5.1 Workload

Similar workload considerations will apply to PDR units as for HDR units, but typically the unit will be used several days per week and one patient per unit treated at a time. The treatment may be delivered continuously around the clock or during standard hours, for example 8 am–8 pm, so staffing considerations may be a factor in the choice of treatment delivery. Each room might treat around 50 patients per year. These units are primarily used for treating gynaecological cancers but have the same flexibility as HDR units for treating other cancer sites.

10.5.2 Layout

The treatment room is best sited near the oncology wards to facilitate nursing care. PDR afterloading requires a suitably shielded treatment room in which the patient is confined to bed whilst connected to the afterloader. The walls, floor and ceiling all provide primary shielding when the source is within the patient. The room will require a door providing adequate shielding to meet dose constraints and a short maze is effective in reducing the shielding in the door.

The emergency source container needs to be located in the room whilst a treatment is in progress and should be sited close to the treatment unit, with its lid open so that in the event of the source sticking, the applicator and transport tube can be disconnected from the unit and placed into the container.

A secure area in which to store the unit between treatments will be required. This may be located outside of the treatment room depending on the space available. The local CTSA should be consulted at an early stage of facility design and their advice obtained on the latest security standards which need to be applied. These are outlined in the National Counter Terrorism Security Office document *Security Requirements for Radioactive Sources* (NaCTSO 2011).

In designing the layout the primary radiation risk to be considered is from a source sticking in an applicator. The position of the treatment unit, emergency container and patient bed need to be carefully considered; in particular the operator needs to be able to approach the treatment unit without going near the patient. The source stick could occur after the patient has been lying in bed for several days and they may not be able to walk out of the treatment room or transfer to a wheel chair. In an emergency situation once the applicators or source have been removed, the patient may need to be transferred out of the room on the bed in a timely manner with minimum obstruction. Careful planning of the layout

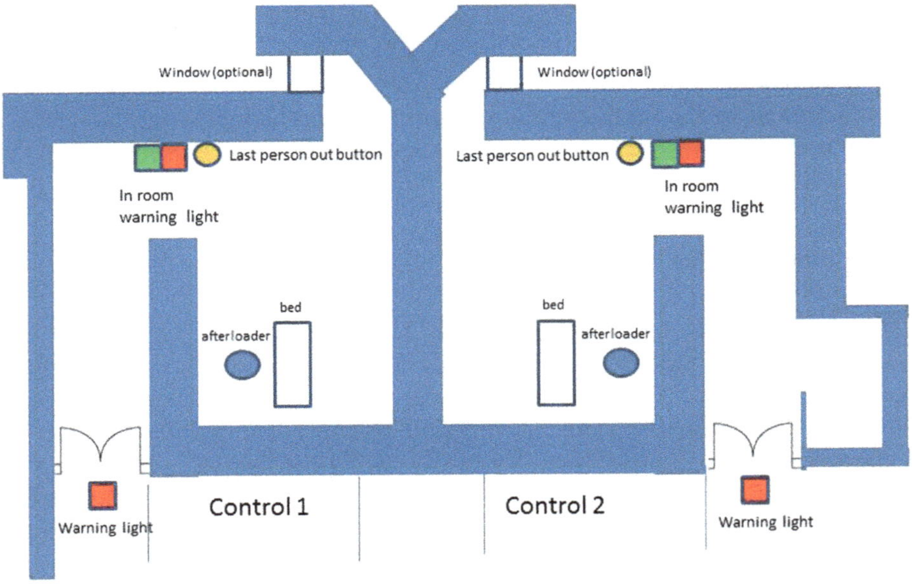

Figure 10.4. A PDR treatment facility with two treatment rooms.

should facilitate this and thus minimise the radiation exposure risk to the patient and staff.

A typical PDR treatment facility with two treatment rooms is shown in figure 10.4.

10.5.3 Shielding calculations

The position of the afterloader in the room will be restricted by the position of the patient bed. The shielding methodology in section 10.4.3 can be used. This might typically result in wall thickness of 35–50 cm of concrete depending on layout, usage and external occupancy. In this case the treatment time per treatment would be the time that the source was exposed. This is the product of the treatment time in hours and the length of the pulse delivered in hours. For example, if the treatment took 15 h to deliver and the pulse in each hour was 10 min long, the source would be exposed for $(10/60 \times 15) = 2.5$ h. If more than one patient is treated per week, these will need to be added to give the cumulative time per week as the value of T in equation (10.1).

Since some PDR units can be upgraded to HDR units, it may be sensible to consider whether the shielding would be sufficient to cope with the use of a more active source and the treatment schedules employed for HDR. The increased security requirements for HDR need to be considered as does the siting of the facility. HDR treatments are often situated within a radiotherapy department. With careful planning a treatment schedule could facilitate a PDR unit in a radiotherapy department whereby the patient is treated in the radiotherapy department and transferred back to the ward overnight.

10.5.4 Engineering controls

The following controls are required:

- Emergency off buttons sited at suitable locations inside the treatment room and at the remote console at the treatment room door. If the computer console is inaccessible during treatment hours it is unnecessary to have an emergency stop on the console.
- Room warning lights need to be provided at the entrance to the treatment room. A panel (remote control) which shows the operating status of the unit should be installed outside the room and this will indicate whether a treatment pulse is in progress, count down the time to the end of the pulse and show how much of the treatment time remains. There should be sufficient time between pulses for nursing or clinical staff to undertake any clinical procedures that are required without the need to pause the treatment. Ideally staff should avoid entering the room within 5 min of the next pulse starting unless they can be in and out without delaying the next pulse starting. The panel should also have an external means of starting and interrupting treatment and returning the sources to the safe during the pulse in a medical emergency.
- Starting a treatment must be controlled by key operation and there should be an audible alarm once treatment has commenced. Some manufacturers may have different alarm tones for different situations and all alarms should be audible at the nursing station.
- Interlocks on the doors to prevent inadvertent access during source exposure. Treatment should not restart by closing the door but by key-enabled resetting at the remote control unit and the last person out button if used.
- A radiation detector with an audible alarm, independent of the treatment unit, in the treatment room as an independent means of knowing that the source has returned safely to the safe when treatment is interrupted or is complete. It must be set to detect the source when it is out of its shielded position, wherever it is in the room. The detector must be linked to a display at the control, remote and nursing station control panels. As with HDR, the independent monitor may also be linked to an in-room traffic light system with green for safe and red for danger. This gives good indication of the source status; with a PDR unit there can be the added option of an orange light which is on for the 5 min before the hourly treatment pulse commences. As the patient is in bed for a long time, the light panel should be visible from the entrance door but ideally not visible to the patient.
- CCTV to monitor the patient during treatment from the nursing station.
- A control unit at the nursing station which shows the same source/treatment status information as the remote control unit at the treatment room door. It should have an audible alarm but no treatment start or interrupt abilities.
- A light system suitably placed and visible from the nursing station indicating the 5 min countdown to the start of a treatment pulse and when treatment is in progress.

The afterloader should also be fitted with the following safety devices by the manufacturer:

- a battery back up to return the source to the safe and safely terminate the treatment in the event of failure in the electricity supply and
- a manual means of returning the source to the safe if the source sticks in an applicator in an exposed position.

The console controlling the afterloader needs to be sited in a secure area adjacent to the treatment room. Once the treatment has commenced all interruptions and re-starts will be initialised at the treatment door remote control unit. During normal treatment conditions the control console area will usually be secured and inaccessible. An area should be incorporated into the layout design to allow the equipment required for an emergency response to be stored adjacent or near to the treatment door such that it is easily accessible.

The nature of the PDR treatment means the patient is lying in bed for a prolonged length of time. The room should be fitted with a TV, DVD player, radio, etc, and decorated in a patient friendly way. A PDR treatment room can have windows; access to which must be controlled via Local Rules, not only for radiation protection purposes, but also to protect patient privacy. 'Round the clock' treatments may finish overnight; if the nursing staff do not have access to the secure storage area, an interim system to secure the PDR unit may be required and reflected in written procedures. These requirements should be addressed at the initial layout planning stage of the facility.

10.6 Permanent implants: iodine-125 seeds

Iodine seeds are used for the treatment of prostate cancer. Sterile seeds are permanently implanted in the prostate using either hollow needles preloaded with seeds and spacers inserted at pre-planned positions or with individual seeds implanted using a 'gun'. Implants are carried out under general anaesthetic using ultrasound imaging for correct positioning of the seeds. Checks on the number of seeds implanted are often made post implant using a mobile radiographic or fluoroscopic unit.

Iodine-125 seeds have a very low x-ray energy, approximately 35 keV, and are easily shielded. The main facilities required are suitable safe storage, e.g. a locked safe within a locked storage facility and a device to ensure seeds can be loaded into applicators with minimum extremity exposure to staff. These devices are usually specific to the brand of seed used and can be obtained from the seed manufacturers. A small local shield to allow the operator to use this device and manipulate the seeds when any difficulty occurs is required. Seeds need to maintain their sterility so checking source activity and loading of seeds is usually undertaken in a theatre environment, in one of the support rooms rather than the main theatre. For needle loading, centres may also have a sealed sources laboratory to prepare seeds for implant or disposal; this is kept clean for this purpose. The room should be sufficiently spacious for the staff to work comfortably. The theatre space will be a controlled area for the duration of the seed loading and implantation and should be supplied with appropriate warning signage.

Table 10.5. Measured external dose rates from a typical iodine-125 seed implant in a large volume prostate gland.

Number of seeds	Total activity (GBq)	Dose rate (μSv h^{-1})			
		Perineum (patient in implantation position)	Anterior	Lateral	Estimate 1 m lateral from patient midline
90–110	1.3	180–340	40–100	20–50	<3

The implant typically uses 70–120 seeds. The patient will usually have an overnight stay in hospital following implantation and should have a single room on or near the oncology ward. During this period, the patient should urinate through a sieve to catch any expelled seeds, although this is not common. Some patients will be catheterised and the catheter bags must be monitored before emptying, and emptied through a sieve if the bag contains any seeds. Any expelled seeds should be put in a shielded container and returned to a suitable and secure location at the earliest opportunity.

Whilst the nursing staff need to be aware of the hazards relating to the care of the patient, the high dose rate area around a patient is extremely localised and does not require any special facilities or procedures, other than avoidance of unnecessary time at the patient's bedside. All persons entering the room might be monitored as they leave.

The exact dose rate varies considerably with the size of the patient and the number and activity of the seeds used. An indication of dose rates for a large volume implant is given in table 10.5 based on measurements from a sample of patients.

Monitoring of finger doses may be done at intervals or with new staff.

10.7 Eye plaques

External brachytherapy using ruthenium-106 plaques is used to treat patients with an intraocular melanoma. Suppliers of these plaques are limited. There are a range of plaques available and the shape required will depend on size and position within the eye of the lesions to be treated. The plaques are sealed sources of a few tens of MBq and are clinically useful for a year, after which time they can be returned to the manufacturer. Ruthenium-106 emits high energy beta radiation, with a maximum energy 3.54 MeV and measuring extremity doses may be sensible for staff new to the procedure. The external dose rate hazard at 2 m from the plaque is negligible.

Plaques are usually inserted in the eye and sutured in place in an operating theatre with the patient under general anaesthetic. 'Dummy' (inactive) plaques can be used to assist in determining the optimal position of the plaque to minimise the surgeon's extremity doses. The theatre and room on the ward will be designated as a controlled area whilst the patient/source are present. Contingency plans are needed to consider the loss of the source.

Patients will then spend up to four days as an in-patient on the ward whilst the plaque is *in situ*. Ideally during this time they will be nursed in a single room to minimise doses to other patients and staff. Whilst the plaque is in place appropriate warning signage will need to be posted at the entrance to the room. Eye care procedures will be carried out by nurses several times a day and take a few minutes each time.

Arrangements for the security of the sources will need to be considered when they are not in use and it may be necessary to have an interim source safe within theatres where the sources can be stored if radiotherapy staff are not present when the plaque is removed. Plaques will need to be sterilized between uses so suitable provision for sterilisation is required within the sealed sources laboratory.

Strontium-90 and iodine-125 eye plaques are also available and require similar precautions.

References

Archer B R, Thornby J I and Bushong S C 1983 Diagnostic x-ray shielding design based on an empirical model of photon attenuation *Health Phys.* **44** 507–17

Beddar A S *et al* 2006 Intraoperative radiation therapy using mobile electron linear accelerators. Report of AAPM Radiation Therapy Committee Task Group No 72 *Med. Phys.* **33** 1476–89

Debenham B J, Hu K and Harrison L B 2013 Present status and future directions of intraoperative radiotherapy *Lancet Oncol.* **14** e457–64

Eaton D J 2015 Electronic brachytherapy-current status and future directions *Br. J. Radiol.* **88** 20150002

EPR 2016 *The Environmental Permitting (England and Wales) Regulations* SI 2016/1154 (London: The Stationery Office)

EC (European Commission) 2013 *Laying Down Basic Safety Standards for Protection Against the Dangers Arising from Exposure to Ionising Radiation* Council Directive 2013/59/Euratom (Brussels: European Commission)

IPEM (Institute of Physics and Engineering in Medicine) 1997 *The Design of Radiotherapy Treatment Room Facilities* Report 75 (York: IPEM)

IRMER 2000 *The Ionising Radiations (Medical Exposure) Regulations* SI 2000/1059 (London: The Stationery Office)

IRR 1999 *The Ionising Radiations Regulations* SI 1999/3232 (London: The Stationery Office)

MARS 1978 *Medicines (Administration of Radioactive Substances) Regulations* SI 1978/1006 (London: The Stationery Office)

NaCTSO (National Counter Terrorism Security Office) 2011 *Security Requirements for Radioactive Sources* (London: NaCTSO)

NCRP (National Council on Radiation Protection and Measurements) 1976 *Structural Shielding Design and Evaluation for Medical Use of x-rays and Gamma Rays of Energies up to 10 MeV* Report 49 (Bethesda, MD: NCRP)

NCRP (National Council on Radiation Protection and Measurements) 2005 *Structural Shielding Design and Evaluation for Megavoltage X- and Gamma-Ray Radiotherapy Facilities* Report 151 (Bethesda, MD: NCRP)

Papagiannis P *et al* 2008 Radiation transmission data for radionuclides and materials relevant to brachytherapy facility shielding *Med. Phys.* **35** 4898–906

RCR (Royal College of Radiologists) 2012 *The Role and Development of Brachytherapy Services in the United Kingdom* (London: RCR)
RSA 1993 *Radioactive Substances Act* SI 1993/0012 (London: The Stationery Office)
Shultis J K and Faw R E 2000 *Radiation Shielding* (La Grange Park, IL: American Nuclear Society)

Chapter 11

Radiation shielding and safety for particle therapy facilities

R L Maughan, M J Hardy, M J Taylor, J Reay and R Amos

11.1 Introduction

The goal of this chapter is to provide a concise overview of the basic principles underlying the general radiation safety practices around a particle therapy facility, in particular the design of radiation shielding and to highlight the differences compared to designing shielding in a conventional photon radiation therapy department. The chapter concentrates on the needs for shielding proton therapy installations but the general principles also apply to heavier particle shielding requirements. The most comprehensive report on the shielding design and radiation safety of charged particle facilities for therapy has been published by the Particle Therapy Co-operative Group (PTCOG 2010) and is available in electronic format. Other major publications providing guidance on radiation protection for charged particle accelerators are NCRP Report 144 (NCRP 2003) and the IAEA Technical Report Series No. 283 (IAEA 1988). Many aspects of designing radiation shielding for a proton or heavier ion facility are similar to those encountered in shielding design for a conventional x-ray therapy department. However, there are some important differences and this chapter will consider how, why and where these differences occur.

This chapter also sets out the information required to specify a facility to equipment vendors and radiation protection specialists so the design meets its clinical aims for a large number of years and meets the requirements of radiation protection legislation. This includes:

- an understanding of the regulatory requirements for radiation dose constraint in order to establish the design criteria,
- an outline knowledge of the building design and its proposed usage necessary to determine occupancy factors and

doi:10.1088/978-0-7503-1440-4ch11

- a knowledge of the proposed workload of the planned facility, including the clinical sites to be treated to determine beam energy and beam angle usage.

All these factors have a significant impact on the final shielding design and as there may be large uncertainties associated with these, particularly over the expected 20 or 30 year life span of a particle therapy facility, it is especially important to pay close attention to them.

All existing particle therapy centres use either cyclotrons (isochronous cyclotrons or synchrocyclotrons) or synchrotrons to accelerate protons or ^{12}C ions. The exact type of accelerator used affects the shielding conditions in and around the accelerator vault, but not necessarily those for the treatment rooms. A cyclotron produces a single energy and the beam energy is generally reduced to give only the penetration required for a particular treatment before it is transported to the treatment room. This energy reduction is achieved by use of a degrader/energy selection system (ESS). The beam losses in the cyclotron and the ESS can be significant producing large neutron fluences which require substantial shielding walls around the cyclotron and ESS; these can be as thick as 4 m of concrete. By contrast synchrotrons do not require an ESS, since the energy of the synchrotron pulse can be varied from pulse to pulse and the accelerator structure is such that internal losses are small. Consequently shielding walls around synchrotrons are considerably thinner, typically 1.5–2 m, with a corresponding reduction in the construction cost. However, synchrotrons generally have larger footprints than cyclotrons and the overall length of the shielding walls around the synchrotron vault may be significantly longer than for a cyclotron. This reduces the concrete volume advantage and partially negates the cost saving.

In recent years there has been a significant trend towards pencil beam scanning (PBS) as the preferred mode of proton beam delivery and most vendors have developed, or are developing, PBS systems. The advantages from a shielding perspective are considerable since PBS makes much more efficient use of the proton beam than a passive scattering system. In a passive scattering system there are considerable beam losses in the modulator wheel or ridge filter, the scatterers, the beam shaping aperture and the compensator; all these losses produce unwanted neutrons. Most of the materials used in these devices produce considerably more neutrons than stopping the beam in tissue (i.e. the patient). In a PBS system these losses are drastically reduced and practically all the beam loss in the treatment room occurs in the patient. There is a twofold gain since not only is the number of neutrons produced per proton entering the room reduced but the number of protons entering the room is also reduced. With fewer protons entering the room the shielding requirement around the accelerator may also be reduced. As a rough estimate the number of protons required for a PBS system is 10–20 times less than for passive scattering, reducing the shielding requirement by 3–4 half value layers (HVLs) which is approximately 60–100 cm of concrete. The layout of a typical single room PBS based facility is shown in figure 11.1, and the layout of a multiple gantry room facility is shown in figure 11.2.

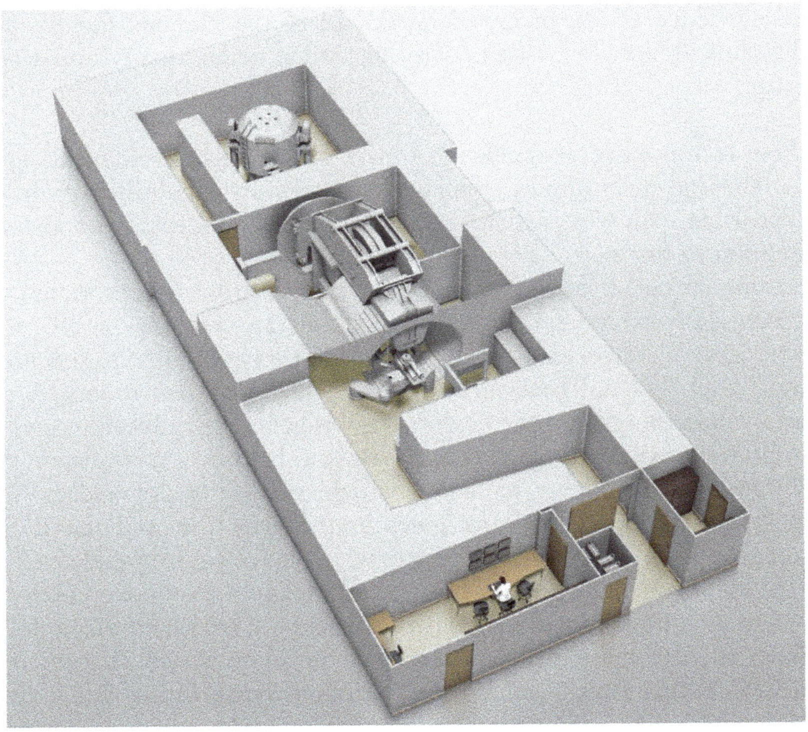

Figure 11.1. Cut away schematic of a typical single room treatment facility for PBS only. (Courtesy of IBA, SA, Belgium.)

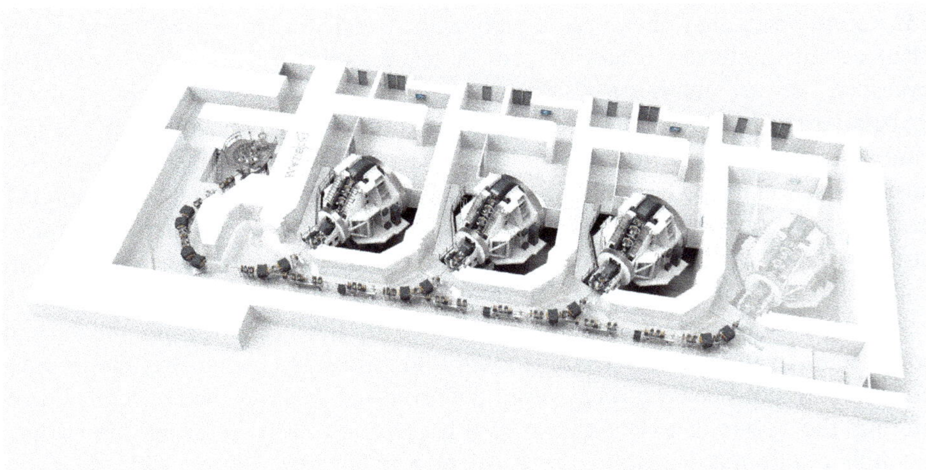

Figure 11.2. Cut away schematic of a typical multiple gantry room treatment facility for PBS only. In this example, the fourth gantry room has the potential for clinical treatments in the future but is intended for research use at the start of the facility's life. (Copyright 2017 Varian Medical Systems, Inc. All rights reserved.)

This chapter also address other radiation safety requirements including radition interlocks for the accelerator vault and treatment rooms, area and personnel monitoring, and the handling of radioactive materials which may be produced within the facility during the course of clinical operation.

11.2 Sources of extraneous radiation

The primary difference between particle beams and x-ray beams is that in order for particle beams to penetrate human tissue (or water) to a depth of 30–35 cm higher energies are required: 230–250 MeV for protons and about 400 MeV per nucleon for ^{12}C ions. The primary beam can be attenuated and stopped by only 12–15 cm of concrete, the most commonly used shielding material, but in stopping the beam the particles undergo many neutron producing nuclear interactions. In practice few, if any, of the primary particles reach the shielding walls; they are stopped in beam modifying devices and in the patient and this is where the secondary neutrons are produced. A broad range of neutron energies are produced from thermal energies (0.025 eV) up to the maximum particle beam energy. Thus, the shielding design is a neutron shielding problem and if we provide sufficient shielding for the neutrons there will be sufficient shielding for all other possible radiations. Another aspect of radiation safety around a particle therapy facility is that of the activation of materials that are struck by the proton beam. This issue will be dealt with in more detail in section 11.12.

There are two main categories of interaction to consider:

1. Those interactions which are not useful for treatment. These occur within the accelerator, degrader, beam line and beam modifying devices. As these interactions result in a loss of protons in the beam, their interaction is termed 'beam losses'. Beam losses are generally quoted by manufacturers as a percentage value and it is critical to understand what this value is a percentage of.
2. Treatment interaction. The patient is also a significant source of proton nuclear interactions and is the most significant source of neutrons in the treatment room for a scanning beam facility (see figure 11.5).

These interactions are considered in greater detail below.

11.2.1 Beam interactions within the accelerator during the acceleration process

In a synchrotron based system there may be a considerable number of interactions in the injection process, but these occur at energies below 3–4 MeV and, therefore, produce no significant neutron fluence. As the energy delivered by a synchrotron can be adjusted from pulse-to-pulse between 70 and 250 MeV, the beam losses and associated neutron production during acceleration vary considerably depending on the extracted energy. Losses during the acceleration process generally occur at lower energies (about 50 MeV) and again the neutron fluence produced is relatively insignificant.

However, in a cyclotron internal losses during acceleration can be considerable. Typically internal losses are in the range of 40%–75% for cyclotrons with room temperature magnets and 10%–20% for those with superconducting magnets. These losses generally occur through interactions of the beam with the magnet pole pieces or the dee structure when the beam diverges from the median plane. They are less in superconducting magnets since the higher magnetic field strengths attained allow for the pole piece gap to be larger than in room temperature magnets. These losses can also critically depend on beam tuning and conditioning of the radio frequency (RF) system, so careful attention to these details may help in reducing losses and, consequently, activation. Thus the neutron spectra of interest here are those produced by proton interactions with the magnet steel [p (Fe,X) y] or the copper dees [p (Cu,X) y]. The proton interactions can occur at any point along the acceleration path from very low energies to the maximum beam energy. These interactions are distributed isotropically around the proton orbits. Therefore they are most conveniently accounted for by distributing them in the median plane about the four cardinal angles. For calculations directly above and below the cyclotron such angular distribution is unnecessary since the relevant neutron production for these two directions occurs at a 90° angle to the beam direction.

11.2.2 Beam interactions with the beam extraction system or deflector

Both synchrotrons and cyclotrons experience this type of beam loss. In cyclotrons these losses always occur at the maximum beam energy, while in synchrotrons they occur at the extracted energy which can vary between the minimum and maximum extractable energies, which are typically 70 MeV and 250 MeV, respectively. The deflector is generally an electrostatic device constructed of copper. These interactions produce a neutron spectrum typical of p-Cu nuclear interactions. Neutron production at the deflector is greater in cyclotrons compared to synchrotrons for two reasons. First, the cyclotron always operates at the maximum energy while a synchrotron does not. Second, the efficiency of the energy selector system used with the cyclotron requires that when the ESS is used to provide low energy beams, currents of up to 300 nA may be extracted leading to much higher neutron production at the deflector. For comparison, the required beam extraction for high energy treatment beams is 1–3 nA, which is comparable to the beam extraction required from a synchrotron at all energies. These considerations also affect the activation of the deflector, so that activation of the deflector in a cyclotron is a greater problem than activation of the deflector in a synchrotron.

11.2.3 Beam interactions with the energy selection system

These losses only occur in cyclotron based facilities. The ESS is comprised of a wedge shaped degrader, often in the form of a rotating wheel, followed by a collimator for geometric clean-up of the beam, quadrupole magnets, divergence slits, dipole magnets to act as an energy spectrometer, more quadrupole magnets and a final slit for energy selection. A schematic of a typical EES arrangement is shown in figure 11.3. In most systems the ESS is situated as close as possible to the accelerator immediately after beam extraction, but some systems use a degrader for each room. The dipole magnets and the final energy selection slits act as an energy spectrometer.

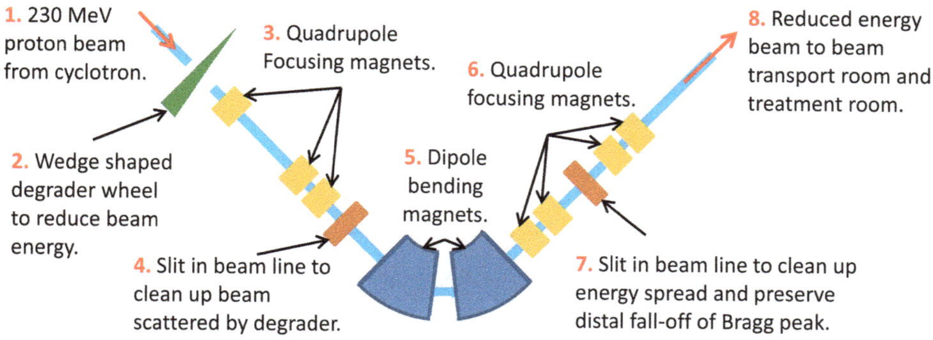

Figure 11.3. Schematic representation of an ESS for use in a cyclotron based proton therapy facility.

In passing through the degrader energy straggling is introduced to the beam, increasing the energy spread of the beam and, hence spoiling the sharpness of the distal edge of the Bragg peak. By using an energy spectrometer the final slit width is set to reduce this energy spread and restore the sharpness of the distal edge of the Bragg peak. Not all system suppliers choose to use a final energy clean-up slit and tolerate the degradation of the distal edge fall-off at low energies. The beam energy loss in the degrader and the beam fluence stopped in the collimator and slits lead to a considerable neutron fluence being produced around the ESS. In practice the transmission efficiency of the ESS can be 0.5% or less, when energies as low as 70 MeV are to be transported to the treatment room. The beam first interacts with the degrader which reduces the beam energy from its maximum energy (up to 250 MeV) to the desired energy, with the lowest energy being 70–100 MeV. The degrader is often constructed of a variety of materials to reduce neutron production depending on the energy degradation required. Aluminium, carbon and beryllium, or combinations of these materials are often used, and fabricated in the form of a linear or circular wedge. Beryllium, however, represents a conventional safety hazard because of its toxicity, which leads to a fire risk issue and may therefore be subject to local regulations. There is only partial energy loss in the degrader so the neutron spectrum corresponds to that produced by the full energy beam and energies down to that at which the beam emerges from the degrader. These spectra therefore have a neutron distribution that contains a higher proportion of high energy neutrons. Other components of the ESS where significant beam losses occur are the collimator, the first slit and the second slit.

The exact transmission properties of the ESS depend on the details of its design and the beam delivery mode (passive scattering or modulated scanning) and vary from vendor to vendor. However, even when the highest energy is transported, there are losses with about 75% geometrical transmission through the first slit and 99% transmission through the second slit for passive scattering. If the energy is reduced to 100 MeV geometrical transmission through the first slit is reduced to only about 5% with about 30% transmission through the energy slit for an overall ESS efficiency of only around 1.5%. The above figures are typical of passive scattering but even greater losses occur for modulated scanning, since the beam energy is varied on a spot by spot basis and to avoid variations of ESS efficiency with energy, at high energies this efficiency is deliberately reduced to ~10% by adjusting the geometrical slits. Thus, neutron production around the ESS is considerable and combined with the cyclotron beam loss results in this area requiring the most shielding in a cyclotron based proton therapy facility. The collimators and slits are typically constructed from tantalum or nickel.

11.2.4 Beam interactions in the beam transport line

The beam transport line transports the beam to each of the treatment rooms and beam losses along it are small and sporadic. During the beam tuning process small amounts of beam may impact on beam stops that are inserted into the beam line at various points along the beam line before the beam is delivered in to the treatment room. The beam often strikes these stops for periods of less than one second and the beam intensity is often reduced during this operation. Beam transport efficiency from the ESS or synchrotron is very high and losses are distributed along the beam line; the losses are dependent on the energy of the beam that is transported. Typically, the proton beam interacts with materials such as iron, tantalum or nickel. Losses are typically less than 5%.

11.2.5 Beam interactions with the treatment nozzle

The extent of beam losses in the treatment room depends critically on the type of beam delivery system that is used. There are three modes of beam delivery commonly in use in proton therapy facilities: passive scattering, uniform scanning (sometimes known as wobbling) and modulated scanning (often referred to as PBS). Passive scattering can be achieved through single or double scattering; single scattering is used when small fields (~5 cm diameter) are required and double scattering for large fields (up to 22–25 cm diameter). A simple schematic of a passive scattering system is shown in figure 11.4. The beam is single or double scattered to provide a beam of the desired lateral dimensions. The beam energy entering the treatment room is adjusted

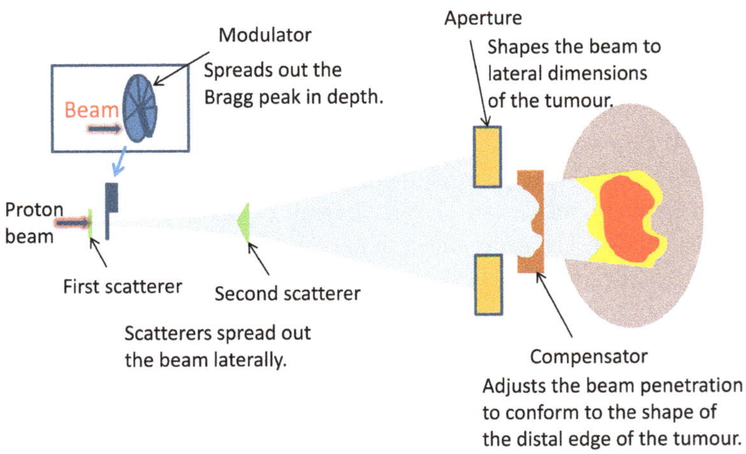

Figure 11.4. Schematic of passive double scattering proton beam delivery system.

to provide a range that is sufficient to penetrate to the distal edge of the treatment volume. A range modulator is used to spread out the Bragg peak across the full extent of the tumour in the transverse or depth dimension. The range modulation is often provided by a wedge shaped rotating wheel but a ridge filter may also be used. The ridge filter is a static device comprised of multiple wedge shaped beam modifiers spaced out across the field dimensions; these spread the beam penetration across the desired treatment depth while providing sufficient multiple scattering to ensure that the wedge structure across the dose distribution in the lateral dimension is 'washed out'. Once the beam has been spread in the lateral and transverse dimensions it is collimated using a custom-made aperture to conform to the lateral dimensions of the tumour shape. Finally a tissue compensator is used to contour the dose distribution to the distal edge of the treatment volume. Neutrons are produced in each of these beam modifying devices. The modulator or ridge filter, and compensator are constructed from hydrocarbon-like materials, typically acrylic plastic or hard wax. The apertures are most often machined from brass or cast from Lippowitz metal; some systems use multi-leaf collimators (MLCs) constructed from iron or tungsten. Scatterers are often a composite of acrylic plastic and lead. Plastic materials produce less neutrons per incident proton than the heavier metals.

The arrangement for uniform scanning is shown in figure 11.5. A single scatter is used to produce a large beam spot, ~5 cm in diameter, and a pair of magnets is used to scan the beam in the lateral x and y directions. The modulator wheel is stepped through the beam energies required to produce the spread out Bragg peak (SOBP) allowing one layer to be scanned before moving on to the next. The beam is scanned across a rectangular field larger than the treatment volume's lateral dimensions and therefore an aperture is required to conform the beam to the lateral shape of the tumour. A single energy is transported to the treatment room and, therefore, a compensator is still required. The neutron spectra produced in uniform scanning mode are similar to those produced with passive scattering. In both passive scattering and uniform scanning the beam shape imposed on the distal edge of the

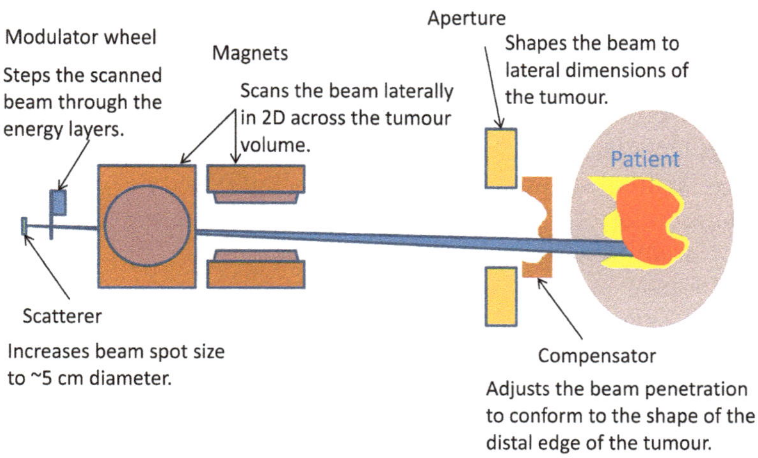

Figure 11.5. Schematic of uniform scanning (or wobbling) proton beam delivery system.

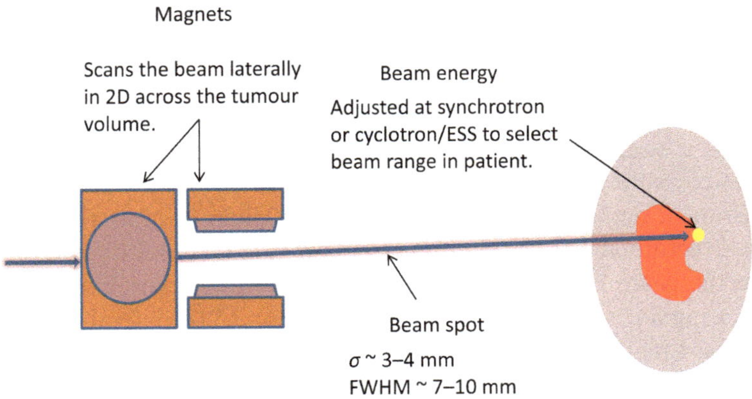

Figure 11.6. Schematic of PBS (or modulated scanning) proton beam delivery system.

treatment volume by the compensator is also imposed on the proximal side of the dose distribution. This results in some healthy tissue on the proximal side of the tumour receiving unwanted dose.

A simplified schematic of a modulated scanning system is shown in figure 11.6. A narrow unmodified pencil beam with a pristine Bragg peak is scanned in the x and y directions to deliver the dose as a series of small dose voxels. The beam may be delivered as a series of spots in a 'stop and shoot' mode or as a raster scan. The beam energy is adjusted to deliver dose to points on the distal edge of the treatment volume; spots are only delivered where the dose is needed. The energy of the beam is reduced at the ESS to 'pull-back' the beam so that the next layer can be delivered. When the most proximal layer is delivered dose voxels are again only delivered where they are needed and, hence, the dose distribution conforms to both the distal and proximal shape of the tumour. In PBS mode no beam modifying devices are required and hence neutron production occurs almost entirely as a result of proton interactions in the patient. All beam delivery systems require dose monitoring and, as in conventional x-ray therapy, this is provided by multiple parallel plate ionization chambers. These chambers have not been included in the simple schematics of figures 11.4–11.6. The chambers are designed to be very thin resulting in minimal energy loss, with corresponding negligible neutron production in comparison to other neutron producing interactions.

Another potential source of radiation in the treatment room may be a range shifter. Range shifters are used in two main applications:

1. In some cyclotron systems the ESS is replaced by an in-room range shifter to adjust beam penetration in the patient.
2. In PBS mode a range shifter must be used if dose is to be delivered to the patient's skin surface, since the minimum energy transported in the room with an ESS is 70 or 100 MeV corresponding to a minimum range in the patient of 4.5 and 7 cm, respectively.

From a shielding perspective the PBS application is not a problem, since the range shifters used are plastic which is essentially tissue equivalent and, therefore, it is not necessary to model the shifter separately from the patient. In the first application, however, the range shifter is generally a set of automatically insertable metal leaves and the neutron yields may needed to be accounted for based on the vendors operating specifications for the range shifter, particularly the incident beam current for various energy outputs and any local shielding that is incorporated into the design.

11.2.6 Beam interactions in the patient

Ultimately a high proportion of the beam stops in the patient. From a practical perspective proton interactions with human tissue can be approximate by proton interactions with water, which means that neutron production originates from proton interactions with ^{16}O.

From the above it can be seen that a wide variety of neutron producing nuclear reactions may occur when a proton beam interacts with the materials found in a proton therapy facility. It is important to obtain specific information from the vendor concerning the magnitude of the beam losses at specific points in their system and the materials in which these losses occur. When high energy protons interact with matter the resulting neutron emission is not isotropic but is forward peaked. Therefore, not only is spectral information at the 0° angle (relative to the direction of beam incidence) required but also at other angles; preferably additional spectra at 90° and 180° should be available as a minimum. With such a wide range of data required for computing shielding thicknesses it is desirable to consider some options for simplifying the calculations.

11.3 Design and build process considerations

When purchasing proton therapy equipment, the vendors generally supply detailed layout drawings, including architectural quality drawings that include recommended shielding wall thickness, often based on the intended use and throughput of the facility. If the system is one that has been previously installed the characteristics of the radiation shield may be well established. However, this is often not the case and in any case the operator is ultimately responsible for the building design and construction and for ensuring that the shielding surrounding the facility is adequate from a regulatory point of view. Therefore, although it may not be necessary to design the shielding walls from scratch, it is always necessary to perform calculations that confirm the adequacy of the vendor proposed design. Some of the techniques available for making these calculations are outlined later in this chapter.

Of the considerations required to tailor a design for an individual centre, regulatory requirements are likely to be the most significant, greatly influencing shielding and safety features. Local conditions, such as space limitations, may require adjustments to the shielding design; e.g. it may be necessary to incorporate high density shielding materials into parts of the design. Use of the facility also has a large impact on design, as ultimately it is the annual dose that is of concern under most regulations. As a large number of energies are used even for one patient, an understanding of the intended case mix is important, along with understanding of throughput, the intended use of surrounding areas, and the degree of flexibility required of the facility for future changes and technological and clinical advancements. An understanding of the uncertainties within the process is important so they can be dealt with in a controlled manner without excessive conservatism and increased concrete cost.

There is a large array of information needed in order to perform calculations estimating the annual doses to the staff and public in areas in and around the facility, and it is efficient to gather as much of the information as possible prior to beginning calculations. To aid this process, table 11.1 outlines much of the preliminary data required. There are a number of sources of this information, with the source depending upon the nature of the information. Accelerator manufacturers are a good source of information, and can offer guidance and specific assurances about their particular equipment performance (e.g. beam loss data). However, caution must be exercised in using some quoted data from equipment manufacturers such as wall thicknesses, as they may be designed for a different workload and regulatory environment. With such a large array of information sources, it is important in the design and build process that the responsibility for providing information is clearly set out to all parties, along with deadlines to ensure the design and shielding calculations can be completed within the timescales required by the project.

In addition to supplying information, equipment manufacturers may be able to offer experience of other builds and links to other centres that they have supplied with equipment. This can be helpful when considering the possibilities for the design and it can be useful to have equipment suppliers' representatives at design meetings. In addition, equipment suppliers should advise on the specifications of the build with respect to equipment requirements for a successful design, such as temperature control, flatness of the beam line floor and duct positions. Including manufacturers, architects and engineers as well as radiation protection specialists in the design process is essential from the outset to ensure that all of the requirements of the design can be met. Any change to the design at a later date needs to be referred back to this design team to ensure that there is no unforeseen adverse effect of the change on other requirements. Such issues are best defined in a change control process and incorporated in the purchase agreement. It may also be useful to have an external independent radiation protection expert review the radiation shielding and radiation safety plans for the facility. In fact these vendor building requirements should be carefully defined in a 'Building Interface Document' which forms part of the formal contractual agreement between the equipment vendor and the customer. Installing a proton therapy system will inevitably involve very close collaboration between the customer, the equipment vendor, the building contractor and sub-contractors. The customer should appoint a project manager who ensures that the appropriate customer representative (physician, physicist, radiation safety officer, administrators or other interested party) is available to appropriately answer questions that arise.

Table 11.1. Information needed in order to perform calculations estimating the annual doses to the staff and public in areas in and around the facility.

Item No.	Information	Source	Comments
1	**Dose rate criteria**		
1.1	Annual staff dose limit	Legislation	May choose pregnant staff limit to avoid need for staff role alteration.
1.2	Annual public dose limit	Legislation	
1.3	Area designation criteria	Legislation	User may want to avoid designation outside of accelerator, beam line and gantry rooms.
1.4	IDR limit in public areas	Guidance	May help with future flexibility of facility.
2	**Design considerations**		
2.1	Proposed design thicknesses	Architect	Need to account for duct work in walls.
2.2	Position and width of conduits within walls	Architect	
2.3	Footprints of equipment	Manufacturer	Also establish flexibility in this.
2.4	Room geometry in general	Architect	
2.5	Wall materials	Builder	
2.6	Floor/ceiling materials	Builder	
2.7	Build tolerances (mm)	Builder	
2.8	Isocentre position	Architect/ Manufacturer	
3	**Beam characteristics**		
3.1	Beam losses	Manufacturer	If possible, these values should be guaranteed by the manufacturer, from measured data and provided in terms of a range of values.
3.2	Position of beam loss	Manufacturer	If the equipment is non-standard, this information may be needed from the accelerator physicist.
3.3	Maximum energy	Manufacturer	
4	**Usage assumptions**		
4.1	Beam-on time per room	User/experienced centre	
4.2	Number of patients per year	User/experienced centre	
4.3	Average patient dose (Gy)	User/experienced centre	
4.4	Average number of fractions	User/experienced centre	

4.5	Fraction of clinical use for patient specific quality control (QC) tests	User/experienced centre	
4.6	Fraction of clinical dose for overnight maintenance	User/experienced centre	
4.7	Fraction of clinical use for run-up	Manufacturer	
4.8	Fraction of clinical use for general QC	User/experienced centre	
4.9	Accelerator current (nA)	Manufacturer	Loss information can be used to calculate current at any point for a particular energy. Average current/ charge may also be useful.
4.10	Beam-on time	User/experienced centre	
4.11	Number of protons per year	User/experienced centre	Can be calculated from knowledge of items 4.1–4.10 or scaled from another centre's data.
4.12	Energy use factor	User/experienced centre	
4.13	Energy to use in energy banding	User/experienced centre	May be different for gantries and accelerator.
4.14	Number of energy bands	User/experienced centre	
4.15	Orientation factors	User/experienced centre	
4.16	Occupancy of adjacent areas	User/experienced centre	
4.17	Assumed occupancy and location of radiographers in gantry room	User/experienced centre	
5	**Future-proofing**		
5.1	Number of patients in any potential extra rooms	User/ commissioning body	Some centres built with unused capacity.
5.2	Potential increase in patient throughput	Manufacturer/ research papers	
5.3	Potential hypofraction dose per fraction (Gy)	Research papers	Becoming common in photon therapy.
5.4	Percentage of patients at this higher fractionation	Research papers	

(*Continued*)

Table 11.1. (*Continued*)

Item No.	Information	Source	Comments
5.5	Potential for increase in average dose per fraction	Calculation	Calculation of above cf overall patient numbers.
5.6	Increase in set up time for hypofractionation	User/experienced centre	Increased on treatment imaging?
5.7	Potential increase in use of particular gantry angle	User/experienced centre	Based on change in patient demographic, e.g. more pelvis treatments.
5.8	Potential for energy mix to change	User/experienced centre	Based on change in patient demographic, e.g. more pelvis treatments.
6	**Contingency factors**		
6.1	Uncertainty in loss information (and other vendor information) %	Vendor	
6.2	Uncertainty in assumptions %	User	
6.3	Uncertainty in calculations %	Physicist	
6.4	Uncertainty in build %	Builder	
6.5	**Total uncertainty (added in quadrature) %**		$= \sqrt{((6.1^2) + (6.2^2) + (6.3^2) + (6.4^2))}$

11.4 Regulatory requirements and design criteria

The design of a radiation shield is generally driven by local regulations which define the acceptable radiation levels that may be received by radiation workers and members of the general public (see chapter 3 for general principles). At the time of writing, new national legislation in European countries, following from the latest European Basic Safety Standard (EC 2013), is required to be enacted by February 2018, meaning most particle therapy centres in the early stages of planning in Europe will be required to comply with this legislation from the outset.

It is valuable to review previously used designs, however, much experience of particle facility design is international, particularly from the USA and Japan, and it is important to understand the dose constraints that those facilities have been designed to. Table 11.2 gives some commonly used regulatory limits recommended by the ICRP (2007), the NCRP (1993) and the United Kingdom *Ionising Radiation Regulations* (IRR 1999, ACoP 2000); the UK regulations closely reflect the ICRP recommendations. In designing a shield around a particle therapy facility situated in a hospital environment it is often desirable to adopt a conservative approach and

Table 11.2. A comparison of ICRP and NCRP recommendations on exposure limits for occupational workers and the general public with the UK *Ionising Radiation Regulations* (new limits not yet enforced in brackets).

Quantity	Recommending organisation		
	ICRP	NCRP	UK IRR99
Occupational exposure limits			
Effective dose limits			
Annual	20 mSv averaged over defined periods of 5 years	50 mSv	20 mSv in any calendar year
Cumulative		10 mSv × age	100 mSv in any 5 year period subject to a maximum of 50 mSv in any year
Dose equivalent annual limits for tissues and organs			
Lens of the eye	150 mSv	150 mSv	150 (20) mSv
Skin	500 mSv	500 mSv	500 mSv
Hands and feet	500 mSv	500 mSv	500 mSv[a]
General public/non-radiation workers			
Effective annual dose limits			
Continuous or frequent exposure	1 mSv	1 mSv	1 mSv
Infrequent exposure	–	5 mSv	5 mSv[b]
Dose equivalent annual limits for tissues and organs			
Lens of the eye	15 mSv	15 mSv	15 mSv
Skin	50 mSv	50 mSv	50 mSv
Hands and feet	–	50 mSv	50 mSv[a]

[a] In the UK the dose limit is specified for hands, forearms, feet and ankles.
[b] In the UK this regulation 'applies to any person (not being a comforter or carer) who may be exposed to ionizing radiation resulting from the medical exposure of another and in such a case the limit on the effective dose for any such person shall be 5 mSv in any period of 5 consecutive calendar years'.

design so that most areas can be unsupervised and accessible to the general public; in the UK this limits the effective dose for continuous and frequent exposure to 0.3 mSv per year.

11.5 Workload, use and occupancy factors

Shielding calculations of the type discussed later estimate values for the instantaneous dose rate (IDR) at points of interest around the shield, but this is only a part of the calculations required to assess regulatory compliance. Estimates of annual dose to individuals and areas are required to determine compliance. This is determined by other factors which include the workload, the energy and angle use factors and occupancy factors. Determining workload and use factors can be more problematic than calculating IDR and also involve greater uncertainties. As proton therapy is a rapidly growing modality, which is being applied to an increasing number of clinical indications, it can be challenging to accurately determine energy and gantry angle use factors. Estimations of the future use of the facility and the uncertainties in the build process are also important. Assumptions and estimations used in calculations should be clearly documented and reviewed at a defined frequency to ensure the on-going applicability of the calculations.

11.5.1 Beam energy

Proton and particle therapy is based on the principal that the particle loses a large proportion of its energy at the end of its track, and will not interact beyond a certain depth, which is defined by its energy. This is seen as a Bragg peak in the dose depth curve (see figure 11.7(a)). As there is a small range over which a high dose is given, a typical treatment will require a range of energies to produce a high dose over the entire depth range of the tumour. This results in an SOBP (see figure 11.7(b)). Thus

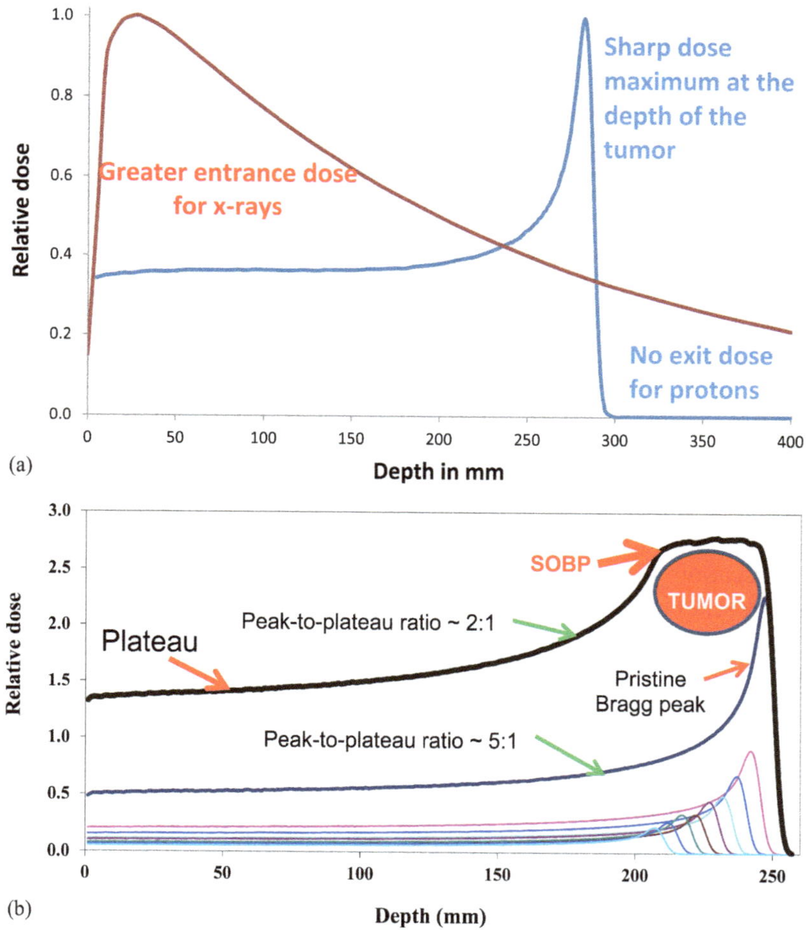

Figure 11.7. (a) Illustrating the superior depth dose characteristics of a proton beam in comparison to a photon beam. There are three important features to note: the reduced entrance dose for the proton beam, the sharp high dose Bragg peak and the absence of exit dose for the protons. (b) Showing how a series of weighted pristine Bragg peaks are summed to create a SOBP that encompasses the tumour volume. A consequence of spreading the Bragg peaks is a degradation of the peak-to-plateau ratio of the dose distribution.

there is an array of incident energies used for a particular patient, and this array may be similar for a particular group of patients. Hence, the energy required to treat a head and neck lesion may be as low as 100 MeV (~7 cm range), while a pelvic lesion may require the maximum energy of 230–250 MeV, with a corresponding range of between 32 and 35 cm. There are considerable shielding implications here as a higher energy beam will produce substantially more neutrons than a low energy beam and the neutrons will also be of much higher energy. It is, therefore, important to allow for this in shielding calculations by introducing a use factor for energy (U_E) and selecting several energies. If the expected case mix is well defined, analysis can be carried out to determine the expected use of particular energy ranges. The energy use factor should also be considered separately for quality control tests, maintenance procedures and research work for both the room in which the activity is taking place and for the accelerator vault.

The actual energy used for the calculation will be a single energy, therefore it is important to decide what energy within the energy band should be used. It would be safe (and somewhat conservative) to consider the highest energy of the band for treatment room calculations, and the lowest energy of the band around the ESS (as beams of these energies will require the most degradation). It is usual to use three to four energy ranges for a proton facility. Typically the highest and lowest energies and some intermediate energy are used, for example 100 MeV, 175 MeV and 250 MeV may be good choices. The number of different energy use factors (or bands) used will determine the energy resolution and hence accuracy of the calculation. However, a balance will need to be struck between accuracy on one hand, and the reliability of the assumption about energy mix and calculation speed on the other (each energy band will require a separate calculation). Alternatively, it can be assumed conservatively that each treatment is made with the worst case neutron production. This results naturally in higher shielding cost, but ensures maximal future flexibility. The estimation of the energy use factors is also dependent on the beam delivery technique employed (passive scattering, uniform scanning or modulated scanning) and on the expected patient population. In passive scattering and uniform scanning a single energy is generally transported to the treatment room and the beam losses occur in the modulator, the beam scatterers, the collimator aperture, the compensator and the patient. In modulated scanning the dose is delivered in 'energy layers', which range from the energy required to deliver protons to the maximum depth in the patient to that required to deliver dose to the minimum depth. The dose to each layer is weighted to produce a uniform dose across the target volume with the heaviest weighting to deepest layers. However, a consequence of these different modes of operation is that the energy use factors appropriate for a double scattering room will be different than those required for a modulated scanning system even if the patient populations are the same. Therefore assigning each of the expected patient populations a single energy use factor for the treatment site may not be appropriate, especially for modulated scanning, where the energy use factors should take into account the range of energies delivered to the room and their weightings.

11.5.2 Beam use

Beam use is a complex factor when considering particle therapy facilities because, unlike x-ray or electron treatments, the dose rate is dependent upon the energy used. As the accelerator is capable of a maximum current (analogous to dose rate for charged particles), the lower the energy required at the nozzle, the lower the current. Ultimately, therefore, to establish an annual dose rate, it is the number of protons used per year for each energy, or the proton charge per year per energy that is required. There are a number of ways of establishing this ranging from a rough estimate of beam-on time and average current to an in-depth analysis of treatment plans. The projected number of patients and average dose per fraction will have a large impact on this value. Finally quality control testing exposures, proton production for servicing purposes and research purposes should also be taken into account, but consideration of when this will happen should be made to establish if this only affects a specific group of staff on a certain shift.

11.5.3 Orientation factor

For proton gantries a use factor must be assigned for each gantry angle (U_θ) appropriate to the patient population. This is the same concept as for conventional x-ray therapy, except that some proton facilities have gantries with restricted rotation (180° or 220°) or fixed beam rooms with horizontal and/or vertical or inclined beam lines. The nature of particle therapy dose deposition curves also means that fewer angles are needed for treatment than with x-ray therapy, so that opposed beams are far less common than in x-ray therapy and arc therapy is not currently used and may not be desirable. Existing centres with similar patient groups may be a good source of this information. Once the centre is fully operational, this assumption can be confirmed via the record and verify system or treatment planning system.

11.5.4 Occupancy factors

Occupancy factors (T) are determined in the same way as for x-ray therapy. Often a long corridor is situated along one side of the facility to allow patient access. In some larger proton therapy facilities corridors extended around two or three sides of the shielded area and this can be a good design feature from a shielding point of view, as corridors are assigned an occasional occupancy factor in the range 0.025–0.4, depending on local regulations. However, consideration should also be given to the projected annual dose in high occupancy areas beyond this corridor. If a floor is to be built above or below the facility this will often include office space or examination rooms where staff have full 8 h occupancy, requiring an occupancy factor of one. Because the expected longevity of proton therapy installations it is likely that the use of adjacent areas may be reassigned and redeveloped multiple times during the facility lifetime. For this reason it is prudent to assign occupancy factors of unity to most of the adjacent areas, apart from corridors and equipment/utility rooms. It is also prudent to assign an occupancy factor of one to adjacent gantry rooms and control desk areas as adjacent gantries are most likely staffed during a treatment occurring in the gantry in question, as the beam can usually only be used in one gantry at a time. The most significant contribution of dose to the control desk area is usually from the gantry that control desk is assigned to. However, contributions from other gantries to this area may need to be accounted for depending on the design. Again, occupancy of one is prudent as there are often staff carrying out tasks in this area most of the time. Areas outside the accelerator vault, beam line, gantry and treatment rooms should be designed such that they do not require designation as either controlled or supervised area as defined in the *Ionising Radiation Regulations* (IRR 1999).

11.5.5 Work patterns and staff positioning

Most proton therapy facilities are planned to operate over an extended day with many centres scheduling patient treatments for 16 or more hours per day and requiring shift work to provide adequate staffing. Therefore, in calculating shielding requirements a workload based on 8 h work period should be used. In addition, physics staff and engineers may be present during extended beam-on periods, and suitable assessment of this should also be made.

An attempt should also be made to establish the position of staff in common scenarios, such as setting up a patient on the treatment couch, as it is unlikely the member of staff will be exposed to the highest dose rate in the room (usually at the wall). Therefore an assumed position is likely to be more realistic, for example 2 m from the treatment couch. In-room imaging is also a possibility with some equipment, which may lead to a second common staff position within a gantry room.

11.5.6 Future-proofing

Due to the expected lifetime of proton facilities (30–40 years), the field is likely to develop and assumptions used that may be realistic today may not be suitable in the future. It is therefore prudent to attempt to predict what changes may happen in order to build a contingency for these into the design. Of course, this is extremely uncertain and has cost implications and a balance between the cost of the facility and the potential future flexibility will need to be struck. Many of the changes may be quantifiable and hence included in the design. Table 11.1 lists some of the potential changes one may want to consider. It is possible to increase dose rate above the currently accepted norm of 1–2 Gy min^{-1}, especially at the higher energies in cyclotron based facilities when ESS limitations are not an issue. It is also possible that technological advancements may mean switching times between energies and rooms may decrease in the future. However, these changes may prove to have limited impact on annual dose as beam-on time is small compared to patient set-up time and other clinical processes. Synchrotrons generally have limitations on the number of protons that can be accelerated in a single pulse due to space charge constraints and this combined with the duty cycle places an upper limit on the achievable dose rate. Hypofractionation and radiosurgery applications may create great pressure on vendors to provide higher dose rates as well as increase the dose per fraction, leading to usage factors that may be 2–4 times higher than now. The high cost of proton therapy has also increased pressure for more efficient workflow to accommodate greater workloads. Some centres are designed to accommodate expansion with additional treatment rooms. Such expansion may have no implications on individual room shielding, but could lead to a significant increase in accelerator and ESS (if applicable) shielding requirements.

11.5.7 Uncertainties

There are a number of uncertainties in the process of designing the shielding and it is prudent to take these into account as an additional part of the dose calculation. Uncertainties are caused by having to make usage assumptions, calculation model simplifications, loss information (and other equipment information), build tolerances and future use. Adding the uncertainties in quadrature has been used as a method for establishing an overall uncertainty with the intention of the uncertainties not over-impacting upon the expected dose as they would do if each was considered in isolation. The overall uncertainty can be applied to the calculated doses to establish a range of expected doses, which can then be compared to the legislative requirement. Options to reduce the potential impact of these uncertainties include adding additional shielding, gaining a better understanding of individual parameters in order to reduce individual uncertainties, and contingency planning (e.g. leaving space for additional shielding) should the upper end of the dose range be realised.

11.6 Construction materials

Concrete is the most commonly used material in constructing radiation shielding. It has the advantages of being both relatively inexpensive and easy to handle in a construction environment. The exact specifications of the concrete are of interest in designing a proton therapy facility. Ordinary concrete is generally considered to have a density of 2350 kg m^{-3} (147 lb ft^{-3}) and a water content of ~5.5% after curing. Water content is important because its hydrogen content is a major contributor to neutron scattering, energy loss and attenuation. In ordinary concrete about 3% of the water is chemically bound, while the remaining 2.5% is in free form and may evaporate over time with a long half-life (tens of years). Concrete can also absorb water so that some equilibrium situation is established which depends on local ambient conditions.

Other materials can also be used as shielding materials. Earth is often used to reduce cost or when installations are below ground. High density concrete may also be used if space is a consideration. An alternative in this situation is to include steel plates in the shielding to reduce shielding thickness around local hot spots. NCRP Report No. 144 (NCRP 2003) recommends that any iron or steel shielding should be backed by at least 0.6 m (2 ft) of concrete, since the cross-section for the interaction of neutrons with iron falls rapidly below about 5 MeV. More detailed information on shielding materials may be found in PTCOG (2010) and NCRP (2003).

Activation of shielding materials should be considered, and can be an issue for decommissioning. Certain impurities within concrete, such as Europium, produce long lived radioactive isotopes. Some companies offer concrete free of elements that will produce long lived isotopes. Activation of other materials used in the construction should also be assessed for potential activation, e.g. floor and ceiling duct work. Centres have used a variety of activation mitigation strategies, including using fly-ash free concrete, using a layer of metal reinforcement-free concrete lining prior to the main concrete (which includes metal reinforcement) in the cyclotron vault, using low cement concrete and using marble or limestone aggregate in the concrete mix close to the ESS. It is, however, currently uncertain what mitigation, if any, is required as no facility has yet been fully decommissioned. Monte Carlo modelling of activation coupled with knowledge of local regulations and available decommissioning processes can help guide this decision. Some useful information is available from the decommissioning of accelerators used in research and other commercial applications (Ulrici and Magistis 2009, IAEA 2003).

11.7 Theory of radiation transport: solving the Boltzmann equation

Ideally, to solve the radiation attenuation problem the energy and angular distributions of all particles throughout the entire shield whatever its composition and geometry need to be known, i.e. the angular fluence needs to be known:

$$\Phi_i(x, E, \Omega, t), \tag{11.1}$$

where Φ_i is the number of particles of type i per unit area, per unit solid angle, per unit time at location x with energy E at time t travelling in direction Ω.

From the angular fluence, the scalar fluence rate can be determined by integrating over direction and energy

$$\Phi_i(x, t) = \int_{4\pi} \mathrm{d}\Omega \int \mathrm{d}E \; \Phi_\mathrm{i}(x, E, \Omega, t). \tag{11.2}$$

Radiation protection quantities such as dose equivalent rate, $H(x, t)$, can be calculated at a location by integrating the product of scalar fluence rate and the appropriate coefficient for converting fluence rate to that quantity, $[g(E)]$, over energy and angle and summing over all particles i,

$$H(x, t) = \Sigma_i \int_{4\pi} \mathrm{d}\Omega \int_0^\infty \mathrm{d}E \; \Phi_i(x, E, \Omega, t) g_i(E). \tag{11.3}$$

The primary tool for determining the angular fluence and thus solving for the dose equivalent rate is the Boltzmann equation, which can be used to describe the distribution of a collection of particles in terms of their momentum and location in time and space. The Boltzmann equation is very difficult to solve and many specialized approximate analytical solutions have been derived. Computational methods based on Monte Carlo methods are widely used to obtain solutions. More detailed information on radiation transport, the Boltzmann equation, methods for its solution and computer codes used in Monte Carlo solutions may be found in NCRP (2003). Analytical solutions of the shielding problem often use data that have been generated in part using Monte Carlo methods. For instance, data on dose equivalent rate at depth in a concrete shield as a function of incident neutron energy are available from several sources, but in order for these data to be useful knowledge of the incident neutron spectrum is required. At the proton energies used in therapy such spectral data can be reliably calculated using a number of Monte Carlo codes, for example MCNP (Briesmeister 2000), Geant4 (Agostinelli *et al* 2003) and FLUKA (Fasso *et al* 2001, Ferrari *et al* 2001).

11.8 Practical shielding calculations

The first step in performing the shielding calculation is to calculate the instantaneous dose equivalent rate (IDR_{calc}) through the shield using either an analytical model, possibly combined with Monte Carlo data, or a full Monte Carlo analysis. Workload, use factors and occupancy factors may then be factored into the calculations to calculate TADR and TADR2000. The equation to be solved to calculate the IDR_{calc} is of the general form

$$\frac{\mathrm{d}}{\mathrm{d}t}H_{\mathrm{d},n} = \Phi N_{\mathrm{p}}\frac{B_n}{d^2} = \mathrm{IDR}_{\mathrm{calc}}, \tag{11.4}$$

where $\frac{\mathrm{d}}{\mathrm{d}t}H_{d,n}$ is the dose equivalent rate at the point of interest; N_{p} is the number of protons incident on the target per unit time; Φ is the neutron fluence rate (neutrons proton^{-1} per sr); B_n is the shielding transmission factor (dose equivalent cm^2); and d is the distance between the neutron source and the calculation point (m).

The time average dose rate (TADR) for a particular gantry angle and energy band $\mathrm{TADR}_{\theta,\mathrm{E}}$ can then be calculated from the IDR (which has been calculated for these conditions) by using equation (11.5):

$$\mathrm{TADR}_{\theta,\mathrm{E}} = \mathrm{IDR}_{\mathrm{calc},\theta,\mathrm{E}} \times W_{\mathrm{d}} \times U_{\theta} \times U_{\mathrm{E}}/8. \tag{11.5}$$

where W_{d} is the daily workload factor (the time in hours that the beam is on during an eight hour shift for all gantry angles and energy bands), U_{θ} is the gantry angle use factor (the fraction of beam time at a particular gantry angle), U_{E} is the energy factor (the fraction of beam time within the energy band). TADRs for all energy bands and gantry angles should be summed to give the total TADR.

The TADR2000 is an hourly dose equivalent rate average over 2000 h taking into account workload, use factors and occupancy, and may be obtained from the product of the TADR and the occupancy factor, T:

$$\mathrm{TADR2000} = \mathrm{TADR} \times T \tag{11.6}$$

The annual dose is then obtained by multiplying the TADR2000 by the 2000 h in the working year:

$$\text{Annual dose} = 2000 \times \mathrm{TADR2000} \tag{11.7}$$

The major challenge in shielding calculations for a proton therapy facility is to determine the shielding transmission factor and the neutron fluence rate.

In many circumstances shielding transmission can be estimated using a simple equation including terms for exponential attenuation and the inverse square law and of the general form

$$H(E, d, \theta) = H'(E, \theta) \times e^{-d/\lambda(E,\theta)}/r^2, \tag{11.8}$$

where $H'(E,\theta)$ is a source term and $\lambda(E,\theta)$ is the attenuation length. Both these terms depend on the secondary particle energy spectra which in turn is dependent on the incident particle type, its energy (E), the target material and the angle between the point of interest and the direction of the incident particle (θ). d is the thickness of the shield and r is the distance between the source and the point of interest outside the shielding wall.

When equations of this form are used to create models of shielding for the high energy accelerators (>1 GeV) associated with high energy physics, many neutral secondary particles may be emitted, so the source term may be complex. However, at the lower accelerating energies associated with proton and ion therapy ($\leqslant$400 MeV) the secondary particles are restricted to neutrons and photons and therefore the situation is much simpler and data are often presented in a tabular or graphical form as a function of mono-energetic neutron energy and fitted to an equation for the dose equivalent transmitted through the shielding of the form:

$$H(d) = H_0 e^{-d/\lambda}, \tag{11.9}$$

where H_0 is the dose equivalent at zero depth, d is the shield thickness and λ is the attenuation length.

Graphical data on dose equivalent transmission rate through a concrete shield as a function of shield thickness for a range of mono-energetic neutrons incident normally on the shield at energies between 0.1 MeV and 400 MeV may be found in figure 4.5 of NCRP Report 144 (NCRP 2003). Tabulated data of the attenuation length in concrete for incident mono-energetic neutron energies between 5 MeV and 1 GeV are available in table 4.2 of IAEA Technical Report Series No. 283 (IAEA 1988). Both these data sets are derived from calculations of Alsmiller *et al* (1969) in the neutron energy range 50–400 MeV, supplemented by data from other sources to extend the energy range: Roussin *et al* (1971, 1973) and Wyckoff and Chilton (1973) for the NCRP and IAEA reports, respectively. The calculations employ a method known as discrete ordinates for solving the Bolzmann equation. In this method the calculations are simplified by approximating the neutron angular distributions using a limited number of discrete angles.

These data provide a simple method for calculating shielding requirements for mono-energetic neutron beams. Unfortunately the neutron fluence produced by the neutron sources found within a particle therapy centre is never mono-energetic. Therefore it is highly desirable to have some knowledge of the neutron fluence as a function of energy (the neutron spectrum) produced by the various neutron sources described in section 11.2. The neutron spectrum represents the term ΦN_p in equation (11.4) summed over energy, or $\Sigma_E \Phi N_p$.

There are little or no measured spectral data at the energies of interest in proton therapy and modelling the spectra using Monte Carlo codes is the most practical solution. Spectra should be calculated for a range of energies and for multiple scattering angles relative to the incident beam for each target material of interest. Typically these materials may include iron and copper for interactions in the cyclotron, aluminium, carbon and beryllium for interactions in the degrader, nickel and tantalum for interactions in the ESS slits, acrylic plastic and brass for interactions in the nozzle components, and finally interactions with water or tissue to represent the patient or the phantom. Calculations of this type combining Monte Carlo neutron methods to derive analytical models based on equation (11.8) have been performed by several authors (e.g. Agosteo *et al* 2007, Sheu *et al* 2013). They found that the data could be better fitted by a double exponential of the form

$$H(E, d, \theta) = \left[H_1(E, \theta) \times e^{-\frac{d}{\lambda_1(E,\theta)}} + H_2(E, \theta) \times e^{-\frac{d}{\lambda_2(E,\theta)}}\right] / r^2 \qquad (11.10)$$

and tabulate values of the pseudo-source terms (H_1 and H_2) and the attenuation lengths (λ_1 and λ_2) as a function of incident particle energy and angle relative to the incident beam direction for protons incident on a stopping target. Agosteo *et al* (2007) have performed calculations of this type for protons between 100 and 250 MeV incident on a stopping iron target shielded by concrete; later extending the calculations to iron and concrete/iron shields (Agosteo *et al* 2008). Sheu *et al* (2013) used a similar approach, H' and λ determination in a double exponential model, to calculate shielding requirements using concrete, iron and lead shields for proton energies of 100–300 MeV and also for a wider range of target materials: iron, carbon and tissue. They extended their work later to include proton incident on a thick copper target as an additional source (Lai *et al* 2015). In this approach the calculated neutron fluences for various shield thicknesses are folded with ambient dose equivalent conversion factors (ICRP 1996, Pelliccioni 2000) to yield the dose equivalent behind the shield.

Avery *et al* (2008) used a different approach to combining Monte Carlo calculations with analytical methods. Rather than calculating H' and λ in equation (11.8) directly for a specific neutron producing target, they take existing dose equivalent transmission data (B_n in equation (11.4)) at mono energetic neutron energies and as a function of concrete thickness from NCRP Report 144 (NCRP 2003) and weight this with a Monte Carlo calculated neutron spectrum for a specific neutron source. This yields a term $\Sigma_E \Phi N_p \times B_n$, which is equivalent to the term $H'(E, \theta) \times e^{-d/\lambda(E,\theta)}$ in equation (11.8) and can be parameterized in terms of H' and λ. They considered several neutron sources: protons incident on stopping targets of Fe, Ni, Ta and water at energies of 100, 175 and 250 MeV, and evaluated neutron spectra in angular bins centred at 0°, 90° and 180° relative to the incident proton beam. Spectra from non-stopping carbon targets for 250 MeV protons incident on the target with emergent energies of 175 MeV and 100 MeV at angles of at 0°, 90° and 180° were also evaluated. These data were used to estimate shielding requirements around the energy degrader used in a cyclotron based proton therapy facility.

These data can be used to estimate shielding requirements although there are considerable discrepancies in dose equivalent rates estimated using these different data sets. Comparing data for protons incident on a thick iron target the data of Agosteo *et al* (2007) and Sheu *et al* (2013) agree within a factor of three for all energies and angles, with the Sheu *et al* data generally giving the higher values. The Avery *et al* (2008) data give a similar level of agreement across all energies in the forward direction (0°) but at 90° these data give dose equivalent rate estimates that are up to seven times greater and at the backward angle (180°) these discrepancies are even greater by a factor of up to nearly 100 in the worst case. The discrepancy in the large angle calculations is due to the fact that the spectra calculated by Avery *et al* (2008) using the Geant4 Monte Carlo code yield considerably higher neutron fluences than are calculated by others using the MNCPX code. Although this level of agreement may seem alarming it may not be significant in practice since in a proton therapy centre it is hard to imagine a situation in which the shielding will be dependent on a neutron source at 180°. In fact, in many situations there are multiple neutron source directions which contribute to the dose equivalent at the point of interest (e.g. a gantry treatment room or around the cyclotron) and the shielding requirements are often driven somewhat by the maximum IDR which is of course highest at the forward angle. Other uncertainties in workloads, use factors, occupancy factors and beam intensities may be of similar magnitude or even greater, as discussed in section 11.5.

A comparison of measurements of the instantaneous dose equivalent rate made around the University of Pennsylvania's shielded rooms with the calculations using the method of Avery *et al* (2008) for the facility for some worst case scenario situations are presented in table 11.3. The data show that these measurements agree within factors of 0.3–7 with the calculations, with both over- and under-estimates occurring, which suggests the measurements would agree well with calculations of Agosteo *et al* (2007) and Sheu *et al* (2013). The observed large variation probably arises from simplifications to the modelling of the installed equipment and self-shielding elements of the design, which can vary considerably with gantry angle, rather than from deficiencies in the basic shielding calculation approach. It is important to note that the measurements made at the University of Pennsylvania were made with a pristine Bragg peak at 230 MeV and 6 nA of beam delivered to the treatment nozzle; in practice the beam is energy modulated and for PBS operates at a current an order of magnitude less (typically ~0.25 nA). Other systems, however, may still operate at the higher beam currents in PBS mode (5 nA) and there may be the ability to operate at higher dose rates in the future.

11.9 Monte Carlo calculation methods

Several authors have made full Monte Carlo calculations which model the architectural layout and the neutron sources in greater detail, although rarely are these sources modelled in complete detail. In particular, modelling allows penetrations through the shielding (which are many and complex for proton beam facilities, see figure 11.8) to be included and the designer to use the proton beam interactions to generate the secondary radiation fields (rather than making assumptions about these). The output

Table 11.3. A comparison dose equivalent rates measured around the University of Pennsylvania's proton therapy facility with calculations for worst case scenario situations, i.e. highest energy pristine Bragg peak and least favourable gantry angle.

Location	Calculation details			Total equivalent dose rate (μSv h^{-1})		Ratio calculated to measured
	Energy MeV	Scattering angle	Target material	Calculated	Measured	
Treatment control room	250	0°	H_2O	12.1	23	0.5
Floor above treatment room	250	0°	H_2O	6.9	5.3	1.3
Corridor outside treatment room	250	90°	H_2O	1.4	1.7	0.8
In adjacent treatment room	250	0°	H_2O	51	7.4	7[a]
In corridor adjacent to cyclotron and ESS	250 reduced to 100 in degrader	90°	C	7.1	1.4	5.1

[a] Self-shielding of gantry components (e.g. counterweight) not included in calculation.

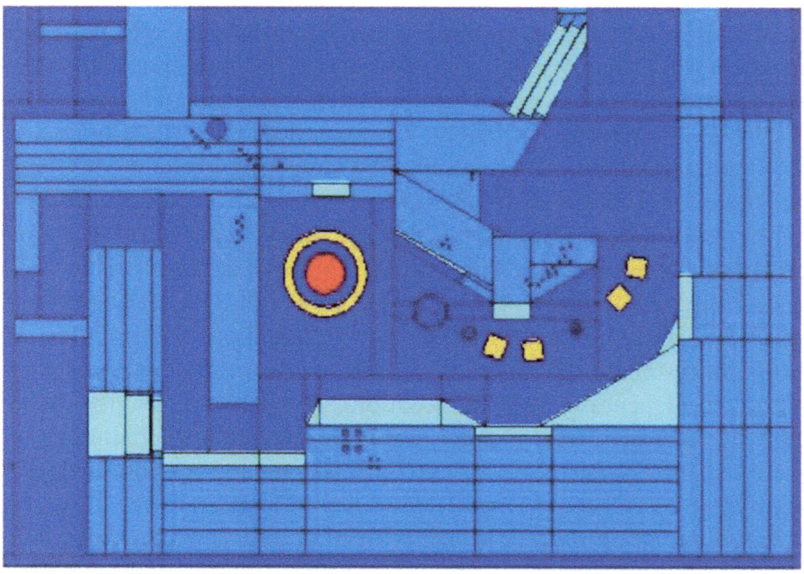

Figure 11.8. Plan view of a cyclotron accelerator hall for a proton beam facility showing the main beam line components, penetrations and temporary blockwork. (Courtesy of Aurora Health Physics Services Limited, UK.)

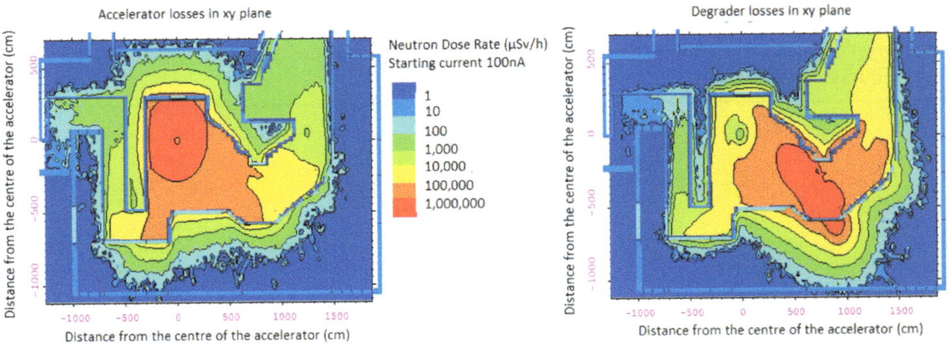

Figure 11.9. Dose rate plots through the plane shown in figure 11.8 for two different radiation sources in the accelerator vault for a nominal starting current. (Courtesy of Aurora Health Physics Services Limited, UK.)

from Monte Carlo simulations can also provide more information than empirical methods; dose or dose rate plots can be generated at planes of interest through the facility (see figure 11.9) and neutron energy spectrum information can be obtained to allow appropriate measurements to be made. However, Monte Carlo methods require expert attention both for the design of the model and interpretation of the results. It is not possible to create an absolutely true to life model for complex facilities (and for lower energy facilities such as linear accelerators, including internal room structures such as wall cladding can significantly affect neutron dose rates). Care should also be taken when comparing Monte Carlo predictions with measured doses. For example, small differences in the density of the materials used to construct the facility compared to that assumed in the model can make a significant difference in the expected dose rate. Designers will generally apply the most conservative assumptions when creating the model to ensure the relevant design parameters are met. The nature of the data generated by specific facility modelling, however, does not generally lend itself to be applied to other facilities. As a result, few data are available in the literature. However, there are a number of papers which compare the Monte Carlo modelling results with observed dose rates. For example, De Smet *et al* (2014) have published a paper comparing extensive Monte Carlo calculations with measurements made with an extended response neutron rem counter (WENDI-2, ThermoFisher Scientific, Waltham, MA, USA) (Olsher 2000). For calculations outside the shield the calculations overestimate the observed dose equivalent rates by a factor of between two and seven depending on the location. Available codes for Monte Carlo calculations include MCNPX, Geant4 and FLUKA (see also chapter 6).

The Monte Carlo N-Particle code (MCNP) is a general purpose code for neutron, photon and electron transport. The code, written in Fortran90 and C, is employed in many areas of radiation detection and protection and is a particular favourite for radiation shielding calculations in the nuclear energy industry. In MCNP, thermal neutrons are described by two models $S(\alpha,\beta)$ and free gas. Using evaluated cross-section data files, all of the associated reactions for neutrons above thermal energies are accounted for. MCNP uses continuous-energy nuclear and atomic data libraries with the primary sources stemming from the Evaluated Nuclear Data File (ENDF;

McLane *et al* 1995), the Advanced Computational Technology Initiative (ACTI; Frankle and Little Computational Technology Initiative 1996), the Evaluated Nuclear Data Library (ENDL; Halbleib *et al* 1992), the Evaluated Photon Data Library (EPDL; Adams 2000) and the Activation Library (ACTL; Koppel and Houston 1978) compilations from Livermore. The variance reduction capabilities of MCNP makes it highly suitable for shielding calculations; however, its inability (up to version 5) to transport protons has meant its use as a radiation shielding and protection tool for proton therapy facilities has been limited. This was solved with the release of MCNPX in 2011 which included all of the features of MCNP4C3 along with the ability to transport protons. The latest incarnation, MCNP6, is a merger of MCNP5 and MCNPX with some additional features, such as the explicit tracking of all charged particles in magnetic fields and complete photon-induced atomic relaxation. MCNP is validated by its development team over a wide range of energies and applications.

Geant4 (Agostinelli *et al* 2003) is an open-source Monte Carlo framework written in C++. It was originally developed for high energy physics but has found many applications in the areas of space science, nuclear energy and medical physics. Geant4 is only a framework and the user must create their own application specifying the necessary physics processes and creating the required geometry. The physics processes offered within the framework are fairly comprehensive covering an energy range spanning from eV to TeV and include electromagnetic, hadronic and optical processes. For most processes a range of models, both theoretical and data driven, can be implemented giving the user complete control to tailor and optimize the physics for a particular application. The modular open-source nature of the framework, however, allows users to create their own physics processes and implement their own models. This flexibility, however, could lead to a high level of risk for non-experts. A number of nuclear cascade models are available (e.g. Bertini, binary ion and intranuclear) to simulate proton–nuclear reactions which are of great importance for proton therapy centre investigations. A full range of particles are available along with the processes to propagate them through complex geometries incorporating electromagnetic fields. A number of event biasing options are available, including adjoint Monte Carlo, making Geant4 highly suitable for radiation shielding calculations. Geant4 is a result of a worldwide collaboration of physicists and software engineers. The physics processes incorporated into Geant4 are extensively validated by the collaboration and the user community.

FLUKA (Fasso *et al* 2001, Ferrari *et al* 2001) is a freely available general purpose tool for calculations of particle transport and interactions with matter. FLUKA can simulate the interaction and propagation of around 60 different particles, including protons, photons and electrons from 1 keV to thousands of TeV, neutrinos, muons of any energy, and hadrons of energies up to 20 TeV. Like Geant4, FLUKA can handle very complex geometries, using an improved version of the well-known Combinatorial Geometry (CG) package. The FLUKA package provides a large number of options to the user, including biasing, and the code utilizes microscopic models for particle transport whenever possible. FLUKA is well suited for proton centre studies as it allows easy determination of activation products as well as IDRs. FLUKA is validated by the development team with contributions from the user community.

It is prudent to remember that the calculation of IDR is only a part of the shielding assessment and whichever method is used, analytical or Monte Carlo, there are always assumptions and simplifications that are involved. The uncertainties involved in both methods may be outweighed by other factors such as workload, use factors and occupancy factors in the long term (i.e. the 30–40 year life time of the facility), and both methods are equally prone to error assumptions. Monte Carlo calculations may offer advantages in certain circumstances. They are time consuming and a significant expense, but may prove cost effective if concrete pour volumes are sufficiently reduced or if building designs are very complex. Analytical calculations when used in a spreadsheet format may offer quick assessments in preliminary studies which can help to consolidate the design before more detailed Monte Carlo calculations are made. Of course analytical calculations are always improved by including Monte Carlo elements, such as neutron spectrum calculations, and such approaches have often proven adequate in the past. Analytical methods can also be complementary to Monte Carlo calculations, as they are a good method of cross-checking the assumptions made in both evaluations.

11.10 Mazes and ducts

There are two general rules for the design of mazes and ducts to provide adequate radiation attenuation along a penetration (Fasso *et al* 2001). These rules are

1. 'Never place any penetration so that a primary particle or photon beam can point directly towards it or so that it allows an unshielded path for secondary radiations or particles from a significant beam interaction point.'
2. 'For any adequate labyrinth, the sum of the shield-wall thickness between the source of radiation and the exit point of the penetration should be at least equivalent to that which would be required if the labyrinth were not present.'

If these rules are followed the radiation fluence at the entrance to the maze or duct on the source side is only scattered radiation and in the case of a particle therapy facility this radiation is scattered neutrons.

Two types of wall penetrations must be considered in a proton facility, these are:

1. Entrance mazes to the treatment rooms, the cyclotron and ESS area, the research room and in the beam transport room.
2. A series of small conduits for cables, water pipes, etc.

11.10.1 Mazes

The maze calculations are the most critical since the ratio of the cross-sectional area of the penetration to its length determines the dose transmission, and this ratio is generally much larger for a maze than small conduit penetrations. Optimizing the cross-sectional area of the maze is important as easy access of patients on a stretcher, for in-patients or in emergency situations, is critical and may limit the ability to 'minimize' this parameter.

Penetrations and mazes are designed in several sections (or 'legs') which run generally at right angles. Transmission through the first leg is the greatest with transmission through subsequent legs becoming progressively less. Mazes in particle therapy centres are generally designed with between three to five legs. Maze calculations may be made using either analytical or Monte Carlo techniques or a combination of the two (Maerker and Muckenthaler 1967, Maerker *et al* 1968). Tesch (1982) studied the attenuation of neutron dose equivalent in concrete mazes using ^{252}Cf and ^{241}Am–Be neutron sources and rem counters. He derived an empirical formula describing the neutron dose equivalent at the exit of a leg maze and multi-leg mazes and compared the results with data from an electron synchrotron, a proton accelerator and a nuclear reactor.

Tesch's equation can be rewritten in terms of neutron dose equivalent transmission through each leg of the maze and offers a relatively simple method for assessing dose equivalent at the maze exit. The transmission through the first leg of the maze (T_1) is given by

$$T_1 = \frac{H(r_1)}{H_0} = 2 \times \left(\frac{r_0}{r_1}\right)^2. \qquad (11.11)$$

This an inverse square term with a factor of two allowance for scattering. The transmission through the *i*th leg of the maze (T_i), where $i > 1$ is given by

$$T_1 = \frac{H(r_1)}{H_{0i}} = \frac{\exp\left(\frac{-r_i}{0.45}\right) + 0.022.\ A_i^{1.3} \exp\left(\frac{-r_i}{2.35}\right)}{1 + 0.022.\ A_i^{1.3}}, \qquad (11.12)$$

where:

H_0 is the dose equivalent at the entrance to the first leg of the maze,

$H(r_1)$ is the dose equivalent at the exit to the first leg of the maze,

H_{0i} is the dose equivalent at the entrance to the *i*th leg of the maze,

$H(r_i)$ is the dose equivalent at the exit to the *i*th leg of the maze,

r_0 is the distance from the source to the entrance of the first leg of the maze on the source side in metres,

r_1 is the distance in to the first leg of the maze measured along the maze centre line in metres,

r_i is the centre line length of the *i*th leg of the maze in metres, and

A_i is the cross-sectional area of the *i*th leg of the maze in m^2; the product of the maze width (w_i) and height (h_i) in the *i*th leg.

A graphical description of the geometrical parameters used in equation (11.12) is given figure 11.10.

The total transmission through the maze is given by

$$T_{\text{Total}} = \prod_{i=1}^{n} T_i \qquad (11.13)$$

and the total dose equivalent at the exit to the maze is

$$H_{\text{Total}} = T_{\text{Total}} \times H_0. \qquad (11.14)$$

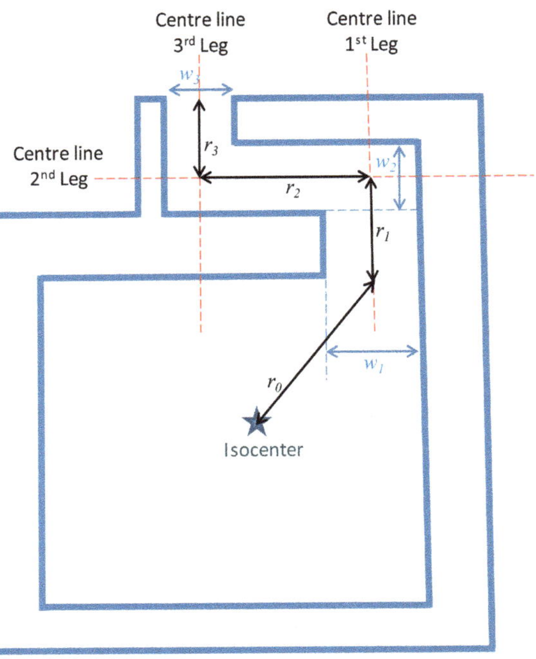

Figure 11.10. Schematic showing the distances and widths required for maze calculations using equation (11.12). The heights of the maze in each leg are h_1, h_2 and h_3 with corresponding widths of w_1, w_2 and w_3, respectively, then the cross-sectional area of the maze in each leg is $A_i = h_i \times w_i$.

This total dose equivalent, H_0, may be determined using analytical methods employing equations such as (11.8) and (11.10).

Using this methodology at the University of Pennsylvania, the calculated IDR at the entrance to a gantry treatment room for a 250 MeV beam and 6 nA beam delivered to the room was 10.6 μSv h^{-1}; this includes both the dose through the shielding wall and the maze leakage. The maximum measured value under similar conditions was 50 μSv h^{-1}, with a significant variation in the dose measured across the maze entrance from left to right. Tesch (1982) recommends that these equations be used for mazes of cross-sectional area ~2 m^2; the University of Pennsylvania mazes have a cross-sectional area of ~6 m^2, suggesting a possible source of this discrepancy.

11.10.2 Ducts

Large ducts (e.g. heating, ventilation and air conditioning (HVAC) ducts) leading into the treatment rooms and accelerator and beam transport rooms may be incorporated into the entrance mazes to these areas for convenience. There are a number of small ducts that must pass through the shielding (e.g. from treatment room to beam transport room, from treatment room to treatment control area, from cyclotron/ESS room to power supply room, etc). These ducts are mainly electrical conduits with diameters of ~6 or 10 cm or water pipes with diameters of 2.5 cm. Electrical and water ducts are usually partially filled with material, water or electrical cables. The lengths of the conduit and pipe runs in the walls are such that the ratio of the run length to the square root of the cross-sectional area of the ducts is very large (25–200) and, thus, transmission factors are very low (10^{-5} or lower). Leakage through these small ducts is well below the lowest leakages calculated for any of the mazes and is, therefore, negligible for a single duct. The main concern is the placement of the conduits in the shielding walls and how the voids that their volumes create reduce the effective thicknesses of the walls. Although the maximum diameter of any duct running between critical locations where personnel may be working is only 6 cm, there are some areas where a relatively large number of conduits pass through the wall in close proximity; there may be areas where groups of between 10 and 20 are involved. To facilitate ease of cable pulling, electrical conduits should not include right angle bends on the legs; 45° bends are preferable. Occasionally, penetrations without bends may be necessary, for example if RF transmission lines must pass through a wall bends may be undesirable because of the power losses involved. In such cases the duct should not pass perpendicularly through the wall but be angled at 45°–60° and in such a manner that the maximum acute angle defined by the source and the duct entry and exit points is used. In these areas the following guidelines in addition to those given above may be applied:

1. When there are multiple conduits or groups of conduits passing through a wall in close proximity, separate the conduits by four diameters between their centres, and position the conduit runs running parallel with the sides of the wall and as close to the centre of the wall as possible.
2. When running groups of conduits through a wall, do not arrange them in more than two rows.
3. In drawing a line across a shielding wall at less than 20° off the perpendicular, you should never be able to pass through more than two 6 cm conduits.
4. Do not place conduits in maze walls opposite the maze entry or exit.

If these guidelines are followed, the effect of groups of 6 cm diameter conduits should be to reduce the effective wall thickness by approximately 3 cm (or the radius of the pipe). Such a reduction has a minimal and practically negligible effect on the dose equivalent transmission.

11.11 Room interlocks and monitoring

Once the shield has been designed another important aspect of the radiation safety in the facility is the interlock system. Typically, the system should be of the classic search and evict (last person out) design. Some unique issues may arise with a particle therapy system compared to a conventional system due to its size. Generally the accelerator and, in the case of a cyclotron, the ESS, are housed in a separate area from the treatment room. Even in a 'one room' system there may be multiple areas within the one room. This is also true for the treatment room particularly the gantry rooms where there may be upper and lower levels which may be closed off creating separate areas. Each area must include its own search and evict system. A search button must be activated before the exit door from the area is secured with search buttons being placed so that every area can be seen from at least one button position. On activating the search button a visual warning (flashing light) and possibly an audible warning (depending upon manufacturer) should be initiated and the door must be secured in a preset time, typically 15–30 s, depending on the size of the room and the ease of exit. Depending on local regulations, audible warnings may be omitted in treatment rooms to avoid distressing the patient. In some systems shielding walls are used within a single area to provide protection for sensitive electronics housed there. In this case multiple sequential search buttons may be required to ensure that personnel perform all appropriate timing requirements and adequate search before securing the area.

The radiation room interlock system is generally an integral part of the vendor supplied system, but the system should be carefully reviewed by the purchaser to ensure that it complies with local regulations. The vendor typically decides which machine functions should be controlled by the interlocks. Generally in a multi-room system room interlocks will control bending magnet power supplies that allow the beam to be deflected into that room and beam stops which block beam access to the room in the beam transport rooms.

Any safety system will also include emergency stop or crash buttons throughout the facility. Careful consideration should be given to which system functions the crash buttons control, local regulations as always require compliance, and a full system power shut-down may require a significant time for a restart (1–2 h). Accelerator functions that can be easily controlled are the ion source, the RF power and the beam extraction system.

An option within radiation areas in the UK (which is a requirement in the USA) is some form of independent radiation detector which will give an audible and visual alarm when radiation is present in the area. Whilst the audible alarm is often omitted in patient areas for the patient's comfort, it is usual to have a significant siren in any technical area at least when the interlock for the area is being set. The visual warning signals produced must be sufficient to ensure that they can be easily viewed from anywhere within the area. Many manufacturers recommend that these monitors be neutron monitors. However this may not be necessary in a particle therapy facility, because whenever neutrons are produced a prompt gamma ray dose always accompanies them. Gamma ray production is significant around the accelerator and an ESS, but in the treatment room neutron and gamma ray production are less and careful location of the detectors may be necessary. Monte Carlo calculations may be used to verify the feasibility of the system. Gamma ray monitors are considerable less expensive than neutron monitors by a factor of approximately five. Another way of reducing these costs is to install gamma monitors that allow for remote read-outs, so that the remote units are used to provide adequate monitoring of an area. For example, in the treatment area of a gantry room the main monitor is installed in the treatment room itself, but a remote unit is installed in the maze close to the entrance door to prevent personnel entering the room if the beam remains on in case of a door interlock failure. Of course, the chance of multiple failures is remote but the essence of a robust safety system is multiple redundancies. Another advantage of using gamma ray rather than neutron detectors is that many of the master units give a digital indication of the residual radiation dose. A potential problem with this is that it may include the effects of detector activation, but the extent of this maybe estimated using a portable radiation monitor for comparison.

11.12 Radiation hazards resulting from activation

Well-designed shielding should provide adequate protection from radiation leakage through the shielding for personnel working around the facility. Another potential source of radiation exposure in a particle therapy facility originates from radio-isotopes, which may be produced by the particle beam striking materials in the beam's path. In the treatment room this radiation derives mainly from induced activity in the treatment nozzle and is generally not produced at hazardous levels.

11.12.1 Solid material activation

There are a large number of isotopes that may be produced from a wide variety of reaction channels, which including reactions such as X(p, n), X(p, 2n), X(p, 4n), X(p, t), X(p, nd), X(p,α tn) to list just a few of the many possibilities. Just which reactions occur and which predominate depends on the energy thresholds for the reactions, the variation of the reaction cross-sections with energy and the energy of the proton beam, which of course slows down as it penetrates the material. Data on proton interactions with specific target nuclei or materials can be found in the nuclear physics literature in the form of excitation functions (i.e. plots of the reaction cross-section as a function of incident proton energy), the half-lives of the product nuclei and their decay modes, including the energies of emitted γ-rays and β-rays. Such data can be useful in assessing the potential hazard from the induced isotope, but direct measurement of the activation from an irradiated material in a practical situation may be more useful. Unfortunately few data of this type are currently published in the literature. Walker *et al* (2014) have published some information on the isotopes produced after bombarding a brass aperture. The brass studied contained 61.5% Cu, 35.4% Zn, 3.1% Pb and 0.35% Fe. The emphasis of this paper is on how long brass apertures need to be stored before disposal. Their data show that 1 day after irradiation the predominant isotope is ^{64}Cu with a half-life of 12.7 h.

In a proton therapy facility target materials that may be of concern are copper (dees and deflector) and iron or steel (magnet pole pieces) in the cyclotron; carbon, hydrogen and oxygen are present in most common plastics or wax used for constructing compensators, and plastics may also be used in modulator wheels and ridge filters. Copper, zinc and lead are present in brass apertures, whilst cadmium, bismuth and lead are present in Lippowitz metal apertures. Finally there is beryllium and carbon (graphite) present in the energy degrader and tantalum present in beam defining collimators. Many of the isotopes produced are short-lived and decay rapidly presenting no long term hazard. Others have very long half-lives and will build up slowly during the lifetime of the facility. The exact quantity of the isotope produced depends on several factors, (i) the cross-section for the particular nuclear reaction producing it, (ii) the variation of that cross-section with energy (known as the excitation function for the reaction) and (iii) the intensity of the proton beam striking the target and its duration. Data on excitation functions for some of the more important reaction channels may be found in the nuclear physics literature (Shahid *et al* 2015, Matsushita *et al* 2016).

In and around the ESS of a cyclotron there may be a very high neutron flux, especially around the degrader when the lower energies are accelerated, therefore excitation functions for neutron induced nuclear reactions may also be significant. Interactions with plastics in beam shaping components and graphite in the degrader itself produce mainly ^{11}C, which has a relatively short half-life of 20 min and presents no long term hazard, decaying to negligible levels in a matter of hours. If a beryllium degrader is used this is more problematical since ^{7}Be may be produced with its half-life of 53 days.

A selection of some of the more important reaction channels and the isotopes produced are listed in table 11.4, together with the half-lives of the products, the target nuclei, their threshold energies, the decay modes and γ-ray energies produced. The table is not intended to be comprehensive but is included to illustrate the complexity of the activation process.

11.12.2 Water and air activation

The chilled water used to cool the accelerator and ancillary equipment is provided by a closed circuit chiller system. This can be a potential problem particularly with a cyclotron when extracting high currents at high duty cycles (i.e. in multi-room facilities, during acceptance, commissioning or extended QA). The water in this system becomes activated with ^{15}O, which emits gamma rays of energy 511 keV, resulting from positron annihilation and has a half-life of 2 min. The storage tank, which is part of this chiller circuit, can be a significant source of x-ray radiation. Depending on the location of the chiller room within the facility it may be necessary to provide shielding of walls and doors; a few millimetres of lead or a few centimetres of concrete should be sufficient.

Water in phantoms may also become active. But the accumulated activity is small since therapeutic dose rates are used, the duty cycles are not high and the half-life of ^{15}O is only 2 min. Therefore, any risk is marginal and can be easily mitigated by a 10 min wait.

Some relevant information on the neutron activation of air is available in the literature on neutron therapy facilities. Ten Haken *et al* (1983) identified the main isotopes produced as ^{11}C ($\lambda_{½}$ = 20 min), ^{13}N ($\lambda_{½}$ = 9.9 min), ^{15}O ($\lambda_{½}$ = 2 min), ^{39}Cl ($\lambda_{½}$ = 56 min), ^{41}Ar ($\lambda_{½}$ = 1.8 h) and ^{16}N ($\lambda_{½}$ = 7 s). They recommended that the HVAC system in irradiated areas be vented to the exterior and investigated the optimum number of room air changes per hour. An additional precaution is to vent through a stack at the highest level in the building. The stack should be modelled to ensure that the stack height is sufficient to adequately disperse the plume of radioactive air. Stack monitoring may also be required depending on local

Table 11.4. List of some more important isotopes produced through proton interactions with materials in a proton therapy facility.

Nuclide produced	Half-life	Target	Natural occurrence (%)	Decay-mode	Energy of emitted γ (keV)	Contributing reaction	Reaction threshold (MeV)	Ref.
^{64}Cu	12.70 h	^{65}Cu	30.83	EC(43.9)	1345.8	^{65}Cu(p,d)	7.805	a
				β^+ (17.6)		^{65}Cu(p,np)	10.064	
				β^- (38.5)				
^{58}Co	70.86 d	^{63}Cu	69.17	EC(85.1)	810.76	^{63}Cu(p,αd)	14.22	a
				β^+ (14.9)	863.95	^{63}Cu(p,αnp)	16.488	
						^{63}Cu(p,t^{3}He)	28.778	
						^{63}Cu(p,pdt)	34.359	
						^{65}Cu(p,αtn)	25.970	
						^{65}Cu(p,αd2n)	32.325	
						^{65}Cu(p,αp3n)	34.584	
^{60}Co	1925 d	^{63}Cu	69.17	B$^-$ (100)	1173	^{63}Cu(p,p^{3}He)	19.162	a
		^{65}Cu	30.83		1332	^{63}Cu(p,2pd)	24.744	
						^{63}Cu(p,n3p)	27.004	
						^{65}Cu(p,αd)	14.100	
						^{65}Cu(p,αpn)	16.359	
						^{65}Cu(p,t^{3}He)	28.643	
						^{65}Cu(p,pdt)	34.222	
						^{65}Cu(p,nd^{3}He)	34.997	
^{62}Zn	9.19 h	^{63}Cu	69.17	EC(91.8)	548.4	^{63}Cu(p,2n)	13.477	a
		^{65}Cu	30.83	β^+ (8.2)	596.6	^{65}Cu(p,4n)	31.574	
^{11}C	20.2 m	^{12}C	98.9	β^+	511	^{12}C(p,pn)		b
^{10}C	19.3 s	^{12}C	98.9	β^+	718.3	^{12}C(p,p2n)		b
^{7}Be	53.28 d	^{9}Be	100	EC	477.8	^{9}Be(p,p2n)		

[a] Shahid *et al* (2015).
[b] Matsushita *et al* (2016).

regulations and environmental conditions. Methods for estimating isotope production resulting from air activation and methods for monitoring this activation may be found in NCRP Report 144 (NCRP 2003).

11.12.3 Risks from activation

The most significant risk for radiographers (radiation therapy technologists) would be with a nozzle delivering passively scattered beams. In such a nozzle the radiographer is required to handle active components when removing and installing the patient specific brass shaping aperture, wax or acrylic compensator, and in some systems the acrylic modulator wheel or ridge filter. However, in spite of this there has been no report in the literature of radiographer in a particle therapy centre receiving a dose above the locally established as low as reasonably achievable (ALARA) limit. At the University of Pennsylvania where a tungsten MLC is used in place of a brass aperture, our experience has been that no radiographer has received a monitor badge reading above the minimal detectable limit (100 μSv) over a three month period. Whilst the MLC negates the need to handle the activated brass apertures, the radiographers must still insert the plastic compensators for each field. The experience is similar for physicians and medical physicists. The physicist staff making QA measurements are handling plastic phantoms and often working with beams at higher duty cycles than are encountered in routine clinical operations.

The situation for the engineering staff servicing and maintaining the accelerator, however, is significantly different. This is particularly the case for cyclotron or synchrocyclotron based systems which use ESSs. The engineers servicing the accelerator regularly have to work in a radioactive environment and the activation levels inside a cyclotron and around the ESS associated with a cyclotron system may be considerable. Of course these hazards are from gamma and beta emitters, and careful photon/beta dose monitoring and component handling are of utmost importance in these cases to ensure that maintenance personnel are not exposed to radiation hazards. It is common practice to allow a 'cooling off' period if maintenance or repair requires that a cyclotron magnet be opened to allow access to the accelerating and extraction components. As many of the most prolific produced isotopes have half-lives up to 10–15 h an overnight delay is advisable. A radiation survey upon entry to the cyclotron vault can provide valuable information on which areas to avoid, and on the dose rate from components that are required to be handled. Such survey information can be valuable for use in assessing the risks associated with major maintenance work, and equipment suppliers may be able to provide this information in the operational planning stages to aid prior risk assessment. In cyclotrons components that may be sources of significant activation are the dee system, the extraction system (deflector) and the pole pieces of the magnet; these are particular problematic since the beam is at full energy (230–250 MeV) at this point. In addition, contamination control procedures may be required for work within the cyclotron and hence staff may require to wear appropriate protective equipment. The ESS, in particular the degrader component, is another potential source of significant activation. For this reason it is common to include some local shielding in this area often in the form of a portable lead shield 2.5–5.0 cm thick. Extraction systems in synchrotrons may also be a source of significant activation, although at a lower level than in cyclotrons for the reasons explained in section 11.2.

11.12.4 Radioactive solid waste

Typically, large amounts of radioactive waste are not produced from the operation of the accelerator and beam line components. In a passive scattering system using metallic apertures it may be necessary to retain the used apertures for a period of time to allow for decay of the radioactive isotopes. The required storage space clearly depends on the daily patient throughput. In large multi-room facilities it may be possible to store radioactive components in a locally shielded area within the lower level of a gantry room. Typically, brass apertures should be held in storage for a minimum of four months before disposal (Walker *et al* 2014).

If a vendor is supplying maintenance support for the facility it may be negotiated in this agreement that the vendor is responsible for storage and disposal of all radioactive waste in compliance with local regulations. Such an agreement could include disposal of waste generated from patient specific modifying devices, such as apertures and compensators, in addition to items associated with the accelerator and beam lines. In addition, a suitably sized and controlled hot store should be planned somewhere in the facility for decay storage of activated items including service consumable such as fluorescent light tubes. A workshop may also be required for handling and working on activated parts, for which careful consideration of the control of activated parts and the possibility of contamination is required. Also, a filtered exhaust air system may be advisable and installation of some form of HEPA filtered work cabinet may be considered.

11.13 Measuring and monitoring techniques and instrumentation

An important part of shielding design is the confirmation of the shield performance after completion of the building and equipment installation. To fully determine the dose equivalents around the shield it is necessary to make measurements of both the photon and neutron dose equivalents. Photon dose equivalent rates are best measured with ion chamber survey meters of which there are many available. Neutron monitoring is more problematic. Bonner sphere type survey instruments have been widely used for this purpose. The basic structure is a gas counter, commonly filled with boron loaded He or BF_3 to detect thermal neutrons, surrounded by a large (~30 cm diameter) polyethylene sphere which thermalises the incident fast neutrons before they reach the gas detector, which has a relatively high efficiency for thermal neutron detection. However, the energy response of these detectors falls off rapidly at energies above 10 MeV. This problem has been overcome by including a heavy metal shield in the polyethylene moderator to provide additional slowing of the fast neutrons and this extends the useful range in to the GeV region. The WENDI-2 detector mentioned above is of this type. The only drawback of these detectors is that they are large and heavy and, therefore, unwieldy in use. Another option for a survey meter is a device based on recoil proton detection; the PRESCILA detector (Olsher *et al* 2004) uses an array of ZnS(Ag) scintillators coupled to a side view bi-alkali photomultiplier tube. This device is much smaller and lighter than the WENDI-2, but its upper energy response is limited to ~100 MeV. This energy response is sufficient for most proton facilities where the maximum beam energy is limited to 250 MeV, but neutron production above 100 MeV may be substantial in facilities accelerating heavier ions to typical energies of 400 MeV per nucleon. Energy calibration of these devices is also a problem since calibration must be performed at lower energies and in practice an ^{241}Am–Be or a ^{252}Cf source producing neutrons with a mean energy of only ~4 MeV is often used for calibration. The sensitivity of the WENDI detector is ~0.84 cps μSv^{-1} h^{-1} measured with a ^{252}Cf source compared to the PRESCILA detector sensitivity of ~0.58 cps μSv^{-1} h^{-1} measured with an ^{241}Am–Be source. However, at the time of writing these devices are the best available options for portable neutron dose equivalent survey meters which give instantaneous readings. A conventional Bonner sphere has a maximum neutron energy response of 12–15 MeV and a sensitivity of only 0.05 cps μSv^{-1} h^{-1} measured with an ^{241}Am–Be source.

Another important aspect of radiation monitoring is the personal protection of individuals working in the facility, which is generally achieved by issuing 'film' badges to those considered to be occupationally at risk. For monitoring photon doses conventional film, thermoluminescent dosimeters (TLD) and optically stimulated luminescent dosimeters (OSLD) are widely used materials in these badges, for which the minimum level of detection is in the range 10–100 μSv depending on the radiation quality. For monitoring neutrons only, CR39 track etch detectors are widely used. Versions of the CR39 are available to detect a range of thermal, intermediate and fast neutrons across the 0.25 eV–40 MeV energy range, with a dose measurement range from 200 μSv to 250 mSv. Typically badges are worn for a 1–3 month period. Another possibility for the engineering personnel who may be expected to receive significant badge readings during certain maintenance procedures, such as internal cyclotron maintenance, is to issue electronic gamma ray monitors which provide an instantaneous readout which can be continually monitored during the working shift. Some of these electronic devices may also allow instantaneous dose rate and total accumulated dose alarm level to be set. Film badges may also be used for environmental area monitoring outside the shield area.

11.14 Summary

The objective of this chapter has been to give a concise introductory overview of the basic principles underlying the design of the radiation shielding and radiation safety practices for a particle therapy centre, with particular emphasis on proton therapy. The importance of fully understanding and adhering to local safety regulations has been stressed. Shielding a particle therapy facility is primarily a neutron shielding problem. The neutrons are produced when the primary particle beam interacts with materials in its path and the major sources of neutron production in a particle therapy system have been outlined. Practical methods for calculating shielding requirements have been discussed including analytical methods, Monte Carlo calculations and combinations of these two techniques. Some guidance on radiation monitoring around the facility, the use of survey meters and personal monitoring, is also given. More detailed information on the shielding of particle therapy centres can be found in NCRP Report 144 (NCRP 2003) and the PTCOG Report 1 (PTCOG 2010). These references should be considered essential reading for anyone planning the radiation shielding for a particle therapy facility. In particular the PTCOG report contains a considerable amount of information on shielding heavy ion (e.g. ^{12}C) facilities.

Finally, each centre should perform a comprehensive radiation risk assessment of all work activities that involve radiation within the particle therapy facility to ensure that all reasonable steps are taken to minimise risk to staff, patients and the public. Such an assessment requires a review of radiation safety interlocks associated with the accelerator vault and the treatment rooms, radiation monitoring in these areas and personnel monitoring for staff working in the facility (radiographers, physicians, physicists and engineers). It also requires a review of potential radiation risks from activated materials within the facility and a plan for how to handle these materials.

References

ACoP 2000 *Work with Ionising Radiation: Approved Code of Practice and Practical Guidance on the Ionising Radiations Regulations 1999* L121 (London: The Stationery Office)

Adams K J 2000 Electron upgrade for MCNP4B *Los Alamos National Laboratory Internal Memorandum* X-5-RN(U)-00-14 wwwxdiv.lanl.gov/PROJECTS/DATA/nuclear/pdf/X-5-RN-00-14.pdf (Accessed: 11 November 2016)

Agostinelli S *et al* 2003 Geant4—a simulation toolkit *Nucl. Instrum. Methods Phys. Res.* A **506** 250–303

Agosteo S, Magistris M, Mereghetti A, Silari M and Zajacova Z 2007 Shielding data for 100–250 MeV proton accelerators: double differential neutron distributions and attenuation in concrete *Nucl. Instrum. Methods Phys. Res. B* **265** 581–98

Agosteo S, Magistris M, Mereghetti A, Silari M and Zajacova Z 2008 Shielding data for 100–250 MeV proton accelerators: attenuation of secondary radiation in thick iron and concrete/iron shields *Nucl. Instrum. Methods Phys. Res.* B **266** 3406–16

Alsmiller R G, Mynatt F R, Barish J and Engle W W 1969 Shielding against neutrons in the energy range 50 to 400 MeV *Nucl. Instrum. Methods* **72** 213–6

Avery S, Ainsley C, Maughan R and McDonough J 2008 Analytical shielding calculations for a proton therapy facility *Radiat. Prot. Dosim.* **131** 167–79

Briesmeister J F (ed) 2000 *MCNP: A General Monte Carlo N-Particle Transport Code LA-13709-M* (Los Alamos, NM: Los Alamos National Laboratory)

De Smet V *et al* 2014 Neutron H*(10) inside a proton therapy facility: comparison between Monte Carlo simulations and WENDI-2 measurements *Radiat. Prot. Dosim.* **161** 417–21

EC (European Commission) 2013 *Laying Down Basic Safety Standards for Protection Against the Dangers Arising from Exposure to Ionising Radiation* Council Directive 2013/59/Euratom (Brussels: European Commission)

Fasso A, Ferrari A, Ranft J and Sala P R 2001 FLUKA: status and prospective for hadronic *applications Electron-Photon Transport in FLUKA: Proceedings of the Monte Carlo 2000 Conference* ed A Kling *et al* (New York: Springer) pp 955–60

Ferrari A, Ranft J and Sala P R 2001 The FLUKA radiation code and its use for space problems *Phys. Med.* **17** 72–80 PMID: 11770541

Frankle S C and Little R C 1996 Cross-section and reaction nomenclature for MCNP continuous-energy libraries and DANTSYS multigroup libraries *Los Alamos National Laboratory Internal Memorandum* XTM:96-313 www-xdiv.lanl.gov/PROJECTS/DATA/nuclear/pdf/scf-96-313.pdf (Accessed 11 November 2016)

Halbleib J A, Kensek R P, Valdez G D, Mehlhorn T A, Seltzer S M and Berger M J 1992 ITS: the integrated TIGER series of coupled electron/photon Monte Carlo transport codes version 3.0. *IEEE Trans. Nucl. Sci.* **39** 1025–30

IAEA (International Atomic Energy Authority) 1988 *Radiological Safety Aspects of Proton Accelerators (Technical Report Series* No 283) (Vienna: IAEA)

IAEA (International Atomic Energy Authority) 2003 *Decommissioning of Small Medical, Industrial and Research Facilities* (*Technical Report Series* No 414) (Vienna: IAEA)

ICRP (International Commission on Radiological Protection) 1996 *Conversion Coefficients for use in Radiological Protection against External Radiation* Report 74. Ann ICRP 26: 3/4

ICRP (International Commission on Radiological Protection) 2007 *2007 Recommendations of the International Commission on Radiological Protection* Report 103. Ann ICRP 37: 2-4

IRR 1999 *The Ionising Radiations Regulations* SI 1999/3232 (London: The Stationery Office)

Koppel J U and Houston D H 1978 *Reference Manual for ENDF Thermal Neutron Scattering Data* General Atomics report GA-8774 (Revised and reissued as ENDF-269 by the National Nuclear Data Center at the Brookhaven National Laboratory) www.nndc.bnl.gov/ (Accessed: 11 November 2016)

Lai B-L, Sheu R-J and Lin U-T 2015 Shielding analysis of proton therapy accelerators: a demonstration using Monte Carlo generated source terms and attenuation lengths *Health Phys.* **108** S84–93

Maerker R E and Muckenthaler F J 1967 Neutron fluxes in concrete ducts arising from incident epicadmium neutrons: calculations and experiments *Nucl. Sci. Eng.* **30** 340

Maerker R E, Claiborne H C and Clifford C E 1968 *Neutron Attenuation in Rectangular Ducts (Engineering Compendium on Radiation Shielding)* ed R G Jaeger (New York: Springer)

Matsushita K, Nishio T, Tanaka S, Tsuneda M, Sugiura A and Ieki K 2016 Measurement of proton-induced target fragmentation cross sections in carbon *Nucl. Phys.* A **946** 104–16

McLane V, Dunford C L and Rose P F 1995 ENDF-102: data formats and procedures for the Evaluated Nuclear Data File ENDF-6 *Brookhaven National Laboratory report 35* (BNL-NCS-44945) www.nndc.bnl.gov/ (Accessed: 11 November 2016)

NCRP (National Council on Radiation Protection and Measurements) 1993 *Limitation of Exposure to Ionizing Radiation* Report 116 (Bethesda, MD: NCRP)

NCRP (National Council on Radiation Protection and Measurements) 2003 *Radiation Protection for Particle Accelerator Facilities* Report 144 (Bethesda, MD: NCRP)

Olsher R H 2000 An improved neutron rem meter *Health Phys.* **79** 170–81

Olsher R H *et al* 2004 PRESCILA: a new, lightweight neutron rem meter *Health Phys.* **86** 603–12

Pelliccioni M 2000 Overview of fluence-to-effective dose and fluence-to-ambient dose equivalent conversion coefficients for high energy radiation calculated using the FLUKA code *Radiat. Prot. Dosim.* **88** 279–97

PTCOG (Particle Therapy Co-Operative Group) 2010 *Shielding Design and Radiation Safety of Charged Particle Therapy Facilities* Report 1 http:/ptcog.web.psi.ch (Accessed: 11 November 2016)

Roussin R W and Schmidt F A R 1971 Adjoint Sn calculations of coupled neutron and gamma-ray transport through concrete slabs *Nucl. Eng. Des.* **15** 319–43

Roussin R W, Alsmiller R G and Barish J 1973 Calculations of the transport of neutrons and secondary gamma rays through concrete for incident neutrons in the energy range 15 to 75 MeV *Nucl. Eng. Des.* **24** 250–7

Shahid M, Kim K, Naik H, Zaman M, Yang S-C and Kim G 2015 Measurement of excitation functions in proton induced reactions on natural copper from their threshold to 43 MeV *Nucl. Instrum. Methods Phys. Res.* B **342** 305–13

Sheu R-J, Lai B-L, Lin U-T and Jiang S-H 2013 Source terms and attenuation lengths for estimating shielding requirements or dose analyses of proton therapy accelerators *Health Phys.* **105** 128–39

Ten Haken R, Awsschalom M and Rosenberg R 1983 Activation of the major constituents of tissue and air by a fast neutron radiation therapy beam *Med. Phys.* **10** 636–41

Tesch K 1982 The attenuation of the neutron dose equivalent in a labyrinth through an accelerator shield *Part. Accel.* **12** 169–75

Ulrici L and Magistis M 2009 Radioactive waste management and decommissioning of accelerator facilities *Radiat. Prot. Dosim.* **137** 138–48

Walker P K, Edwards A C, Das I J and Johnstone P A S 2014 Radiation safety considerations in proton aperture disposal *Health Phys.* **106** 523–7

Wyckoff J M and Chilton A B 1973 Dose due to practical neutron energy distributions incident on concrete shielding walls *Proc. of the Third International Congress of the International Radiation Protection Association* ed W S Snyder, W3A-105 www.irpa.net/irpa3/cdrom/VOL.3A/W3A_105.PDF (Accessed: 8 November 2016)

Chapter 12

Shielding verification and radiation surveys

D J Peet and J Reay

12.1 Introduction

As has been described previously, undertaking the calculations to provide the radiation shielding design is just one aspect of facility design. The shielding design provided by the radiation shielding designer(s) (often a Radiation Protection Adviser (RPA) or other radiation safety professionals and clinical staff) will have been converted into architectural and engineering drawings by the construction team. It is also possible (in fact, in the authors' experience, quite likely), that changes will be required to the design as it is developed for construction. This may include changes to key features that were previously agreed, for example the inclusion of lintels, changes to the key dimensions of access routes as a result of changes in clinical or equipment requirements, and changes to the clinical equipment or use of that equipment.

The radiation shielding designer(s) should work closely with the construction design team to ensure all changes that are made are assessed and approved by the shielding designer.

Once construction has begun, it is advisable to appoint someone, often a member of the construction team, to ensure all of the key assumptions and design parameter used in the shielding design remain true. This includes the actual density of the materials used, the dimensions of the shielding provided and an assessment of any deviations from the construction drawings.

In order to have confidence that the facility has been constructed in accordance with the agreed design, the shielding designer should undertake inspections of the facility throughout the construction period. This includes:

- during construction,
- before decoration,
- before installation of equipment and
- after any structural changes or any significant additions to service penetrations.

doi:10.1088/978-0-7503-1440-4ch12

In addition, the shielding design, as built, should be reviewed:

- if any changes are made to the equipment resulting in an increase in dose rate which might impact on the integrity of the shielding and
- after equipment replacement.

Radiation shielding review is an ongoing process and should also be undertaken:

- after installation of equipment and
- if unexpected doses are recorded on personal or environmental monitors.

However, this report is concerned with the design of facilities and will concentrate on those reviews, checks and measurements that are required before the facility is used clinically.

In addition, this chapter concentrates on photon and neutron measurements. Design checks and pre-use radiation surveys for proton facilities are covered in chapter 11.

12.2 During construction

During construction, the primary methods available for ensuring the facility is built in accordance with the design are visual assessment and review of construction quality assurance data. The primary aims at this stage are to assess the build quality against that specified, identify any obvious deviations from the design and any areas in which special consideration should be made once the clinical radiation source has been installed, e.g. voids around structural columns where blocks have been used.

The following items should be checked during construction:

- density of construction materials, e.g. test cube results,
- thickness of walls and slabs,
- position and thickness of primary barrier materials, e.g. steel sheets or high density concrete sections,
- width and height of the maze, particularly where lintels are key in the design,
- construction joints, particularly at corners and where blocks have been used,
- contractor's photographs, where available,
- position and in-filling of removed tie bolts,
- dosimetry cableway,
- air conditioning ducts,
- other service entries,
- layout of surrounding areas and
- lines of sight down the maze from the treatment room and from the maze entrance.

It is also important to ensure that any pre-installation work that is required, e.g. forming service channels, does not compromise the shielding. As a result, the following items should be checked visually before decoration:

- contractor's photographs, where available,
- ceiling arrangements without false ceiling,

- service duct entries,
- surface mounting of alignment lasers, or that the backing plate offers equivalent shielding if the lasers are recessed into the primary barrier,
- position of maze entrance barrier/light curtain and
- surface mounting of all other services or suspension from the ceiling without affecting the integrity of the shielding.

Careful records should be kept of all the information gathered and of any measurements made for future reference.

12.3 Post construction radiation survey—detailed shielding integrity testing

The most effective method of ensuring that a facility meets the design specification is to undertake a radiation survey of the dose rates outside that facility. In some instances, taking dose rate measurements down the maze can also be very informative.

In order to perform a radiation survey, it is necessary to use a radiation source which can penetrate the shielding provided. Due to the thickness of the primary barriers, it is normal practice for radiotherapy installations to carry out the first radiation survey once the equipment has been installed. However, there is some evidence to suggest that the construction of bunkers is not always as planned or specified, and that defects will be present in more than half of the facilities (Reay *et al* 2010). Discovering these defects after the clinical equipment has been installed can be very costly. In the worst case, where the defect cannot be addressed, restrictions may be placed on the clinical use of a facility. In addition, in some instances, there will be limited opportunity for rectifying any problems with bunker construction or the level of shielding provided once the clinical equipment has been installed, e.g. where the space is very limited or the facility is being handed over to the user before the equipment has been installed.

It is therefore sometimes advisable to undertake an assessment of the shielding (or shielding integrity testing) before the installation of the clinical equipment. This testing can be performed as soon as all of the shielding is in place (even if there is no mains power). Critically, this means that any defects or issues are identified before final surface finishes have been applied, making any remedial work less costly.

In other circumstances, equipment may be planned to be installed into a pre-existing facility where the barrier material, thickness, density and or integrity is not well known or understood. In these circumstances the recommended approach is for such an assessment to be undertaken.

In order to perform shielding integrity testing for radiotherapy facilities, it is necessary to use a portable linear accelerator (a betatron). A 7.5 MeV betatron can be used to reliably assess the equivalent of around 2 m normal density concrete. Using a mobile source allows all areas of the shielding to be assessed, not just those which will be accessible using fixed clinical equipment. Mobile sources also allow the position of additional shielding in the primary barriers, such as steel sheet, to be confirmed. Results are typically reported in millimetres of normal density concrete equivalence, but can also be interpreted for other materials, such as steel or high density concrete.

The details of the survey that is undertaken depend on the design of the facility and are usually agreed with both the operator's RPA and the construction design team. However, as with all radiation surveys, the following information should always be recorded:

- records of all transmission and scatter measurements (actual not corrected values),
- background measurements,
- details of who made the measurements,
- the monitoring equipment used,
- the physical set up for each set of measurements and
- the positions of all measurements taken and the readings obtained.

The purpose of post construction testing is to ensure that the facility has been built in accordance with the physical design.

This is not necessarily the same as the tests and checks undertaken as part of the critical examination or the full radiation survey which requires all modes to be set up to enable appropriate measurements to assess worst case situations and to confirm annual dose constraints will be met in normal clinical use. Of particular importance is assessing transmission in flattening-filter-free (FFF) mode.

12.4 Preliminary safety assessment

When the installation engineers reach the point when they require the beam to be on as part of the installation process, a preliminary safety assessment must be made outside the bunker as soon as the equipment can provide a radiation beam to ensure the facility is safe for the remainder of the installation. It can sometimes be possible to carry out the checks required to meet the requirements of the critical examination and the full survey at this point, but it may be more efficient to carry out some simple measurements under a limited range of operating conditions, e.g. limiting the beam direction downwards to ensure the safety of the installation engineers and those in the surrounding area until the full radiation survey is completed.

12.5 Critical examination

A critical examination is required for all installed equipment to demonstrate that the radiation safety features which have been included in the prior risk assessment are providing the level of protection that has been assumed. For radiotherapy facilities, this will always include the radiation shielding, although the installer may not have had any control over the design or construction of the facility.

Although it is the installer of the equipment who is legally required to complete the critical examination (IRR 1999), they may ask the hospital or the construction team's RPA to complete this on their behalf. As the purpose is to ensure all safety features are operating correctly, checks should be carried out in all clinical modes and discussions held about which checks are appropriate to carry out in service mode.

IRR99 Regulation 31 (IRR 1999) by definition requires a critical review of the installation and safety aspects and whilst a prescribed check list can be helpful as described in chapter 7 and in table 12.1, it must not be seen as adequate on its own.

A critical examination is not required for mobile equipment, although in this case safety features should still be examined. Some radiotherapy equipment might be moveable but will still require a critical examination, e.g. a brachytherapy afterloader.

The safety features for most radiotherapy equipment can be complex in design and operation. A linear accelerator for example operates in a number of modes. Some safety features in place in clinical mode can be overridden in service mode. It is important the person carrying out the critical examination has sufficient understanding of these and is able to assess whether they are operating correctly.

The items recommended to be checked are listed in table 12.1 should be considered with comments on the correct outcomes.

The critical examination for diagnostic equipment is described in IPEM Report 107 (IPEM 2012) and clinical acceptance testing of radiotherapy equipment is covered in more detail in IPEM Report 94 (IPEM 2006). The following sections of this report are concerned with the aspects of the critical examination which are relevant for shielding design.

Table 12.1. Checklist for a critical examination for a linear accelerator.

Check	Comments
Controlled Area/Do Not Enter lamps	Check lights work and come on at the correct time and turn off at the correct time.
Last person out button	Check operational and complete visibility of the room from the position of the button.
Maze barrier interlock	Check operational and stops the radiation exposure when opened in all modes and that the exposure does not restart when the barrier is closed.
Exposure initiation	Check operational.
Emergency off buttons	Check that they stop radiation exposure when operated in all modes.
Other safety features	Describe following discussions and a review of the operation manuals.
Room radiation protection	See below (within design limits).
Primary barrier protection	See below.
Secondary barrier protection	See below.
Roof protection	See below.
Head radiation leakage (excluding collimators)	Within IEC specification (IEC 2009).
Neutron protection	Within design limits.

12.6 Radiation surveys

Radiation surveys are required to be carried out to provide accurate information regarding the radiation doses and dose rates outside of the new facility. This allows the operator to demonstrate that radiation exposure is restricted to levels as low as reasonably practicable (ALARP) as required in IRR99 Regulation 8 (IRR 1999).

A survey by radiation protection specialists might also assess radiation leakage through the housing of the equipment but this is considered beyond the scope of this report.

Records of any transmission or scatter measurements should include details of who made the measurements, the monitoring equipment used, the physical set up for each set of measurements, the positions of all measurements taken and the readings obtained. The reading recorded should always be numerical and not recorded as 'background' if equal to the background value.

12.6.1 Radiation monitoring equipment

Radiation surveys should be carried out with suitable equipment. Instruments should be calibrated, have sufficient sensitivity and have a suitable energy response. They may need to be sufficiently robust to be able to operate outdoors. Most will not operate when wet and external assessments may require the use of plastic covers to protect them.

Surveys of all radiation barriers should be carried out. Measurements should be made of the doses and/or dose rates transmitted through each barrier. This may require the use of ladders, scaffolding or a cherry-picker at heights above floor level. A contamination monitor with a scintillation detector can be used to identify areas with the highest dose rates outside a facility. These can be followed up with more detailed dose rate measurements using a dose rate meter.

A dose rate instrument should have a fast response, be able to measure the highly pulsed radiation from a linear accelerator and operate over the dose rate range that is of interest. The ideal instrument to measure x-rays is an ionisation chamber. These are not affected by the pulsed radiation from linear accelerators but have a relatively slow response and can be subject to recombination errors. Semiconductor detectors and scintillation detectors can be used, but an understanding of their response to pulsed radiation and the energies measured is necessary.

Neutrons can be measured with a variety of instruments. Meters usually rely on neutron capture reactions B^{10} (n, α) Li^7 or He^3 (n, p) H^3. Most come with a plastic moderator and a boron filter to correct for the over-response to intermediate energy neutrons.

Instruments are normally calibrated in units of ambient dose equivalence. There are a number of publications describing suitable instrumentation for particular measurements, e.g. HSE (2011), Burgess (2001) and IAEA (2004).

Environmental monitoring is normally carried out when an installation is in full clinical use. Monitors are placed in critical positions for a period of time—typically between one and three months. Monitors for photons and electrons are either thermoluminescent material or optically stimulated luminescent material. Neutron monitors are generally passive monitors using poly-allyl diglycol carbonate (PADC). Care should be taken if personal dosimeters are used as they are calibrated in different units.

12.6.2 Linear accelerator bunker checks

As described above, a preliminary safety assessment must be made outside the bunker as soon as the equipment can provide a radiation beam to ensure the facility is safe for the remainder of the installation. The check is relatively simple and involves measurements at key positions with a fast responding dose rate meter.

12.6.2.1 Assessment of primary radiation barriers

The full radiation survey should include measurements of transmission through the primary barrier made initially at all cardinal orientations. The largest field size rotated through 45° should also be used and checks made to ensure the primary barrier covers this field in cardinal orientations.

Measurements of transmitted dose rates should be made under the following conditions:

- 40 cm × 40 cm field size at 45° collimator rotation,
- no scatter in the beam,
- highest x-ray energy and
- highest dose rate.

Measurements should be made over each of the primary barriers with the beam pointing directly at the barrier under test. Mobile phones or radios can be used to get dose rate meters into the correct position before the beam is turned on. Help to identify the location of the isocentre on each of the barriers can help make the survey more efficient. Noting this position for future checks or measurements (with photographs) can also be helpful.

Measurements on the roof should be made remotely if the roof has been designed to allow the transmission of high dose rates. Many instruments have long cables and remote readouts. The detector can be placed in a plastic container and dragged across the roof.

The meter should be used to measure dose rates through each of the walls at 30 cm intervals at waist, ankle and head height, and at 30 cm and 1 m from the barrier. Dose rates should also be measured at height if possible. Measurements should be made through the centre of the barrier on the roof and off axis to the left and right of the centre. The nearest occupied areas should be measured if measurements are not possible at height above floor or ground level.

Recording the results for these measurements can result in several pages of results as each measurement needs to be recorded with the beam parameters associated with it. Recording results on plans and elevations can be the most efficient way for primary barriers as the maximum readings will usually result from a single beam set up.

Survey results should be compared with those calculated in the design to produce example summary results, as shown in table 12.2.

Table 12.2. Example results comparing measured and calculated dose-rates from a primary barrier survey of a linear accelerator bunker.

Point	Predicted IDR (μSv h^{-1}) 10 MV 2400 MU min^{-1}	Maximum measured IDR (μSv h^{-1})	Comments
External 1	2	1	At head height in the centre of the barrier.
Adjacent bunker 2	0.4	0.2	At isocentre height and in the centre of the barrier.
Roof 3	22	20	Higher dose rates covering roughly 1.5 m × 1.5 m at the centre of the primary barrier.

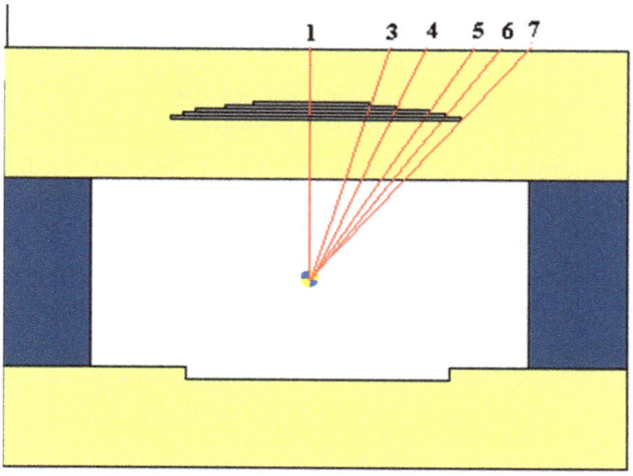

Figure 12.1. Measurement positions with a laminated roof with steel plates.

If a laminated barrier has been constructed with steel plates, more measurements may need to be made to ensure that dose rates remain acceptable at each change in the thickness of steel plates (see figure 12.1)

To fully assess the primary barriers, the gantry may be rotated to ensure measurements are made of the whole primary barrier. This might be especially important if the ground level outside is lower than the finished floor level and high density material has been used in the walls and the base is poured concrete, or if a room in an adjacent building above the level of the bunker roof is a critical point. However, using the biggest possible field size in this situation may cause the primary beam to spill beyond the edges of the primary barrier so more clinically realistic field sizes should be used for such measurements. It is not expected that the largest field size would ever be used for anything other than treatments such as total body irradiation (TBI).

12.6.2.2 Assessment of secondary radiation barriers

Measurements of transmitted dose rates should be made under the following conditions:

- scatter in the beam,
- 40 cm × 40 cm field size at 45° collimator rotation,
- highest beam energy,
- lowest beam energy (maze entrance measurements only),
- highest dose rate and
- beam pointing in each of the four cardinal directions.

The scatter should be large enough to produce a worst case scattering condition without significant self-absorption. A water tank may be too large. Water bottles and or solid water slightly larger than the beam itself is considered to be the minimum scatter required.

Measurements should be made over all barriers with the beam at each angle at the highest energy and lowest energy as described above (relaxing the number of dose rate measurements where readings are low).

Recording the results for these measurements can be quite extensive. Recording results on plans or forms can be used. A summary sheet can be produced for secondary measurements as in table 12.2, although the gantry angle will also need to be specified for the positions where the highest dose rates are measured.

Particular attention should be made to the dose rates at the maze entrance, particularly at the edges. Meter readings should be made at closer spacing for these measurements. Measurements should also be performed at the maze entrance for the lowest x-ray energy, as the scattered doses may be higher at lower energies if scatter from a wall close to the maze entrance is not the dominant component.

Dosimetry cable conduits and any other penetrations should be carefully assessed.

12.6.2.3 Assessment of neutron fluence

At x-ray energies above 8.5 MV, neutron production may result in neutrons being scattered down the maze. Measurements at the end of the maze and at any conduits passing though the walls, e.g. the dosimetry cableway, should be checked with a neutron monitor. Care needs to be taken about the interpretation of the results and the radiation weighting factor used to calculate the effective doses that might be received.

12.6.2.4 Assessment of skyshine

Radiation passing through the roof of the facility may be scattered down as skyshine (see section 5.4). Measurements of dose rate should be taken at a distance from the building at ground level. This is particularly important if nuclear medicine departments or rooms with radionuclide counting equipment are close by.

12.7 Surveys of kilovoltage equipment

Measurements should be recorded outside the room using a dose rate meter. The positions where maximum dose rates are found can be quickly assessed using a contamination monitor.

For primary radiation beam directions, each wall that the unit may point at should be checked using the largest applicator size and highest energy. It should be ensured that the unit cannot point at doors or the ceiling unless they have been designed to attenuate the direct beam effectively.

Measurements should be repeated with a scattering medium and the dose rates outside the walls, floor (if appropriate), ceiling and around the doors should be checked.

Service ducts and the edges of the door should be carefully assessed, particularly the bottom of the door.

12.8 Surveys of brachytherapy facilities

Measurements should be recorded outside the room using a dose rate meter with the source in the expose position. The positions where maximum dose rates are found can be quickly assessed using a contamination monitor.

All walls, ceiling, floor (if appropriate) and doors should be checked with the source exposed in clinically realistic positions. Measurements can also be made with the source as close to each barrier and opening as possible to perhaps indicate source positions which need to be avoided in practice.

Measurements should be repeated with the source in an applicator in a suitable phantom.

Particular attention should be paid to any service ducts, dosimetry channels and the edges of door openings, if a door is required.

12.9 Surveys of CT scanners

Scattered dose rates outside the room should be measured. A large phantom in the centre of the field of view and maximum mAs should be used. If an engineer is present, the table can be fixed and the beam continuously set to rotate around the phantom.

A contamination monitor will identify areas of higher penetration. These can then be checked with a dose rate meter. Cracks or other defects can be further investigated using imaging plates.

12.10 Validation of results

The measurements should be compared with the calculated values from the design. These should then be used to confirm that the dose constraints will be met. If dose rates are higher than expected and constraints might be exceeded, the measurements should be repeated for clinically realistic fields and environmental monitoring should be carried out over a period of time.

A report summarising the results should be prepared and approved by the RPA. The records should be kept carefully for any future changes in use and should be used in risk assessments.

References

Burgess P 2001 *Guidance on the Choice Use and Maintenance of Hand Held Radiation Monitoring Equipment* NRPB R236 (Didcot: National Radiological Protection Board)

HSE (Health and Safety Executive) 2001 *Selection, Use and Maintenance of Portable Monitoring Instruments* (*Ionising Radiation Protection Series* No 7) (London: HSE)

IAEA (International Atomic Energy Authority) 2004 *Workplace Monitoring for Radiation and Contamination. Practical Radiation Technical Manual* No 1 (Vienna: IAEA)

IEC (International Electrotechnical Commission) 2009 *Medical Electrical Equipment—Part 2-1: Particular Requirements for the Safety of Electron Accelerators in the Range 1 MeV to 50 MeV* 60601-2-1, 2nd edn (Geneva: IEC)

IPEM (Institute of Physics and Engineering in Medicine) 2006 *Acceptance Testing and Commissioning of Linear Accelerators* Report 94 (York: IPEM)

IPEM (Institute of Physics and Engineering in Medicine) 2012 *The Critical Examination of x-ray Generating Equipment in Diagnostic Radiology* Report 107 (York: IPEM)

IRR 1999 *The Ionising Radiations Regulations* SI 1999/3232 (London: The Stationery Office)

Reay J, Hill R and May A 2010 Shielding integrity testing for ionising radiation facilities *Scope* **19** 6–8

IOP Publishing

Glossary

Absorbed dose	The mean energy imparted to matter by ionising radiation. The unit of absorbed dose is the joule per kilogram and is given the specific name gray (Gy).
ACoP	*Approved Code of Practice* (to the Ionising Radiations Regulations), gives practical advice on how to comply with the regulations.
Activity	The number of nuclear transformations that occur in a quantity of a decaying radionuclide per unit time. The unit of activity is one transformation per second and is given the specific name becquerel (Bq).
Afterloading	A technique used in brachytherapy to avoid handling high activity radioactive sources directly. Applicators into which the source(s) are introduced during treatment are positioned accurately in the patient before treatment commences without the sources present. The sources may then be quickly introduced into the applicators before the operator leaves the treatment room. This technique considerably reduces the potential radiation dose to the hands of the radiation oncologist.
ALARA	*As low as reasonably achievable*, a term introduced by the ICRP to describe the basic principle of optimisation of radiation protection. It is intended to minimise the likelihood of exposures occurring, the number of individuals exposed and the magnitude of any dose incurred to levels as low as reasonable achievable, taking social and economic factors into account.
ALARP	*As low as reasonably practicable*, the Ionising Radiations Regulations (IRR 1999) use the term 'reasonably practicable' because it was found that 'reasonably achievable' (see above) cannot be defined in law.
Background radiation	Natural background radiation arising from natural sources, cosmic radiation, radon and fallout. The average background dose in the UK is 2.7 mSv/year (Public Health England).
Barrier	A wall, floor or ceiling of radiation attenuating material needed to reduce the dose equivalent on the far side of the barrier from the radiation source to an acceptable level.
Barytes concrete	A high density concrete in earlier use for bunker shielding and now superseded by other high density concretes incorporating iron ores that are easier to handle.

doi:10.1088/978-0-7503-1440-4ch13

Beam stopper Shielding mounted on a treatment unit opposite the radiation source which substantially reduces the intensity of the radiation reaching the wall of the treatment room.

Brachytherapy The treatment of cancer using sealed source(s) of radioactivity placed in or in close proximity to the tumour. Treatment can be intra-cavity or intra-luminal when the source(s) are introduced through a body cavity or opening, interstitial when implanted into the tumour and external when the sources are placed on the skin or surface of the eye.

Bunker A shielded treatment room containing a radiation generator, e.g. a linear accelerator or cobalt-60 unit, producing megavoltage radiation. The term 'vault' is used in the USA.

CCTV *Closed circuit television system*, usually used for monitoring the patient during treatment. May also be part of the security surveillance of high activity radioactive sealed sources used in brachytherapy.

Collimator A device used to shape the outline of the radiation beam to match the required treatment outline. See also 'Multi-leaf collimators'.

Control room The room or area outside the treatment room from which the treatment equipment is operated and the patient on treatment is monitored. It should be close to the entrance to the treatment room to supervise and authorise access.

Controlled area A designated area in which (a) it is necessary for any person who enters or works in the area to follow special procedures to restrict exposure to ionising radiation or prevent and limit the probability and magnitude of radiation accidents or their effects, or (b) any person working in the area is likely to receive an effective dose greater than 6 mSv a year or an equivalent dose greater than three-tenths of any relevant dose limit.

Critical examination An examination following the installation of radiation equipment to ensure that the features for radiation protection designed into the facility are present in the completed facility; in particular that (a) the safety features and warning devices operate correctly and (b) there is sufficient protection for persons from exposure to ionising radiation. It is the responsibility of the installer to undertake the critical examination but it is often carried out under the supervision of the employer's RPA with the agreement of the installer. The installer must also provide the employer with adequate information about proper use, testing and maintenance of the equipment. The equipment installer is responsible for the examination being carried out but may not have been involved with the shielding design, in which case agreement on the responsibility for the shielding is necessary.

CTSA *Counter Terrorist Security Adviser*, a member of the local police authority who advises the Environment Agency on suitable security measures for the use and storage of high activity radioactive sources.

CyberKnife® A linear accelerator operating at 6 MV mounted on a remotely controlled robotic arm for the delivery of multiple small non-coplanar beams with high positional accuracy in order to achieve a highly conformal dose distribution. Sometimes termed 'robotic radiosurgery'. The fact that the radiation beam can point in any direction and is not confined to a vertical plane through the isocentre like a conventional linear accelerator means that the primary shielding is more extensive than for a conventional linear accelerator. CyberKnife is a registered trademark of Accuray.

Design IDR The IDR chosen for radiation protection calculations.

Design TADR Normally the design IDR averaged over 8 h working day.

Dose constraint A prospective restriction on the individual radiation dose from a specific source which serves as an upper bound in the optimisation of radiation protection of that source. The recommended value in the UK is 300 μSv/year for members of the public from a single source of radiation but in some circumstances 1 mSv is used for radiation workers. The dose constraint is generally less than the legal dose limit to allow the possibility of exposure from more than one source.

Effective dose The sum of the equivalent doses from external radiation to all the organs and tissues of the body multiplied by the appropriate tissue and radiation weighting factors. The weighting and radiation factors are specified by the ICRP. The unit of effective dose is joules per kilogram and is given the specific name of sievert (Sv).

Electronic brachytherapy Brachytherapy in which the radiation source is low energy x-rays, typically 50 kV. It is employed in treating superficial lesions or intraoperatively.

Employer The entity having legal responsibility for the radiation protection of staff, patients and members of the public. If an employee is carrying out work with ionising radiation, then that person's employer is by definition the radiation employer.

End point energy The highest x-ray energy in the x-ray spectrum from an x-ray unit or linear accelerator corresponding to the effective accelerating potential in kV or MV. Strictly speaking it should have the units keV or MeV, but kV and MV are commonly used.

Engineering controls The combination of interlocks, warning lights and signs designed together with the shielding to prevent the inadvertent radiation of persons during operation of the radiation facility.

Environmental monitoring A collection of passive dosimeters sited at critical points around the exterior of a radiation facility to record the doses received over a period of time, e.g. three months. Such a survey will show if a new facility or an existing facility with revised treatment techniques meets an annual dose constraint. Measurements need to commence when the clinical techniques are fully established.

Equivalent dose The product of absorbed dose to an individual organ or tissue multiplied by the radiation quality factor. The unit of equivalent dose is joules per kilogram and is given the specific name of sievert (Sv).

Euratom directive Directives of the European Union derived from ICRP Reports which lay down the standards of radiation protection and practice in Member States. Directive 96/29 Euratom is the basis of the Ionising Radiation Regulations 1999 and Directive 13/59 Euratom is the basis of the forthcoming Ionising Radiation Regulations 2017.

FFF linear accelerator *Flattening-filter-free* linear accelerator, a beam modality in a linear accelerator without the traditional flattening filter positioned after the target to generate a uniform beam fluence. This allows a higher dose rate in the primary beam and reduces the amount of scatter and leakage from the head of the accelerator. Non-uniform fluence is acceptable when modulated (e.g. IMRT, VMAT or TomoTherapy®) or small field (e.g. SBRT) treatments are being given. The higher dose rate allows hypofractionated treatment times to be reduced for similar treatment plan quality and simplified beam modelling.

Fraction The fraction of the total dose given in a single treatment; often given daily. The radiation dose to the tumour is divided into multiple equal smaller doses (or fractions) to spare normal tissue. The number of fractions with external beam treatments may extend to 30–40 fractions.

Gamma Knife® A device with a large number of cobalt-60 sources in a 'helmet' surrounding the patient's head which collimates the gamma radiation to treat brain tumours and malformations with high spatial accuracy and highly conformal dose distributions (see SRS). Units are largely self-shielding compared to other megavoltage units but require infrequent source changes. Gamma Knife is a registered trademark of Elekta.

Gantry The rotating C-arm on which the treatment head of a megavoltage treatment unit is mounted. The gantry can rotate 360° about its horizontal axis of rotation, enabling the collimated radiation beam to enter the patient at any angle.

Groundshine The amount of radiation scattered beneath the wall of the treatment room into an adjacent area when the radiation beam points toward the junction of the wall and floor. This only normally occurs with thin walls (of high density material).

HVL (or HVT) *Half value layer* (or *thickness*) of shielding material which reduces the exposure rate by a factor of two when normal to the path of the radiation. The values in this report reflect broad beam geometry.

Hypofractionation Delivery of the total dose in a few high dose fractions, typically used for slow-growing tumours such as prostate, or when highly conformal dose delivery leads to sparing of normal tissue and the potential for dose escalation (e.g. SBRT or SRS).

IDR *Instantaneous dose rate*, the direct reading of a dosimeter to enable comparison with calculated dose rates.

ICRP *International Commission on Radiological Protection*, an international body established in 1928 which considers new information on the effects of radiation and the impact of new techniques. It publishes regular reports with recommendations on dose limits and other aspects of radiation protection. Its recommendations are the basis of international guidance and national legislation on radiation protection standards.

ICRU *International Commission on Radiation Units and Measurements*, an international body established in 1925 for the ongoing evaluation of radiation metrology and radiation quantities. It publishes regular reports with recommendations on quantities and units of radiation and radioactivity and acceptable measurement techniques.

IEC *International Electrotechnical Commission*, an international body which develops and publishes standards on the safety and performance of electrical equipment, including medical equipment.

IMRT *Intensity modulated radiotherapy*, a treatment technique in which the beam fluence is modulated around the patient, typically by computerised optimisation, to build up a complex individualised dose distribution across the tumour. This may include fixed gantry angle IMRT (with multiple static MLC segments, or dynamic MLC motion while the beam is on), dynamic rotational treatments (VMAT and helical TomoTherapy®, robotic radiosurgery or intensity modulated proton therapy.

IMRT factor The ratio of the number of monitor units of radiation exposure needed to deliver the prescribed tumour dose with a single uniform radiation field to the number needed to deliver the same dose using smaller intensity modulated IMRT fields. This results in a longer exposure for the same tumour dose and consequently a greater dose from head leakage radiation per treatment leading to thicker secondary shielding.

Interlock A device that terminates the radiation exposure of a treatment unit because further operation is unsafe or out of specification. Interlocks can be external to the treatment unit, e.g. a treatment room door interlock to stop the exposure in inadvertent entry into the treatment room, or internal if the quality of the radiation beam no longer meets its specification. The treatment unit should not resume the exposure when the interlock is reset but needs to be re-initialised.

IRR *Ionising Radiations Regulations*, the UK legislation implementing EC Directives based on ICRP recommendations for the radiation protection of the general public and radiation workers. The regulations were first implemented in 1985, revised and re-issued in 1999 and again in 2018.

Isocentre The point of intersection of the axes of gantry, collimator and patient couch rotation for a megavoltage treatment unit. This is usually 100 cm from the radiation source in a linear accelerator.

Kerma or air kerma *Kinetic energy released in matter*, a dosimetric quantity used when modelling the absorption of radiation. It indicates the energy of the secondary particles released when x-rays interact with matter.

Kilovoltage therapy Treatment performed with x-ray beams under 1 MeV. The term ‘orthovoltage treatment’ is often used for treatments with 150–300 kV beams and ‘superficial treatment’ for treatments with 50 kV–150 kV beams. The term ‘Grenz rays’ is sometimes used for x-rays up to 50 kV.

Leakage radiation Radiation apart from the collimated beam coming from the treatment head of a linear accelerator due to scatter interactions of the beam with the components in the treatment head. It is reduced by shielding within the treatment head and its intensity should not exceed 0.1% of the intensity of the collimated beam as specified in (IEC 2002). In practice it tends to be less than this limit and is further reduced for linear accelerators operating in FFF mode due to the absence of an x-ray flattening filter. The term may also be used to describe the dose rate on the external surface of the shielded container of a radioactive source.

Linear accelerator A device using radiofrequency electromagnetic waves for accelerating electrons before hitting a target to produce high energy x-rays. In current clinical practice, x-rays with end point energies in the range 6–18 MV are employed. By withdrawing the target, a number of electron beams with a range of energies can also be produced.

Linear accelerator head The part of the accelerator housing the target and the collimation system for shaping the outline of the radiation beam. It also contains a bending magnet and flattening filters for x-ray beams or scattering foils for electron beams to give beams of uniform intensity across the radiation field.

Local rules A written system of work that contains the key working instructions intended to restrict any exposure in controlled or supervised areas. The rules should be appropriate to the nature and risk of exposure to ionising radiation. The rules should cover normal work practice and the particular steps to be taken to control exposure in the event of a radiation accident. Local rules for a controlled area should include a summary of the arrangements for restricting access.

Maze A long corridor with a number of bends giving access to a megavoltage treatment room from a public area and designed to reduce the radiation dose rate at the entrance during equipment operation to an acceptable level. The dose rate will fall with a longer maze due to the inverse square law and more right angle bends to reduce the intensity of scattered radiation.

Maze entrance Normally the outer (or external) entrance to the maze for staff, patients and equipment. In describing the radiation protection provided by the maze, reference may be made to the inner maze entrance from the treatment room and the outer maze entrance.

Megavoltage therapy Treatment performed with x- or gamma-ray radiation above 1 MeV, usually with linear accelerators or cobalt-60 units.

MPE *Medical Physics Expert*, an experienced medical physicist in radiotherapy or diagnostic imaging, whose knowledge and experience has been accepted as meeting the requirements for registration by a national accrediting authority.

Monitor Unit (MU) An internal machine unit used in radiotherapy devices to terminate the exposure based on a prescribed dose of radiation as measured by a monitor ion chamber in the treatment head. Each device must be individually calibrated to relate MUs to absorbed dose in a specified reference condition (e.g. 1 cGy/MU at 5cm deep for a 10 x 10 cm field).

Monte Carlo simulation A summation of the simulated radiation pathways in a facility using a knowledge of the cross-sections and probabilities which govern the radiation interactions, the positions of the shielding and other structures and a detailed representation of the radiation source. A sufficient number of paths must be modelled for the results to be statistically significant.

MLC *Multi-leaf collimators*, x-ray collimators comprised of opposing leaves of a heavy metal, e.g. tungsten, that can be moved under computer control to form radiation fields of an irregular shape to match the tumour outline. There can be up to 60 pairs of leaves. These typically have a projected width of 5–10 mm at the isocentre distance but specialist stereotactic units have a projected width as small as 2.5 mm for treating brain tumours.

NCRP *National Council on Radiation Protection and Measurements* (USA), chartered by the US Congress in 1964 to collect, analyse, develop and disseminate in the public interest information and recommendations on (a) protection against radiation and (b) radiation measurements, quantities and units, particularly those concerned with radiation protection. The Council produces regular statements and reports with recommendations on good practice.

NPSA *National Patient Safety Agency*, became part of NHS Improvement in 2016.

Obliquity correction A term used when primary radiation does not strike a shielding barrier at normal incidence and passes through the barrier at an oblique angle. Due to the longer path length in the barrier, the thickness of the barrier may be reduced at this point without increasing the intensity of the beam over that at normal incidence. This is useful when using expensive shielding materials.

Occupancy The fraction of time an area in or adjacent to a radiation facility is occupied by persons during the working day. It is used in the calculation of potential annual radiation doses in a particular location.

OJEU *Official Journal of the European Union*, a publication of the European Union in which all equipment and services above a threshold cost must be advertised for open tendering for their supply. In 2016/17 the threshold was £106 047 for NHS Trusts and £164 170 for NHS Foundation Trusts.

Option appraisal A formal process in which all the features of a piece of equipment or a service are identified and given a weight related to their importance to the purchaser. Individual proposals are then scored against each of the features and the total weighted score used to identify the best buy. For equipment it is important to take into account its performance characteristics and less quantitative issues such as maintenance and training required.

Plaques A term used in external brachytherapy to describe the device holding the sealed radiation source with fixings to attach it to an external body surface for a specified period of time, e.g. the eye.

Primary barrier A section of a wall, floor or ceiling at which the collimated beam from the treatment unit can be pointed directly and designed to attenuate the radiation to an acceptable level on its exterior surface.

Prior risk assessment A comprehensive assessment prior to the introduction of new equipment or a service looking at all the reasonable risks that can be anticipated and deciding the measures needed to reduce their risk of occurrence and severity. The results of the assessment will be an input to the writing of the radiation protection procedures.

QART *Quality Assurance in Radiotherapy*, a quality management system for the delivery of radiotherapy based upon the standard ISO 9001.

RPA *Radiation Protection Adviser*, the person appointed by an employer carrying out work with ionising radiation for the purpose of advising him/her on compliance with the Ionising Radiations Regulations and other relevant legislation and guidance. RPAs must be registered with a national accrediting body but the employer must be sure that the RPA appointed has the relevant experience for the work concerned, e.g. radiotherapy.

Radiation protection survey Measurement of the dose rates around a radiation facility to ensure these meet statutory requirements and to check the adequacy of the design of the shielding.

Radiation workload The cumulative radiation dose delivered by the treatment unit at the depth of maximum dose in patients totalled over the relevant working period, e.g. Gy/week or kGy/year. The basis of shielding calculations to achieve an annual dose constraint.

Reflection coefficient In considering radiation scattered by barriers, e.g. in a treatment room maze, the fraction of the dose at the surface of the barrier which is scattered to 1 m from a 1 m^2 irradiated area at particular angles of incidence and reflection from a specified material.

Remote afterloading An afterloading technique in which the source(s) are passed into and removed from pre-positioned allocators under computer control from a control unit outside the treatment room. The source positions and dwell times at each position are determined by the patient treatment plan. This technique has largely replaced manual afterloading in which the sources were transferred by the radiation oncologist from a shielded container to the applicator, further reducing the potential for a radiation dose.

SBRT *Stereotactic body radiotherapy*, the use of high doses per fraction along with highly conformal often inhomogeneous dose distributions and high positional accuracy to deliver a more radical treatment to tumours which are often small and close to or within organs at risk. This is also called *stereotactic ablative body radiotherapy* (SABR) when the dose is high enough to completely ablate the tumour.

Scatter Radiation scattered from a patient or the walls of a treatment room.

Secondary barrier A wall, floor or ceiling designed to attenuate the leakage radiation from the treatment head and the radiation scattered by the patient during treatment to an acceptable level.

Skyshine The amount of radiation backscattered from the air above a treatment room in the direction of the ground when the radiation beam is upward and has penetrated the roof of the treatment room.

SRS *Stereotactic radiosurgery*, the use of radiotherapy to treat brain tumours and malformations, usually in a single high dose fraction, with highly conformal often inhomogeneous dose distributions and high positional accuracy.

Supervised area A defined area kept under review for the need to be controlled or where an individual is likely to receive a dose of ionising radiation greater than one tenth of any dose limit, but less than three tenths of that limit.

TADR *Time averaged dose rate*, this is usually the IDR multiplied by the expected daily beam-on time and then averaged over 8 h working day for a particular direction. It takes into account the proportion of the time the radiation beam points in the direction concerned (see 'Use factor').

TADR2000 The time averaged dose rate over 2000 h at a specified location. It takes into account the occupancy of the location. TADR multiplied by 2000 (8 working hours/day × 5 working days/week × 50 working weeks/year) gives an estimate of the annual dose at the location.

TBI *Total body irradiation*, a treatment technique which involves irradiation of the whole of the patient, typically for haematological disease. This is usually done with the patient standing, or lying in a horizontal position, at an extended source to skin distance so that the length of the patient is covered by the largest radiation field size.

TVL (or TVT) *Tenth value layer* (or *thickness*) of shielding material which reduces the exposure rate by a factor of ten when normal to the path of the radiation. During attenuation spectral hardening takes place over the first TVL thickness (designated TVL_1) but the spectrum remains appreciably constant over subsequent TVL thicknesses with a shorter constant TVL thickness (termed TVL_e).

TomoTherapy® A linear accelerator operating at 6 MV and attached to a rotating gantry similar to a CT scanner. IMRT is performed by having a multi-leaf collimator across the width of the radiation beam which either blocks or unblocks segments of the beam parallel to the central axis of rotation as the gantry rotates about the patient. Large volumes of the patient may be treated by having the patient couch move through the gantry during the treatment. Treatment times are typically longer than with a conventional linear accelerator. The unit incorporates a beam stopper which

	reduces the primary shielding requirements. TomoTherapy is a registered trademark of Accuray.
Transmission factor	The ratio of the intensity of the radiation at a point on the exterior of a barrier to the intensity at that point if the barrier was not present.
Use (or orientation) factor	The ratio of the time the radiation beam points in a specified direction relative to the total beam-on time per day.
Vault	See 'Bunker'.
VMAT	*Volumetric intensity modulated arc therapy*, a form of IMRT using one or more continuous arcs around the patient during which the gantry speed, dose rate and MLC positions are all varied dynamically to deliver a highly conformal dose distribution in a shorter time than fixed gantry angle IMRT. Typically coplanar arcs are used to reduce the risk of collision but non-coplanar arcs may be used for SRS and SBRT.
Workload	See 'Radiation workload'.

Lightning Source UK Ltd.
Milton Keynes UK
UKHW052121200621
385802UK00003B/50

9 780750 314411